Making Madness Visible

LIVERPOOL STUDIES IN HEALTH, DISABILITY, CULTURE & SOCIETY

Series Editor
Stuart Murray, University of Leeds

Formerly known as 'Representations: Health, Disability, Culture and Society', this series provides a ground-breaking and innovative selection of titles that showcase the newest interdisciplinary research on the cultural representations of health and disability in the contemporary social world. Bringing together both subjects and working methods from literary studies, film and cultural studies, medicine and sociology, Liverpool Studies in Health, Disability, Culture & Society is scholarly and accessible, addressed to researchers across a number of academic disciplines, and practitioners and members of the public with interests in issues of public health.

The key term in the series will be representations. Public interest in questions of health and disability has never been stronger, and as a consequence cultural forms across a range of media currently produce a never-ending stream of narratives and images that both reflect this interest and generate its forms. The crucial value of the series is that it brings the skilled study of cultural narratives and images to bear on such contemporary medical concerns. It offers and responds to new research paradigms that advance understanding at a scholarly level of the interaction between medicine, culture and society; it also has a strong commitment to public concerns surrounding such issues, and maintains a tone and point of address that seek to engage a general audience.

Other books in the series

Articulating Bodies: The Narrative Form of Disability and Illness in Victorian Fiction
Kylee-Anne Hingston

Disability, Literature, Genre: Representation and Affect in Contemporary Fiction
Ria Cheyne

Disability and the Posthuman: Bodies, Technology, and Cultural Futures
Stuart Murray

HIV/AIDS and the Stage: Politics and Performance in Neoliberal Times
Louisa Hann

Decolonizing Disease: Pandemics, Public Health and Pathogenic Novels
Claire Chambers

Making Madness Visible

A Cultural History of How Mental Disorder is Visualised

Alvise Sforza Tarabochia

LIVERPOOL UNIVERSITY PRESS

First published 2026 by
Liverpool University Press
4 Cambridge Street
Liverpool
L69 7ZU

British Library Cataloguing-in-Publication data
A British Library CIP record is available

ISBN 978-1-80596-841-2 (hardback)
ISBN 978-1-80596-842-9 (epdf)
ISBN 978-1-80596-843-6 (epub)

Typeset by Carnegie Book Production, Lancaster
Printed and bound by CPI Group (UK) Ltd, Croydon CR0 4YY

'If sanity and insanity exist, how shall we know them?' David Rosenhan's question of 1973 has been central to the long discourse on madness across history and cultures, and the answer has been sought, first and foremost, in the visual field. How shall we know insanity from sanity? This book is a cultural history of the ways in which we have attempted to make madness visible, and of the tropes that have governed these attempts. At the same time, it is an analysis of how these visualisations serve first and foremost the purpose of othering those suffering from mental disorders. It thus demonstrates how these tropes have shaped and still shape our understanding of mental disorders and our tendency to fear and marginalise those who are deemed different. While this work is a cultural history of visual representations, and thus a history of visual culture, it also demonstrates that the way in which we represent mental disorders as a visible entity has a very real impact on how we treat them.

Contents

Acknowledgements

IT TOOK ME quite some time to put this book together, and from start to finish it would simply not have been possible without Wissia Fiorucci. Her rock-solid belief in me and in this project provided the safe ground I needed to tread on whenever doubts crept in—which, truth be told, was quite often. I owe her far more than this book, though that would require a volume of its own.

This all began a long time ago—I would say about ten years—when, for a combination of positive and some less positive reasons, I turned my attention to photography. I owe this turn to my friend and (former) colleague Francesco Capello, who gave me the encouragement I needed. As academics, we talk a lot about research-led teaching. This monograph, however, is really the product of teaching-led research. In 2019 Barbara Bruschi and Alessandro Perissinotto, whom I am honoured to call friends, invited me to the University of Torino to deliver a module on Storytelling and Mental Disorders. The session on visual storytelling became the very first sketch of this work. I am also grateful to Sergia Adamo at the University of Trieste for giving me further opportunities to test my ideas within the Health Humanities School.

When it came to pulling everything together, Ben Hutchinson (to whom I owe the very title of this book) gave me both mentorship and the discipline to crack on despite everything happening around us. Francesca Billiani has been a mentor, a friend, and a sharp reader. And I must single out Angelos Evangelou: we have shared our academic upbringing, and at a decisive moment he uttered a single, razor-sharp sentence (which shall not be repeated here) that jolted me out of chapter two. Without it, I would still be stuck there. He was also the most attentive of readers and gave invaluable recommendations across the whole manuscript. Thanks also to Michael Mulryan, whose careful proof-reading and copy-editing spared readers from many of my linguistic excesses.

My friends—all of whom have been colleagues of mine at the University of Kent, though some have since moved on to pastures new—Alex Marlow-Mann, William Rowlandson, Larry Duffy, Tobias Heinrich, Maggie Awadalla, Mathilde Poizat-Amar, Caoilte Ó Ciardha, Heide Kunzelmann, Valeska Hass, Ru Su, Mano Suzuki, Christina Kim, Laura Bailey, Ann Alwis, Krista Bonello Rutter Giappone and Shane Weller—have generously provided me with linguistic insights in languages I do not speak, as well as countless crucial suggestions. Additionally, Maya Coianiz, Ryan Perry, Camilla Pasqua, Guido Reverdito and Paola Villani helped me with writing systems I don't read and languages that are no longer spoken.

I am also grateful to my mother, Fulvia Vattovani, former Professor of History of Illumination, whose expertise illuminated (pun intended) everything to do with medieval manuscripts.

Many wonderful people, colleagues, friends and institutions made it possible to source the iconography of this book: the Erfurt University Library, the Free Library of Philadelphia, the Staatsbibliothek Berlin, the Library of Congress, the Biblioteca Casanatense, Dominique Strange, the Wellcome Trust, the Rijksmuseum, the Universitäts- und Landesbibliothek Darmstadt, Cornell's Division of Rare and Manuscript Collections, the Meadows Museum in Dallas, the Civica Raccolta delle Stampe Bertarelli in Milan, Marco Rodolfo Galloni, Il Saggiatore, Gianni Berengo Gardin, Michela Rondi at the Dipartimento di Salute Mentale in Trieste, Yale's Historical Library, Cristina Cilli at the Museo Lombroso, Fiora Gaspari at San Servolo, Chiara Bombardieri at San Lazzaro, the Kunstmuseum in Basel, Universitäts Bibliothek in Heilderberg, Egidio Priani and Giacomo Doni. My great friend Matteo Weber was kind enough to edit and prepare for print several images. And of course the amazing Anita Inverarity to whom I owe the cover of the book.

Finally, no small thanks go to my editor at Liverpool University Press, Michael Ansley, and to my production editor at Carnegie, Lola Moreno LaVey.

A Note on Translations

In this monograph I often cite works that are not originally written in English. If a translation is available I always cite the translated edition. If a translation is not available, I have translated the citation myself, unless stated otherwise.

Introduction

It is 1973 and 'anti-psychiatry' is raging. Coined by David Cooper in 1967, the term anti-psychiatry designates an ample spectrum of psychiatrists, psychologists and psychoanalysts who criticised, to different extents, the premises of psychiatry thus far: namely, that mental illness is a malfunction of the brain, that it poses a risk to society and, in particular, that it needs a secluded and specialised space to be treated, that is to say the mental asylum. In the midst of this turmoil, the American psychologist David Rosenhan publishes in the journal *Science* an article entitled 'On Being Sane in Insane Places', where he lays out the findings of his 'experiment'. Inspired during a lecture delivered by the British (anti)psychiatrist R.D. Laing—famous for his masterpiece *The Divided Self* of 1961 and for taking LSD with his schizophrenic patients at Kingsley Hall—Rosenhan sets forth to debunk the grounds of psychiatric diagnosis. He sends eight of his students to different psychiatric institutions on the west coast of the USA, instructing them to feign symptoms of schizophrenia and, upon admission, immediately start to act 'normally'. All of them are committed with a diagnosis of schizophrenia and all of them are discharged between seven and 52 days after admission, with a diagnosis of 'schizophrenia in remission'. No single member of staff of said institutions realises they are actors, but many of the fellow inpatients do. When Rosenhan announces the results, a single institution, which remains anonymous, challenges him, maintaining that their methods of assessment and diagnosis are fool proof. Rosenhan rises to the challenge and in the following months said institution spots 41 actors of the 193 patients they assess. Rosenhan, however, had sent no one. The publication of 'On Being Sane in Insane Places' sparks outrage, and the results are immediately challenged. Of course, such an 'experiment' can be considered anecdotal evidence at best; however, what is of interest here is the 'neither capricious nor itself insane' question that Rosenhan asks: 'If sanity and insanity exist, how shall we know them?' (Rosenhan 1973, 250). His conclusion is that we simply cannot, at least by means of psychiatry and its diagnostic criteria.

This monograph is a cultural history of our continuous, restless and at times haphazard attempts to know sanity from insanity. My claim is that across history and cultures, we have done so primarily through *visual* means. We try to tell the sane from the insane by making madness visible and by visually *othering* those affected by it. To be more precise, this book is a cultural history of the main tropes that have governed the visualisation of mental disorders, and that made it allegedly possible to visually distinguish the sane from the insane: from ubiquitous props, such as the staff of madness, to the extraction of the stone of folly, to convulsionary dances, and medical imaging of the face first and of the brain later.

Madness troubles borders and blurs distinctions: those between reason and unreason, between norm and deviance, between humanity and animality, between civilisation and wilderness. This is why it needs to be detected, visually othered: to be easier to spot, to manage, to keep it away from 'sane' eyes and society. Even if the visual othering of madness is meant to make the borders more demarcated and the distinctions clear-cut, even at that point, madness continues to resist definition. The more we dive into the history of the visualisations of mental disorders the more we encounter ambiguous visualisations, and the porous nature of the border between sanity and insanity, madness and reason, is revealed. For instance, the seemingly insurmountable walls of the asylum permit a metaphorical exchange, to the point that we will see how the 'cage of fools' becomes the image of the world itself gone mad. It is on this that anti-psychiatry leveraged its visual strategies of communication: by turning the othering of the insane upside down or, we should say, inside-out. Those affected by mental disorders belong to the community, and it is there that treatment and integration need to happen, not behind the closed doors of mental institutions, far from the eye of 'sane' society. In the following chapters I reconstruct the history of this continuous visual movement of definition and blurring at the borders between sanity and insanity. Throughout this study, I explore how visual representations have historically shaped our understanding of mental disorders by constructing the insane as 'other'. Across time, certain visual tropes have persistently defined distinctions between the 'sane' and the 'insane', yet these boundaries are often fluid, subject to negotiation and reinterpretation. Even when imagery seeks to impose clear demarcations, it reveals moments of ambiguity, where meanings shift and categories become unstable. However, mental illness has consistently been depicted as aberrant, deviant and outside the bounds of normative experience, something to be regulated, contained or excluded. This book examines how such representations have not merely reflected prevailing medical and cultural discourses, but have actively shaped them. From early anatomical drawings to institutional photography, images have lent authority to psychiatric diagnoses, reinforcing processes of pathologisation and contributing to the ways in which mental disorders have been understood, classified and marginalised.

Some Notes on Methodology

It might come as a surprise to the reader that the object of study of this monograph is the visual representation of madness and mental disorders in general, seemingly lumping together very different conditions. This is done on purpose, to enable us to account for the varying definitions of mental disorders across history and cultures, while at the same time avoiding retrospective diagnosis, that is to say, projecting our current understanding of mental disorder to eras when this was (at best) completely different. Several conditions and even characteristics that are not mental disorders were in the past considered tantamount to forms of madness. Most prominently epilepsy, the 'sacred disease', as the ancient Greeks called it, despite Hippocrates deeming it as sacred as any other disease (i.e., not sacred at all). Lunatic asylums housed both the insane and the epileptic, who were thought to suffer from a neurosis up until well into the nineteenth century (Berrios 1984). This is just one example of a condition and a representation that we can include in our study by looking at madness in general rather than one mental disorder in particular. There are also conditions that would have not been considered madness at the time, but that we would now consider mental disorders. This is the case for instance with demonic possession, which I will discuss in depth in chapter two. The iconography of possession shows clear similarities with that of epilepsy, mania and hysteria, even though it was regarded for a long time, and across the globe, as a religious and spiritual condition rather than a form of madness or mental disorder. Finally, tracing a history of the visualisation of mental disorders in general enables us to account for disorders and conditions whose definition changed, sometimes radically, over the course of history. Such is, for instance, the case with hysteria, which might compare to what is today defined as a 'conversion disorder' (a mental health condition that causes physical symptoms that the person cannot control). Hysteria has had a long and winding history, being recognised as being caused by anything from the uterus moving around the body and pressing on vital organs, to vapours obfuscating the brain and causing epilepsy (see Scull 2011). In iconography, despite a rather marked and enduring dichotomy between the representation of raging mania vs the composed and diminutive pensive representation of melancholia, there are constant overlaps and borrowings, and we will encounter hysterics represented as melancholics and raging maniacs, as much as we will encounter medical records with diagnoses of 'hystero-epilepsy in lypemania' (i.e., depression). The co-morbidity (simultaneous presence of two or more disorders) that is often lamented in psychiatric diagnosis (van Loo and Romeijn 2015) finds an equivalent in iconography, and further substantiates the choice of looking at madness in general rather than at each disorder individually.

Existing literature is split between works on individual disorders and on madness in general. Works in either category are excellent, and I will work in their wake, drawing from their findings. McDonagh (2008) produced an outstanding cultural history of idiocy, Scull (2011) of hysteria, Bell (2014) of melancholia/depression and Kromm (2002) focused on the visual representation of mania during the Victorian era. On the other hand, several works have traced very convincingly the cultural history of madness and mental disorders in general, including Porter's brief history of madness (Porter 2002), Cross's *Mediating Madness* (Cross 2010) and Scull's *Madness in Civilization* (Scull 2016). The present work differs from the former group of studies in that it looks at many if not all of the disorders that at one point or another in history were considered tantamount to madness (or to what today we would regard as a mental disorder). It also differs from the latter group of studies in that it is entirely focused on the 'visual' (more on this shortly). The main point of reference for this monograph is Gilman's *Seeing the Insane* (Gilman 2014), a seminal work that has been republished without substantial updates numerous times since its first edition in 1981. With this masterpiece, Gilman has produced *the* cultural history of madness and art in the Western world. I share Gilman's premise that the insane are those who are 'seen as "other" by a culture' (Gilman 1984, xiii), and that madness can be employed as an umbrella notion to study the representation of different mental disorders in history. I strive, however, to ground my analysis in the practices that produce the images analysed. Gilman's work appeared at least a decade before the definition of visual culture, and thus at times it might be seen as reducing visual culture itself to a 'free-floating web of meanings unconnected to any social practices' (G. Rose 2016, 218). In this, my approach is closer to Kromm's analysis of mania (Kromm 2002) but adopting Scull's wider historical scope of analysis: from biblical antiquity to the present (Scull 2016).

Primarily, I subscribe to Kromm's notion that visual culture is not a product of the present but has a history. It is well known that 'visual culture' was defined in 1999 as being 'concerned with visual events in which information, meaning or pleasure is sought by the consumer in an interface with visual technology' (Mirzoeff 1999, 3). This definition puts visual culture in a direct relationship with the consumption of visual artefacts, and the circulation of information and technology: it is a contemporary product, dating at best as far back as the invention of photography, but not earlier. As Kromm (2010, 5) has it, if this were the case, visual culture would be 'a unique aspect of our contemporary era [...] intimately related to the proliferation of visual technologies', whereas, according to her, visual culture has a 'historical dimension in relation to visual preferences and developments' (Kromm 2010, 5), a notion with which I agree. This book should therefore be considered, in reference to mental disorders and madness, as a history of visual culture or a cultural history of visual representations.

This brings me to another, crucial, methodological note. What is the visual? Or, in other words, what is the object of study of this book? In Mirzoeff's definition of visual culture, visual nature depends not on the sense of vision (perhaps to the detriment of other senses) or on pictures (however they might have been produced), but on a 'modern tendency to picture or visualize existence' (Mirzoeff 1999, 6). This in turn hinges on

> The realization that *spectatorship* (the look, the gaze, the glance, the practices of observation, surveillance and visual pleasure) may be as deep a problem as various forms of *reading* (decipherment, decoding, interpretation, etc.) and that 'visual experience' or 'visual literacy' might not be fully explicable in the model of textuality. (Mitchell 1994, 16, original emphases)

According to this definition, pictures have always been around, but the 'visual', as something that can create and/or characterise a whole 'culture', is a product of contemporary times.

In line with the premise that visual culture has a history, and a long one at that, I adopt a wider take on the notion of the visual, understanding with it anything that can be perceived exclusively or primarily through the sense of vision, i.e., through the eyes. This includes both human-made artefacts (e.g., paintings, drawings, photographs, sculptures) and items or features that are promptly visible (e.g., bodies, faces), those that can be made visible either by simple means (such as extraction, e.g., blood) or technological ones (e.g., neurons) or can even be believed to be visualisable even if they do not in fact exist (e.g., black bile for humoral medicine). What is central to this wide take is that someone derives, or derived, meaning from something that they encountered primarily through their eyes, even though they might have brought it into the field of vision themselves. They might have made it visible (either by looking for it or crafting it tout court) precisely and exclusively for that purpose. Take the functional magnetic resonance image (fMRI) of a brain for instance: you see the outline of a brain with some parts coloured in various tones ranging from red to blue. Our brain features no such colours. We could describe it as pale pink/greyish with visible deep-blue blood vessels perhaps, but certainly not bright orange. The fMRI image is the image of something that is real but does not exist in that form; it is an artefact that depicts the brain of a living human being in action. It is a way to visualise data, which we then interpret, and from which we derive meaning. The brain and its activity pre-exist this image, but the image has been created on purpose to try and understand something that is otherwise invisible: brain activity. Before the rather recent invention of MRI (1970s), picturing brain activity on the grounds of real data was impossible. In accordance with humoral medicine, it was believed that some mental disorders could be caused by vapours moving around the body: heating up the brain for instance. These vapours needed to be let out in some way, sometimes, as Paracelsus recommended, by cutting holes in various parts of the body. Madness is invisible and has no substance, there is little that can be done about it, so vapours come in very handy as they give substance to madness *and* to its invisibility. They allow us to visualise the invisibility of madness, seemingly a paradox. After letting St. Thomas touch his wounds, Jesus tells him: 'Because you have seen me, you have believed. Blessed are those who have not seen and (yet) have believed' (John 20:29)—or, as the saying goes, 'seeing is believing'. The visual field is the field of knowledge, our primary, and possibly most primeval, way of attempting to make sense of the world. What we cannot see but must know, we try to make visible.

In this book, I thus study attempts to make madness visible: in medicine, in the visual arts and in textual form, when the visual description is the primary way to make sense of mental disorders. The objects of study are as varied as the elements that, taken together, give shape to visual culture. They include drawing, painting, stained-glass decoration, sculpture, etching, prints, photography, but also literature, poetry and medical writing, i.e., textual descriptions of the visual appearance of mental disorders. Examples are selected without the pretence of exhaustiveness, but with the aim of analysing both the objects themselves and their conditions of production and circulation: what Rose calls the sites of the image itself, of production, of circulation and of audiencing (G. Rose 2016, 24). The primary criterion in the selection of my examples is, therefore, the retrievability of the context of the image, which is crucial to situate the image itself within visual culture through meaningful and concrete relationships. I also study, albeit not centrally, performative acts, including theatrical works, cinema and descriptions of performances, such as dances. I am chiefly interested in the synthetic and symbolic nature of the visual, how it can, quite literally, almost at a glance, make madness identifiable and recognisable. I thus might refer to films in which certain scenes draw from tropes or motifs of static visual culture, but will not work on extensive narratives of mental disorders, where films or plays can leverage their textual nature to complicate the discourse of and on madness. Finally I analyse common expressions and the etymology of words relating to madness that I believe are grounded in iconography and the visual—whether it is the English 'stone crazy', the Italian 'fuori di testa' [outside of the head] or the etymology of the word 'fool'/*folle*/*fou*, which derives from the inflated balloon often carried by the insane in iconography.

I strive to adopt what could be regarded as an 'emic' approach in discourse analysis, that is to say, I try to understand visual artefacts that relate to mental disorders from the perspective of those who produced them (see Mostowlansky et al. 2020). In analysing the discourse on madness as visible, I neither identify disorders based on contemporary diagnostic criteria nor look for their representations in history. Rather, I select those representations that were understood as depicting madness both in the eyes of the imagemakers and their intended audiences. This is an emic approach in that it proceeds from the perspective of the subject—Baxandall's 'period eye' (Baxandall 1988)—rather than from the point of view of the observer. It is an approach that does not 'try to discover what could have been said about madness [...] by interrogating the being of madness itself'

(Foucault 2002, 35). On the contrary, it is a study of madness as 'constituted by all that is said in all the statements that [...] described it' (Foucault 2002, 35), with a focus on 'visual' statements. To this extent I focus my attention on the concrete practices that shape the discourse on madness as visible: 'Rendering [madness] visible is [...] part epistemology, part topography, part technology, [...] part network of forces, even part ethics' (Rose and Abi-Rached 2013, 56). The practice of making madness visible rests on numerous factors, including conditions of visibility (e.g., exterior observation, medical imaging), spaces where this visibility is fostered (e.g., church, asylum, lab) and practices of looking (e.g., shared symbolic repositories). An analysis of the practices that place the primary objects of my study in concrete relationships is pivotal for my wide scope.

> When we speak of rendering the mind visible, we do not just mean the act of seeing. We mean the whole configuration by means of which a certain way of seeing becomes possible and can be articulated. The ways of seeing that characterize a scientific practice, or a mode of intervention, do not arise from an isolated act of looking, but from a conjunction of different elements and practices. (Rose and Abi-Rached 2013, 55)

Even though I employ an iconographic approach (Panofsky 1955)—privileging meaning over form—formal considerations that are crucial for contextualisation are taken into account. As Cross (2010, 2) has it, 'the meaning of madness is mediated in and through cultural forms that construct its appearance such that we know that this is what madness "looks like"'.

Central to my methodological approach is the notion of semantic slippage. In contrast to the relatively stable relationship that signifier and signified maintain over time, according to Ferdinand de Saussure's structuralist approach (De Saussure 2013), semantic slippage or slippage of meaning indicates that the relationship is rather unstable, and that the movement of signification is incessant (see, e.g., Campbell 1999). In brief, and at risk of oversimplifying, I understand semantic slippage as the fluidity of how words, symbols or concepts evolve over time, gradually shifting their meanings and accumulating new associations while retaining echoes of their earlier uses, which reveals a dynamic interplay between language, symbols and cultural imagination. Take the 'staff of madness' for instance, which is the object of study in the first chapter. Initially, the staff appears in medieval iconography as a symbol carried by the fool of Psalm 52, often topped with a sack or bladder to signify emptiness, folly and pride. Over time, this object transforms: it becomes the jester's marotte, a staff bearing a carved head that symbolised the duality of the fool's persona. The staff also appears as the witch's broom and as the bindle of the vagrant. What remains constant is that around the staff and its attachments, several 'undesirables' are portrayed: the insane, the witch, the vagrant. The staff and its attachments and variants serve as a marker of 'otherness', a visual shorthand for individuals cast adrift by societal norms.

Thus, we need to pose another crucial question: who represents what and for whom? That is to say, when talking about visualisations of madness, are we talking about medical doctors visualising mental disorders in the patients? Are we talking about the general public or authorities trying to tell the sane from the insane? Or are we talking about those suffering from mental disorders picturing their condition as an act of self-expression? It is not just a matter of delineating the object of study; the question that underpins these is: what purpose does the visualisation of mental disorders serve? It should be clear from the very first lines of this introduction that my claim, similar to Gilman's (2014), is that mental disorder is visualised in order to tell the sane from the insane as easily as possible, that is to say, mental disorder is visualised in order to *other* those suffering from it. Therefore, a large part of the artefacts I study are produced with this in mind. The study of such artefacts reveals shared tropes and motifs of this othering, for instance the already mentioned staff of madness but also the representation of madness as air, as an item that can be extracted (chapter two) or as convulsive movements that take hold of the entire body (chapter three).

The visual othering of madness or the othering of the insane by visual means, I argue, not only serves the purpose of marginalising the insane, marking them as different and making them, as it were, easy to spot. It also serves an ontological purpose:

> Diseases afflicted matter alone, which is to say, the body, leaving the soul (and theology) intact. Insanity seemed, nonetheless, to be a disease that affected the soul. So the problem remained: was insanity an affliction of extended matter or of thinking substance? [...] Theology dictated that the eternal soul must be free from any blemish such as insanity. So the medical task for these doctors was to describe insanity in such a way as to leave the soul intact and free from any permanent damage. Nonreligious and materialist moderns did not face this problem. Since the materialist accepted only Descartes's concern

> with extended matter, for all practical purposes the materialist need not be concerned with a soul, but simply with mechanical causality working itself out in the body. Hence there is no problem with madness that is not a medical problem. Madness afflicts the body, the body is a machine, and that is a problem of medical mechanics. (Thiher 1999, 103)

To what extent does this issue affect the representation of madness across history and cultures? In this book I claim that this is a crucial concern. How can we explain madness as an affection of the soul, but at the same time as something that does not affect its divine nature? How can it affect the soul but be of material origins? Visualising mental disorders is a key strategy. Madness is given a material substrate that can be classed as 'other' to the body but also to the soul of the affected: it is a stone that can be extracted, an infection that can be purged, a malfunctioning part of the brain that can be destroyed. Yet, the visualisation of mental disorders goes beyond the quest for materialising madness. Across history and cultures madness has been represented as invisible and immaterial in the form of air, smoke and vapours, thus representing madness *and* the very necessity of making it visible. This is, for instance, the case with madness represented as air in chapter one, but also in the theorisation of the strategy of 'unmasking' in anti-psychiatry in chapter seven. These same tropes are in fact turned upside down (again, we should rather say inside-out) when we look at movements that try to appropriate this otherness and own it: thus, I look at anti-psychiatry and their strategies of communication in chapter seven and at the emergence of outsider art, that is the art of the insane, in chapter eight. This could be considered a semantic slippage on a macro scale: the incessant movement of signification allows for a reappropriation of discriminatory and segregating notions. This book traces a history of visual othering and marginalisation but also one of reappropriation and ownership, the visual history of madness troubling borders.

Brief Overview of the Chapters

The aim of the book is threefold:

- To argue and demonstrate that our primary way of understanding mental disorders (the 'discourse' on mental disorders in Foucauldian terms) has been, and, to a certain extent still is, visual;

- To reconstruct a history of the dominant tropes of the visual representation, and the understanding, of mental disorders—from antiquity to the present—and the practices that produce them;
- To analyse the extent to which these tropes still govern our contemporary understanding of mental disorders.

Over the course of history we witness a series of consistent representations, governed by recurring (and invariably visual) tropes that shape variable understandings of different mental disorders. This book is thus organised around a succession of case studies, one per chapter. Each chapter analyses a different trope of the representation of mental disorders. The case studies are divided into four parts: the roots of the visual othering of madness; the othering of the body of the insane; medical imaging and medical othering; the inversion of the tropes of visual othering.

In part one, I look at the origins of the visual othering of the insane. In chapter one, I start with images of the fool, and the staff that they invariably carry. By analysing the attachments that appear over the course of history on the staff and its variants, I reconstruct the connection of this prop with air: the fool as an inflated balloon. I thus analyse how air, in different periods of history and across cultures, has been associated with madness, and how at the same time the insane are represented in ways that are very similar to vagrants, witches and other categories of 'unwanted' people. In chapter two I move on to discussing materialisations of madness and representations of extractions. The best-known example is the stone of madness, portrayed in particular in Dutch and Flemish paintings of the fifteenth, sixteenth and seventeenth centuries. I discuss the extent to which this repository of images can be associated with real surgical operations or episodes of quackery, and I present the iconography of trephination, that is to say, boring holes in the skull for medical reasons. The extraction of madness, whether in the form of stones or vapours that are let out, brings it very close to the iconography of another act of extraction, that of exorcism. I thus analyse the similarities and differences between the extraction of the stone of madness and exorcisms.

In part two, I turn my attention to the bodies of the insane, understood either as individual bodies or as the multitude of the insane that invades and corrupts the whole of the social body. In chapter three I argue how the body—individual or social—can be regarded as a boundary, which is troubled by madness, in real life like in iconography. I start by discussing the case of choreomania or epidemics of collective dancing, showing how dance was portrayed as both the malady and the potential cure for it. I then show how such considerations on convulsive and incontrollable movements apply to Charcot's photographic study of (and male gaze on) hysteria in the second half of the nineteenth century. Choreomaniacs are depicted in groups and are contagious; they need to be driven out of cities to avoid the spread of the convulsive dance to the sane social body. The insane are often depicted in large groups. This is the case with the real events called the feast of fools, which took place at the beginning of January between the thirteenth and the sixteenth centuries, especially in France. Here, fools invade the city, elect a bishop, enter the churches and celebrate mass. Such a multitude needs to be contained, and iconography and medicine provide numerous means of containment, including walls and the asylum itself. But such walls are not insurmountable. At least in iconography there is a constant permeability, and the motif of the cage of fools, where the multitude of the insane is contained, soon becomes a metaphor for the whole world: the world is an asylum and we are all mad. Insanity etches itself onto the individual bodies of those suffering from a mental disorder, at least in iconography. To this extent, in chapter four, I trace the history of physiognomics, the pseudoscience of matching personality traits, including insanity, to external characteristics, in particular facial features. I study how this evolves into phrenology, the study of the shape of the skull, for the very same purposes, and how this is adopted, not always very successfully or enthusiastically, in medicine. I conclude the chapter bringing together the study of exorcism and that of convulsionary dances, with an analysis of how insanity is made to emerge in the field of the visible by means of different postures of the body.

Part three is dedicated to medical visualisations of mental disorders. Of course, in the previous parts of the book I have already discussed medicine and medical visualisations; whether as a stone or as vapours it is normally a medical doctor who extracts madness. Charcot was himself a medical doctor, and of course physiognomics and phrenology were employed in medicine. This part, however, focuses exclusively on medical visualisations and how they are not exempt from aesthetic considerations nor from the same biases as modes of representation that I have discussed earlier. In chapter five I focus on photography, in particular portrait photography of asylum inpatients. While photography has been used in almost every mental hospital/asylum worldwide, especially up until the turn of the century when the significance of photography in psychiatry waned, I will narrow the case study to post-unification Italian asylums. As I shall explain in the chapter, this is a perfect case study to exemplify an international reality: photography is adopted acritically and saluted as a tool to visualise scientific truths and to aid therapy. In this chapter, I show how photography shows a continuity with physiognomical and phrenological considerations. In chapter six, I turn my attention to brain imaging and contemporary medical visualisations of mental disorders. Chapters four and five will have paved the way for us to understand the biases and preconceptions that govern the lay understanding of brain imaging in its psychiatric applications. Despite being, at the time of writing, of no use in clinical psychiatry—i.e., no psychiatrist could tell if someone suffers from a mental disorder just by looking at an fMRI of their brain—brain imaging is generally understood as being a photograph, that is to say a truthful and realistic representation of the activity of the brain. As such, it is by and large understood that mental disorders can be realistically pictured by the tools we have at our disposal. This emerges in popular culture (including cinema and scientific communication), but also in tribunals of law, where psychiatric expertise is often reinforced by brain images that, in fact, tell us very little about the mental disorders from which the subject might or might not be suffering.

In part four, I turn my attention to the inversion of these tropes in anti-psychiatry first, and then in the emergence, discovery or recognition of outsider art. In chapter seven, I analyse the visual strategies of what has been labelled, not entirely accurately, 'anti-psychiatry', with a particular focus on Italy between the 1960s and 1970s. As I explain in the introduction to the chapter, I have chosen Italy not only for continuity with chapter five, but also, and especially, because it is a very emblematic case, where radical reformist psychiatric movements had a real and long-lasting impact on policies and mental health care. Italy is, in fact, to date the only country that has banned by law public psychiatric hospitals, and whose involuntary hospitalisation (what is known as 'sectioning' in the UK) is the shortest in the world (one week, to be renewed weekly). The movement that led to such a radical approach is co-imbricated with visual strategies of propaganda, including photobooks that openly engage with, and subvert, the traditional iconography of the mad, as well as performances reminiscent of the feast of fools, analysed in chapter three. In chapter eight, I turn back to the nineteenth century to trace the history of the emergence of outsider art. We could consider it an 'emergence' but also a 'discovery' and a 'recognition'. Arguably, those suffering from a mental disorder, who in the nineteenth century were almost invariably interned in lunatic asylums, had always produced some form of art. But it is only in the second half of the nineteenth century that this starts to be preserved, looked at and studied. We have to wait until the early twentieth century though for it to be acknowledged as art, with two labels: '*art brut*' or 'outsider art'. In chapter eight, I also discuss to what extent the recognition of the art of the insane as art is an inversion of the existing tropes. It might in fact be the case that recognising it as art but still labelling it as 'outsider' perpetrates the enduring notion that those who do not fit the norms should continue to be considered outsiders.

In each of the chapters I find examples of how the tropes under scrutiny, for good or for ill, can still be found in contemporary and, at times, very recent understandings and representations of mental disorders. In concluding this book and summarising my argument, I focus my attention on these contemporary reiterations of the tropes I worked on throughout the monograph. How shall we know sanity and insanity, if such a distinction exists at all? By making madness visible continues to be the answer.

PART ONE

The Fool and the Roots of Visual Othering

CHAPTER ONE

Fools and Vagrants or How to Visualise the Invisibility of Madness

WHERE BETTER TO BEGIN an exploration into the visualisation of mental disorders than with one of the most enduring symbols of madness: the staff. At first glance it may seem like just a club or a walking stick, but upon closer inspection its layers of meaning start to unfold. The staff, I argue in this chapter, not only symbolises madness but also, and perhaps more curiously, seems to connote madness through its connection with air: the invisible, intangible element we can feel but never see. In a way, the staff allows air to do what seems impossible; it represents the unrepresentable. Air, after all, has long been tied to madness through metaphors of emptiness, inflation and the unpredictable force of the wind. As we shall see shortly, the inflated bladder that often appears at the tip of the fool's staff, or the child's pinwheel that replaces the staff in later iconography, are more than just props; they speak to madness as something both weightless and heavy, as light as air but still a burden to carry. This association between madness and air runs deep, stretching back to Hippocratic ideas of winds shaking the rational mind (*phrenes*) and medieval and modern notions of vapours disturbing the body's balance. Across time, air emerges as a powerful metaphor for madness: it is intangible yet omnipresent, invisible yet deeply felt, a force both natural and unsettling.

In this chapter, I also argue that the staff itself often marks those who carry it as *other*. Whether it is a fool wandering aimlessly, a madman clutching a bladder-tipped cudgel or even a witch soaring on a broomstick, the staff links its bearer to 'outsideness'. It is a symbol that connects madness to society's margins, where other figures—vagrants, wild men and wanderers—also dwell. They share visual traits: ragged clothes, unkempt hair, bare feet and, most significantly, a staff burdened with a bundle or an empty sack. In this way, the fool becomes not just a representation of madness but also a symbol of 'outsideness', someone cast adrift from the boundaries of civilised life.

The staff of madness, then, works on many levels. It makes visible what is otherwise invisible—madness as air, as emptiness—while also marking its bearer as fundamentally *other*. The staff embodies the contradictions of madness: intangible yet burdensome, unseen yet inescapable, internal yet imposed from without.

In this chapter, I trace how the staff evolved as a visual marker of the fool and its enduring connections to air and 'outsideness'. I begin with illuminations of the *insipiens*, the fool of medieval Psalters, who carries a staff often tipped with an empty sack or ball: a *follis*. Through Augustine's use of the word *follis* (an inflated sack) as a metaphor for pride and folly, we can see the roots for the word 'fool' (*follia, folie*). From there, I will explore how the motif of the staff transforms over time, appearing as pinwheels, witches' brooms and other variants, always underscoring the relationship between madness and air. Finally, I will show how the object of the staff aligns the fool with vagrants and other outsiders, revealing how madness is viewed together with marginalisation and the unsettling experience of being cast out, adrift and othered.

By focusing on the staff and its many forms, this chapter explores the deep and lasting connections between madness, air and outsideness, themes to which we will return throughout this monograph. In the next chapter I turn to the material: the *stone* of madness. Even there, air and vapours remain central, as we will see in practices of extracting madness to 'vent' its invisible presence. For now, though, we begin with the staff, a deceptively simple object that carries the weight of centuries of folly, otherness and madness.

Insipientes and Their Staff

During the Middle Ages, the most common depiction of the insane, in particular the fool, can be seen in the initial 'D' of Psalm 52 (53 in modern Catholic numbering): *'Dixit insipiens in corde suo: non est deus'* (The fool says in his heart: 'There is no God'). The iconography of the *insipiens*, especially in relation to the professional court fool, the buffoon and the jester, has been the object of several scholarly studies (Gifford 1974; Assirelli 1988; Pietrini 2002; Saffioti 2013; Valente 2018). For the purposes of this chapter—to trace a history of

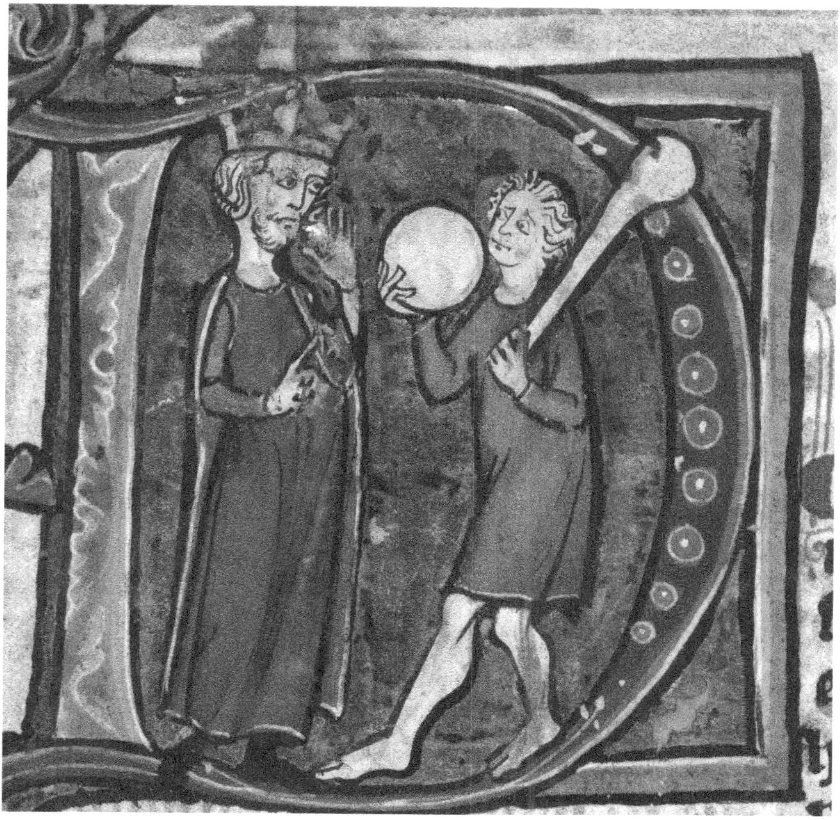

Figure 1: Initial 'D'(ixit) at the beginning of Psalm 53. Psalter and Book of Hours, Use of Saint-Omer. France, N.; 1276. Source: Yates Thompson 43, f. 54. Courtesy of British Library.

the depiction of madness as invisible and the insane as outsiders—I will summarise the characteristics that recur most frequently in the iconography of the fool, something which undergoes a marked evolution from the relatively variable to the quasi-uniform archetype of the jester (around the fifteenth century) (Fig. 1).

Even before the standardisation of the jester, fools shown in the manuscript 'D's do display some recurrent characteristics: they are usually naked, dressed in rags or poorly dressed; barefoot or with only one shoe on; and bald or with the head unevenly shaven. They almost invariably hold a round object in their hands, which they sometimes eat. They are at times portrayed with or alongside a king, who points in their direction (e.g., *Bromholm Priory Psalter*, ms. Ashmole, f. 66,

Bodleian Library, Oxford) or towards the sky (e.g., *Wilton Abbey Psalter,* f. 66v, Royal College of Physicians, London), where there might be an image of God overseeing the exchange (e.g., Ms. *Rawlinson* G 185, f. 43v, Bodleian Library, Oxford). In some manuscripts, the fool is in the presence of a dog (e.g., *La Bible Hystoriaus ou les Hystoires Escolastres,* ms. *Royal* 17.E.VII(I), f. 241, British Library, London) and, in some rare instances, he commits suicide (e.g., Ms. 34, f. 202, Bibliothèque Mazarin, Paris). Invariably, though, the fool holds a staff, to which I will return shortly.

The nakedness or the rags of the fool could be a reference to his inappropriateness and disregard for social conventions; he seems a marginalised social outcast. The slightly later addition of the bald or strangely shaven head (Haseloff 1938, 25) could be a sign of *diminutio* (Ménard 1977), a loss of vitality and strength. Alternatively, Pietrini (2002, 97) suggests it could be a variant of the clerical tonsure, either as a satire or, more likely, to recall vagrant clerics, who, 'outcast by society and harshly condemned by religious authorities [led a] dissipated life'. Towards the end of the tenth century, the Church had decreed that the tonsure should be shaven off vagrant clerics to delete their affiliation to the Church (as per the Archbishop of Sens Gautier Cornut's statute in *Statuta,* XIII, pl. 132, 720).

The most plausible interpretation for the round object they hold is that it represents a loaf of bread (Assirelli 1988, 29). Psalm 52 continues by stating that the *insipientes,* the evildoers who do not believe in God, 'devour my people as though eating bread' (Psalms 53: 4–5). According to Assirelli (1988, 29), madmen in medieval literature are often eager to devour bread, while Pietrini (2002, 83) notes that in the Bible, bread is often a synecdoche for food. Unsalted bread could also be a reference to the lack of taste, drawing on the etymological relationship between *sapientia* (knowledge) and *sapor* (taste), established by Isidore of Seville in his *Etymologiae* (X, 240). The *insipiens* therefore would lack knowledge as much as bread would lack taste/salt, a correspondence that recurs in sayings such as the Latin *cum grano salis* ('with a pinch of salt' to express scepticism) or the Italian *avere sale in zucca* ('to have salt in the pumpkin [head]' to indicate that someone is wise). It is also worth noting that the typical central Italian saltless bread is called *sciocco,* which means both saltless and stupid (Stabile 2008).

Vis-à-vis the king, *insipientes* may be portrayed as his *alter ego,* his counterpart (the fool's staff and round object could be a parody of the sceptre and the orb). The presence of the dog could be explained, following Gross, as a confusion between *panis* and *canis,* an allusion to the stupidity and animality of the fool or even as a satire of the cynics (Gross 1999), whose name derives from the Greek *kynikos*, meaning 'dog-like', reflecting their association with shamelessness, simplicity and rejection of social norms. Could it also be a reference to the canine *Lyssa*, the personification of madness (and rabies) in fifth-century Greek tragedy (Padel 1992, 14)? Another feature, the *insipiens* sometimes committing suicide, like Saul in the Bible, perhaps suggests that not to believe in God means to kill one's soul.

A thirteenth-century medical manuscript by Rogerus de Parma (on whom we will return more extensively in chapter two) dedicates a page to illustrate where to cauterise in cases of insanity (Fig. 2). Bottom right it illustrates migraines (*dolore capiti*), bottom left melancholia, top right epilepsy (considered a form of insanity until well into the twentieth century) and finally, top left, mania. I will return to the other illuminations in chapter three, but for the time being we should note that the maniac is half naked, barefoot, shaven/bald and has a staff: he is an *insipientes*, thus demonstrating that, in medieval iconography, *insipientia*, mania and madness overlapped.

Despite the relative variability of the individual elements within the image of the *insipiens*, one is omnipresent: the staff. This is also the iconographic element that especially interests me, not only because it is the most frequent, but also because it is the one that has survived the longest. As Gilman (2014, 11) says, 'like the leper's clapper, the staff comes to represent the inner nature of the one bearing an outer sign'.

It is perhaps not possible to identify once and for all the origins of the omnipresent 'staff of the mad'. The most plausible explanation is that its origins are as varied as its evolutions and meanings. Gilman (2014, 10–11) describes several potential interpretations: it could have originated from Chronos/Saturn's scythe (Klibansky, Panofsky and Saxl 1964), from Seth-Typhon's flail (Gifford 1974) or it could also be a semantic slippage coming from the bifurcated staff that Brant, in his 1494 book *Ship of Fools*, depicts as the devil's tool to capture souls (Brant 1962, 299). In looking for its origins, I believe Gilman overestimates the prevalence of bifurcated staffs in the iconography of the insane. While there certainly are depictions of madmen with bifurcated staffs, there are many more with clubs, bindles or *marottes*, i.e., non-bifurcated sticks. Also, the two-pronged pitchfork is one of the most prevalent tools of peasants and shepherds in medieval iconography, and therefore the semantic slippage from the tool of the shepherd (transhumant, vagabond par excellence) to the symbol of madness might be more readily explainable in this way.

The simplest form of the staff is that of a club or cudgel, a rough stick ending with a bulge, probably a rudimentary weapon in contrast

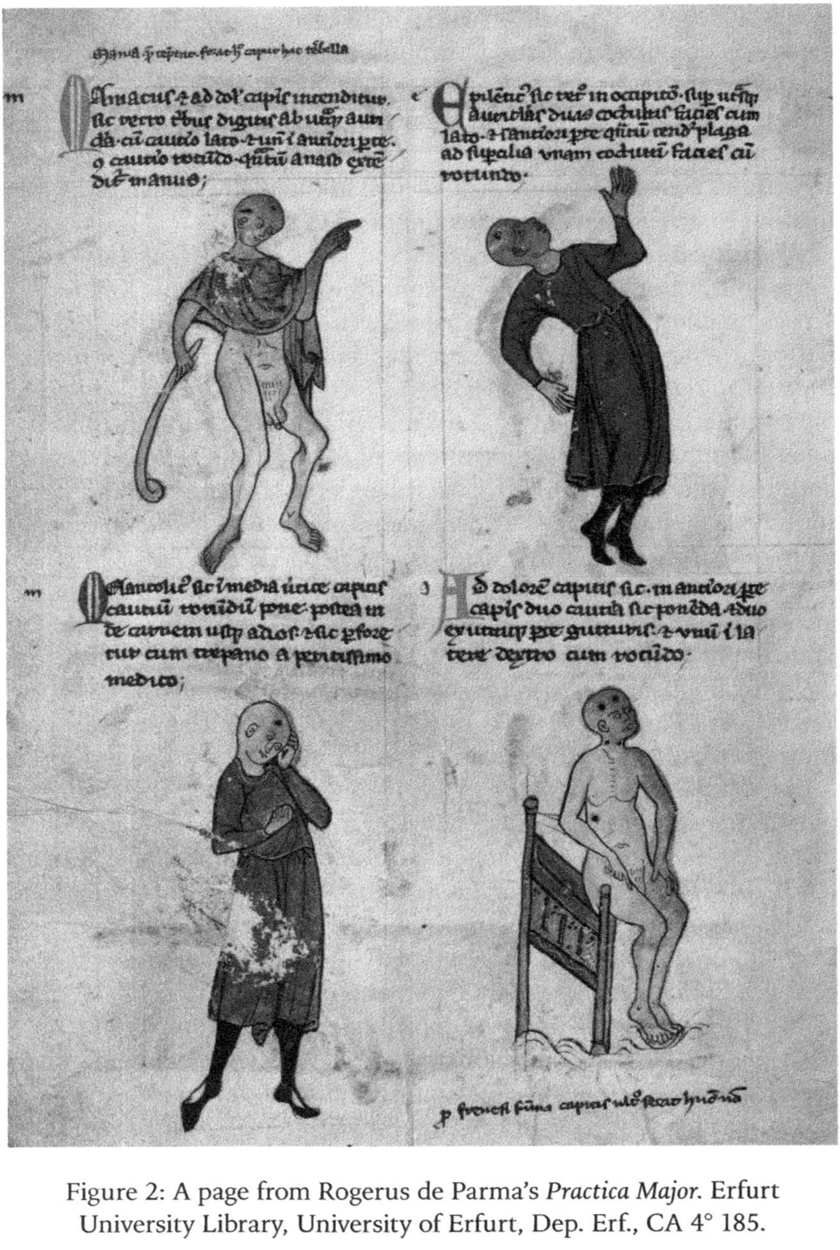

Figure 2: A page from Rogerus de Parma's *Practica Major*. Erfurt University Library, University of Erfurt, Dep. Erf., CA 4° 185.

to the knightly ones (such as swords and maces). Within the illustration inside several drop-cap 'D's from manuscripts, the bulge at the end of the club becomes a head that often resembles the head of the *insipiens* himself, much like the later *marotte*.

Over the course of the fifteenth century, the image of the fool evolves. His depiction appears in contexts other than the initial 'D's of Psalm 52, and his garments and props turn into the iconic image of the jester: court fools dressed in vivid bi-coloured garments, with the typical cap and bells, pictured holding a staff ending in a head, the *marotte*. This is his main stage prop, which he seemingly uses as his own *alter ego*, to stage dialogues and to reach out to the entertained audience (Fig. 3).

Wild men are also depicted with a coarse staff, as if they were using a long branch as a walking stick. At times, there is some overlap in the depiction of wild men, fools and jesters (Amateis 2015). For instance in Thiers (France), the wooden façade of a fifteenth-century house (now occupied by the *Musée de la coutellerie*) features an *homme des bois*, a wild man, carrying a knobstick that ends with a head, much like the *marotte*.[1]

There are also variations as to what is attached to the staff, rather than its shape, the most prevalent of which is an inflated bladder, and indeed a third possible staff of the *insipiens* is that of a short stick with a sack or bladder hanging at its end.[2] Pietrini (2002, 84) notes that this iconography dominates Anglo-Saxon manuscripts, but is almost entirely absent from continental ones. According to her, the bladder is a *bauble*, typical of English fools: an instrument 'whose function was to make noise when it was rotated', normally consisting of an inflated pig bladder containing dried peas (Pietrini 2002, 84). Thus, for her, the bladder is not an attachment to the *marotte* or to the staff, but, when present, makes it a musical instrument in its own right. Pietrini seems to suggest that all staffs with bladders attached fit a description taken from *Gargantua and Pantagruel*, in which Rabelais (1653, 301) describes Panurge giving the jester Triboulet a 'hog's bladder puffed up with wind and resounding because of the hard peas that were within it'. Triboulet

1 An image of the *homme des bois façade* can be seen at: https://commons.wikimedia.org/wiki/File:Thiers_-_l%27Homme_des_Bois_-_JPG1.jpg [accessed 9 Feb. 2024].

2 Of the several potential examples, it will suffice to mention the historiated 'D' in the *Carrow Psalter*. Mid-XIII Century. East Anglia, England. Walters Art Museum, Walters Ms. W.34, f. 113r; see: https://art.thewalters.org/detail/3667/fool-with-bladder-on-stick-eating-cusped-loaf-2/ [accessed 9 Feb. 2024].

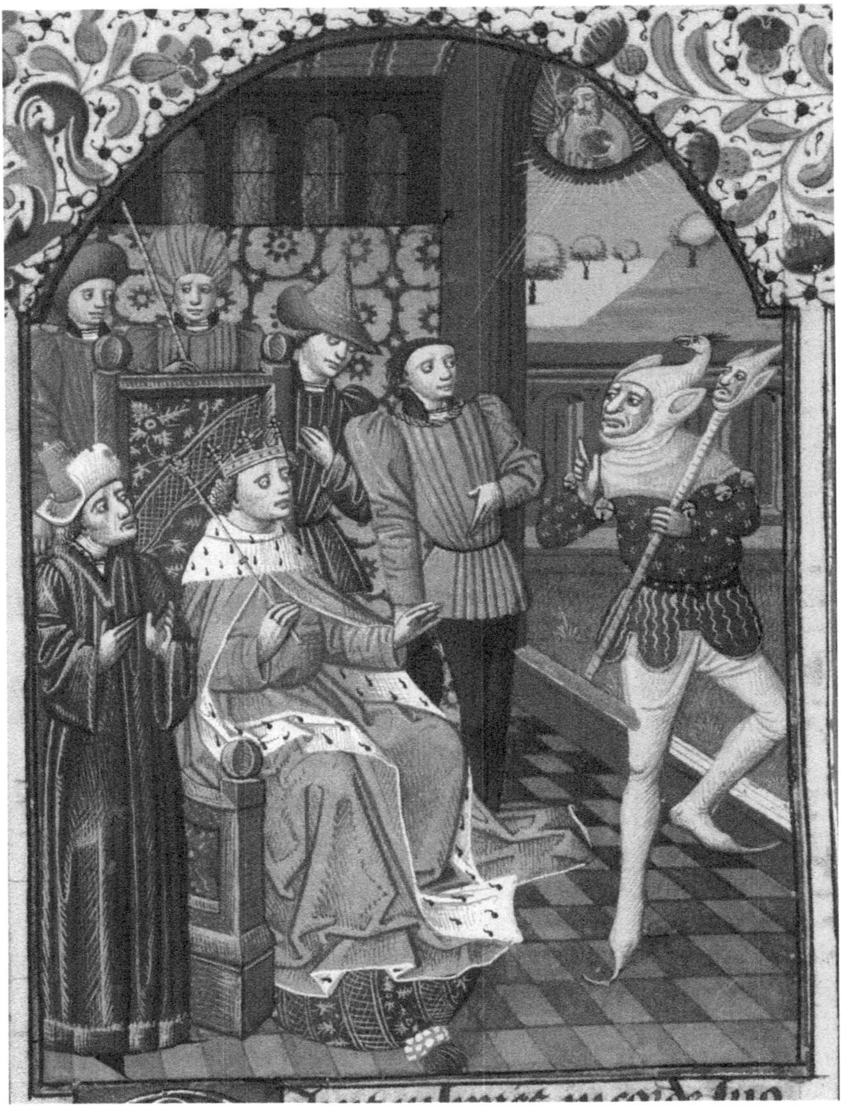

Figure 3: A fool at the beginning of Psalm 53. Bible du XIIIe siècle (1475?), France (Rouen). Free Library of Philadelphia, Rare Book Department, Widener 2, f.290r.

'took a huge delight in the melody of the rickling crackling noise of the peas' (Rabelais 1653, 301). Pietrini's interpretation, however, contradicts Willeford's, who uses the term 'bauble' as a synonym of *marotte*, and maintains that 'attached to the bauble of European court jesters was often a bladder formed into a clear representation of a phallus' (Willeford 1969, 11). This is likely why in the recent exhibition *Figures du fou* at the Louvre (16 October 2024 to 3 February 2025) 'bauble' is simply used as a direct translation of *marotte* in captions, complicating the relationship between the terms. We can rule out the possibility that it represents a bagpipe, as no *insipiens* is depicted blowing into the object, in contrast to a number of Bohemian and Hungarian wall tiles in which court fools are unmistakably playing bagpipes (See Cserey 1974; Gruia 2008; Richterová 1982).

The interpretation of the bladder at the end of the stick as a bauble, a 'musical' instrument that predates the 'profession' of the jester, is certainly plausible. The bladder, however, also survives in depictions of non-jester fools in the modern era. For instance, Mitelli's 1678 *Proverbj figurati* illustrates the proverb 'He who believes himself the wisest, is the craziest', with a badly dressed, semi-barefoot dancing fool, holding a pinwheel in each hand, from each of which hangs one inflated bladder (Mitelli 1967, plate 10).[3] Since the proverb has no reference to the court fool, the image seemingly depicts a madman. His demeanour is not that of a jester and he does not have a *marotte*, but instead he handles two pinwheels with bladders.

In the sixteenth century, when the iconography of the jester is well established, the non-jester fool is indeed often depicted holding a pinwheel: a child's toy operated by blowing air (Pinson 2003). This is the case for instance in Holbein's illustration of Psalm 52 in his 1547 *Icones historiarum Veteris Testamenti* (Holbein 1869). In this illustration, the fool, dressed in rags and with a feather cap resembling Giotto's *Stultitia* in the *Cappella degli Scrovegni*, trips on (or rides) his staff while holding a long pinwheel under his right arm.

In the book on emblems, *Iconologia*, by Cesare Ripa (1593), which we will look at again later, *pazzia* (madness) is described as a 'normal' person (i.e., not bald, not dressed in rags, not barefoot), but instead is riding a long staff and brandishing a child's pinwheel, as if it were a sceptre or mace. Mitelli's plate 10, in fact, pictures the madman by combining pinwheels and bladders. The last plate of Mitelli's book, plate 48, reiterates this use of the pinwheel as a symbol of insanity.

3 The plate can be viewed at: https://www.britishmuseum.org/collection/object/P_1872-1012-3838 [accessed 9 Feb. 2024].

The proverb given is 'The bier gives intellect' (Fig. 4), and the figure who contemplates the funeral bier is dressed in rags and half barefoot, his head is adorned by a hat with feathers and he seems bald under it, all traditional characteristics of the *insipiens*. Most importantly, at his feet, there lies a broken pinwheel; by contemplating mortality, the fool becomes wise. The fool is often depicted in *memento mori* scenes as well. The approach is normally the opposite of Mitelli's though; the fool does not regain intellect by contemplating death, on the contrary death chases the fool, who tries to ignore it (Antoine-König 2024). This is for instance the case in plate XCIIII of Sebastian Brant's fifteenth-century *Narrenschiff*, on which we will return shortly. The plate illustrates chapter 94 of the book *De neglectu mortis* (*On ignoring death*) and depicts a fool (in jester's attire and no staff) chased by a skeleton carrying a bier.

Finally, the staff of the mad also recurs in the witch's broom. According to Gilman (2014, 10), the very first image of a flying witch is in Molitor's 1489 *De lamiis et phitonicis mulieribus*, and depicts a demon flying on a bifurcated stick. However, the actual first illustration of a flying witch predates Molitor's, and is a *marginalis* to the 1451 edition of Martin Le Franc's *Le Champion des Dames*, as noted by Kors and Peters (2001) (Fig. 5). The *marginalis* features two women flying: one on a long stick, the other on a broom, but we still do not know whether the iconographic origins of the witch flying on the broom is from the staff of the *insipiens* or not. We need not stretch it as far as Mann's (2000) pharmacological interpretation to problematise the stick–*marotte*–broom line of iconographic filiation. According to him, witches would trip on alkaloids whose only non-lethal route of administration is vaginal, thus the rubbing on a broomstick. It is sufficient to observe that in numerous images of the *insipiens*, the madman and the jester ride their staffs (e.g., Ms. 76 F 28, f. 81r, *Flemish Psalter*, c.1430, Koninklijke Bibliotheek, L'Aja; see Saffioti 2013, 119), and that not all witches ride brooms.

But why was the staff of madness such an omnipresent prop assigned to the insane? Did fools carry a club to fend off animals or have a walking stick because they were ramblers? Did they have a sack at the end of the stick to carry their scant possessions? That is to say, is the prop of the staff of madness simply a realistic representation of how fools by and large actually appeared in the Middle Ages and beyond? It is certainly possible. But why would they carry a pinwheel or an inflated bladder? Was it because they were all court fools or jesters? I believe the key to understanding the omnipresence of the staff of madness and its variants is in a symbolic reading. In the next

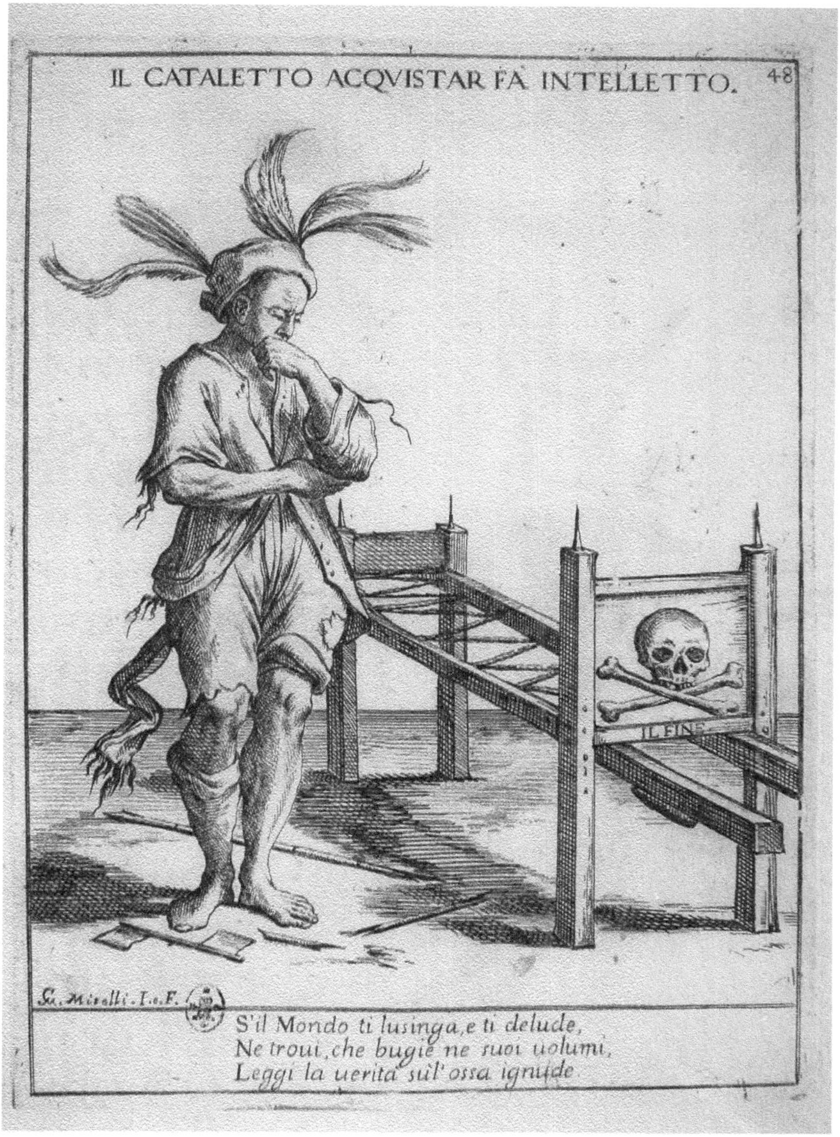
IL CATALETTO ACQVISTAR FÀ INTELLETTO.
48
IL FINE
S'il Mondo ti lusinga, e ti delude,
Ne troui, che bugie ne suoi uolumi,
Leggi la uerità sul'ossa ignude

Figure 4: Mitelli, Proverbj Figurati, plate 48. Courtesy of Biblioteca Casanatense, Roma, MiC, CCC.R.I.XV (tav. 48).

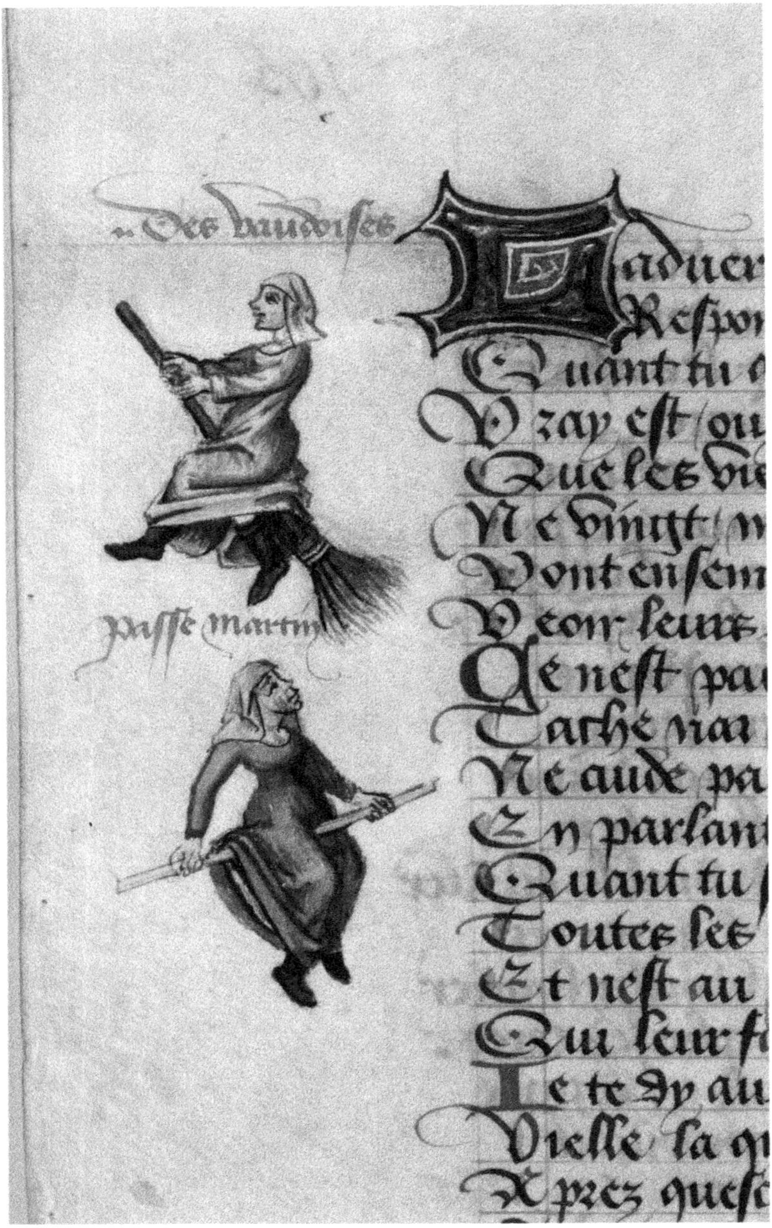

Figure 5: Illumination depicting the two witches on a broomstick and a stick, in Martin Le Franc's "Ladies' Champion", 1451. BNF « Le Champion des Dames, » par « MARTIN LE FRANC, prevost de l'église de Lausane. » (1440). ID/Cote :ark:/12148/btv1b78011897 Folio 105 verso cadré sur "les drôleries des deux sorcières en haut à gauche".

section, I argue, on the one hand, that the staff represents the invisible entity of madness that the insane carry around as a burden, invoking air, either as that which inflates the bladder at the end of their stick or as that which operates their pinwheel. On the other, I will also argue that the insane share the staff as a recognisable feature of their status with several other social outcasts, such as vagabonds.

Folly as Emptiness or Fullness of Air

The visual triangulation between madness, air and the staff pivots on the very etymology of the noun 'fool'. Numerous European languages have cognates of the words 'folly' and 'fool', for instance French with *folie* and *fou* and Italian with *follia* and *folle*. While in English 'folly' and 'fool' are not synonyms of 'madness' and 'mental disorder', in Italian *follia* is, by and large, considered a synonym of *pazzia*: madness. The most widely accepted etymology for the word 'folly' has it deriving from the Latin *follis* (see Pianigiani 1907, 548; Skeat 1888, 215). The first meaning of *follis* was 'bellows', a device used to blow air: an empty bag that is inflated and deflated repeatedly (from which we also get the Spanish vulgar word *follar*: to have sex). Further meanings of the word *follis* are purse, sack, bag and inflated ball, all referring to empty (or air-filled) containers; the metaphorical use of *follis* to indicate the fool, rests on this: the head of the fool is empty but also swollen. The semantic history of this metaphor leads back to early Christianity. In part following Tertullian, who called Anaxarchus' body a 'case' (*follem*) (Tertullian, *Apologeticus*, L.7), Augustine (1991, 244) asks: if there is nothing humbler than God, who let himself be humiliated on the cross for all human beings, 'why do you still rear up, still swell up, you inflated balloon [*follis inflatus*]? God is humble, and are you proud?' This is often quoted as the first written metaphorical use of *follis* in relation to the madness of straying from God's path, in particular in relation to the capital sin of pride (Martino 2008, 30).

Hence, rather than just a realistic depiction of the bauble 'musical' instrument, an item that a court fool might have carried, the bladder at the end of the madman's stick represents a *follis*, both as an inflated balloon and an empty container. It is thus also, and perhaps in particular, a metaphorical signal that the depicted individual is a fool, in that he carries, as a burden/bundle, his *follis*.

Air was long held as the element that animated the body, that is, it enabled the immaterial soul to interact with the material body

(Tertullian's *follem*, the 'case'). According to Stoic philosophers, this happened 'through the agency of *pneuma* (*spiritus* in Latin), or bodily spirits' (Trenery and Horden 2017, 64) (Erasistratus' *pneumatists* based their entire medicine on this assumption: see Nutton 2004, 207). The very word 'psyche' derives from Plato's 'soul', *psyché*, a word which, in turn, originally meant 'breath'. In Homer's *Iliad*, *psyché* is the last breath that humans exhale before dying (e.g., Book V, line 696). *Psyché* does not originally refer to mental processes but is the 'breath of life': 'It [...] behaves sometimes like breath, sometimes like blood. Sometimes it means simply 'life' [...] You have only one, which leaves you at death' (Padel 1992, 30). *Thymós*, the ancient Greek word which we can approximate to 'vital energy', also connects to breath and air. As Onians (2011, 44) says, '*thymos* itself is the breath, which may always be felt as vaporous and sometimes is visible. With it may be compared *fumus*, Sancrit [*sic*] *dhūmaḥ*, "vapour, smoke", Old Slav. *Dymŭ*, "smoke", *duchŭ*, "breath, spirit", etc.'. *Thymos* is not 'mere breath but breath related to blood, not mere air but something vaporous within' (Onians 2011, 48). Ancient Greek gods breathed emotions and thoughts into men (Onians 2011, 56). The ancient Greeks knew perfectly well that without air there was no life (Thivel 2005), even though it is invisible or, better still, visible only through reason: '[Air] is invisible to sight, though visible to reason. For what can take place without it? In what is it not present? What does it not accompany? For everything between earth and heaven is full of wind' (Hippocrates 1923, 231). The notion that air animates the body dominates the medical conception of the psyche throughout the Middle Ages and the modern era. The 'spirits' that animate the body, according to medieval doctors, are the 'inward wits' (Harvey 1975, 2).

'Spirit' is also one of the archetypes that populate the collective unconscious, according to Jung (2010, 385–86); it is 'the principle that stands in opposition to matter [...] the *ligamentum animae et corporis*'. Also, the 'development in man's idea of spirit rests on the recognition that its invisible presence is a psychic phenomenon' (Jung 2010, 390). The archetype of the spirit is 'in keeping with its original wind-nature, [it] is always an active, winged, swift-moving being as well as that which vivifies, stimulates, incites, fires, and inspires' (Jung 2010, 389). We do not need to embrace an archetypal psychoanalytic reading to recognise that the notions of insides, psyche, soul and spirit do indeed have a deeply rooted correlation with air (the very etymology of the Latin noun for soul, *animus*, from which the Italian *anima* derives, can be traced back to the ancient Greek noun *ánemos*, wind).

However, in antiquity and the Middle Ages, reference to the air in the *follis*—and in its metaphorical derivative 'the fool'—does not necessarily stem from the omnipresence of inward wits or spirits; after all, air *qua* inward wits had a neutral if not positive connotation. It was the air that animated the body, and did not necessarily cause madness or illness. The air that causes disease is the air that blows: 'A breeze is a flowing and a current of air. When therefore much air flows violently, trees are torn up by the roots through the force of the wind [...]. Such then is the power that it has in these things' (Hippocrates 1923, 231). The blowing air, wind in particular, can cause madness: 'gusts of passion', such as when 'a raging *pneuma* of madness carries off Io' or '"blasts of hostile winds" are breathed by an impious besieger of Thebes' (Padel 1992, 92); 'winds shake *phrenes* [...] hatred and fury are gusts in the mind. Antigone's soul suffers "blasts of the same winds"' (Padel 1992, 116).

The reference to blowing air as causing madness surfaces in Sanskrit as well, in which both the words *vātula* (inflated with wind) and *vātika* (windy, stormy) mean 'affected by the wind-disease', thus madness (Monier-Williams 1872, 900–902), although *vātika* can also refer to a medical procedure to 'calm the wind' (Scharfe 1999, 615). Both derive from *vāt*, which means to blow gently but also to go, to act favourably towards one setting out on a journey (Monier-Williams 1872, 900). From *vāt* also derives *vāta*, one of the three humours/faults (*doshas*) of the *āyurveda*, the traditional Indian medicine, a humour made of ether and air (Scharfe 1999). This conception not only survives in contemporary *āyurvedic* alternative medicine but also in indigenous medicines such in Tibet's notion of *rLung* (wind/breath), which is involved in both the cause and the treatment of what conventional medicine would consider mental disorders (Deane 2019). We can also find it in the Arabic expression 'dimaghou mehawiya' ('his head is breezy') and of course in the English 'he is full of hot air'.

The *follis* refers also to the act of inflating, of *blowing* madness into humans. This emerges in iconography, for instance in one of the fourteenth-century misericords of the Great Malvern Priory, which depicts a man blowing air up another man's bottom by means of a pair of bellows. The one who is being inflated is naked and his head is that of an ass (or at least he has ass's ears) (Fig. 6). Such an idea is also on display in the iconographic evolution of the staff into the pinwheel: a child's toy which symbolises the changeability, the unpredictability of the mad, but also spins because of the blowing air, the wind (cf. the German idiom *Am Rad drehen*, 'to go crazy', literally 'to spin the wheel' but also the English 'winds of change').

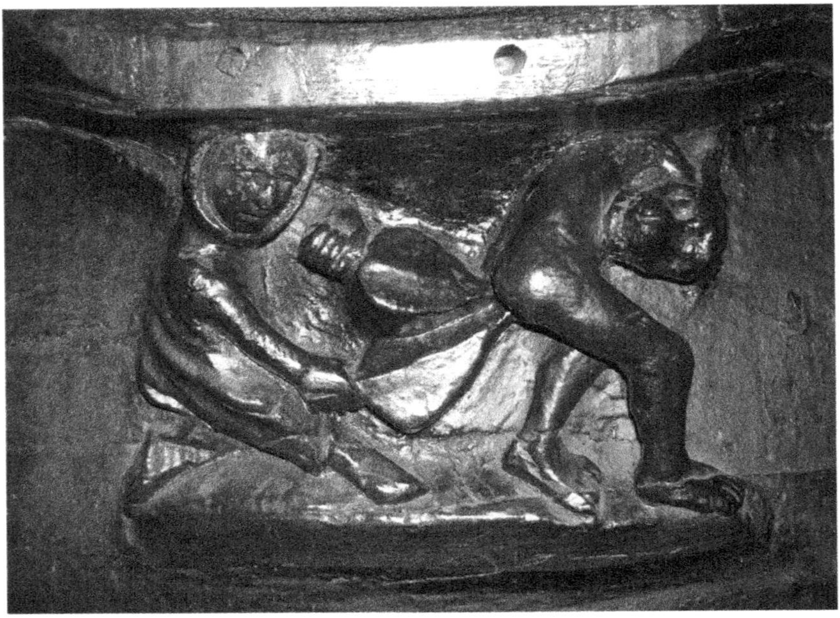

Figure 6: Misericord of the Great Malvern Priory.
2025 © www.misericords.co.uk.

Finally, it is worth noting that it is on a staff/broom that the witch flies *in the air*. 'Air, breath, wind are the soul's elements. Of course it flies', concludes Padel (1992, 97). We could say the same about the witch. The air inflates the mind with emptiness and madness and is symbolised in the staff on which this emptiness is carried. Of course the witch flies in the air on a stick.

In iconography, therefore, the *follis* establishes a complex relationship between inside and outside, a complexity to which we return often in this monograph: the air that causes madness is blown in from outside the fool, but it resides within him. Blowing air also operates the pinwheel and accounts for the inconstancy of the insane. The stationary air inside the *follis*, instead, is a reference to the emptiness that fills the head of the fool. Mitelli's '*pazzo*', who carries a pinwheel with an inflated bladder in each hand, is indeed captioned: 'nothing fills your mind, but vapours' (Mitelli 1967, plate 10). However, in iconography this air is not inside the fool. On the contrary, it is an emptiness that the fool *has*, perhaps as his only possession, and that he carries with him as a burden. Arguably, it is a very 'light' bundle, made of air, which also alludes to the light-headedness and fickleness of the insane. It is a burden nevertheless; the only 'luggage' in the vagabondage of the insane. In this context, I will, shortly, analyse the overlap in the depiction of the insane and the vagabond.

This connection between madness and air persists through history, independently of the idea of the staff of the madman and of folly, repurposing the abovementioned notion of inward wits or bodily spirits. In the sixteenth century for instance, Paracelsus (1979, 150), to whom I will return in the next chapter, recommended cutting open fingers and toes to let air in to cool mania down. If this does not always help, at all or in part, it is only because the matter cannot be cooled sufficiently to let out the distillation.

In 1621, in *The Anatomy of Melancholy*, Burton (2004, 1.II.V, para. 5) maintains that

> The devil many times takes his opportunity of such storms, and when the humours by the air be stirred, he goes in with them, exagitates our spirits, and vexeth our souls; as the sea waves, so are the spirits and humours in our bodies tossed with tempestuous winds and storms.

While on the one hand Burton seems to be referring to the tradition of considering stormy winds as harbingers of mental disorder and its conveyance into one's soul, he is also tapping into the centuries-old medical imagery of 'vapours'. According to Pormann (2013, 240), 'vapours rising from the stomach to the brain are one of the explanations for [melancholia] that we find in a variety of sources'. In 1733, the pioneering physician George Cheyne published *The English Malady: or, A Treatise of Nervous Diseases of all Kinds*. According to Cheyne (1733, 194), 'vapours' (and its synonym 'spleen') is a generic term that was so broadly used in English that 'it is a common subterfuge for meer [*sic*] ignorance of the nature of distempers'. Vapours proper should only be called a first degree of the disorder

> when [...] the symptoms then, besides lowness of spirits are wind, belching, yawning, heart-burning, croaking of the bowels [...] a pain in the pit of the stomach (which is sometimes mistaken for lung case, especially if attended with shortness of breath, and a tickling cough, from a wind in the cavity pressing on the diaphragm, and thereby pressing on the lungs, which is common and goes very justly by the name of an hysterick, or nervous cough) and sometimes inflation, and an actual visible swelling, to a very considerable bigness, in the stomach to be seen. (Cheyne 1733, 196–97)

The *vapours* or *spleen*, later called just the nerves or the 'hyp', i.e., 'milder' affections such as hysteria or hypochondria, referred to disorders 'thought to have their origins in the hypochondrium, or the upper abdomen' (Scull 2016, 163). Although neither air as an external cause nor movements of internal vapours are explicitly mentioned in Cheyne's description, numerous symptoms relate lowness of spirit to air (e.g., bloating, cough), not to mention the name itself: vapours. Most interestingly, Cheyne (1733, 52) explicitly splits the relationship between air and folly: 'It is a common observation [...] that *fools* [...] are seldom much troubled with vapours or lowness of spirits'. Starting with Cheyne, those affected by the air in the form of vapours, the spleen or the hyp will be the higher and middle classes: 'From the eighteenth century onwards, polite society has continued to find in such "nervous" disorders (the vapours, the spleen, and hysteria, [...]) a rich social idiom' (Porter 2002, 86).

As Scull (2011, 8) has it, 'In the seventeenth and eighteenth centuries, there was much anguishing about the distinctions between hysteria, hypochondria, the spleen, and the vapors, though for many informed physicians this was seen as so much hair-splitting, rather than corresponding to a clearly separable set of disorders'. Even in the contemporary era, in the twentieth and twenty-first centuries, studies have been carried out in psychiatry to ascertain the impact of weather, in particular of wind, on mental disorders (e.g., Bos, Hoenders and Jonge (2012); Bulbena et al. (2005)). Never mind that none has proved conclusive, what these studies testify to is that the metaphorical relationship between wind and mental disorders is still prevalent, and remains the potential subject of scientific enquiry.

The Insane as Outsider: Fools and Vagabonds

With its attachments (in particular the *follis*, but also, as we shall see in this section, the human-shaped bulge of the marotte) and in its evolutions (such as the pinwheel and the witch's broom), the staff symbolises, on the one hand, that the insane carry with them insanity as a burden, on the other that that insanity is outside of the insane, it is other to the human. The majority, if not all, of the depictions of fools, the insane and madmen from the early Middle Ages to the modern era feature a staff. This is a crucial characteristic that they share with other 'unwanted' categories, such as witches and wild men. The relationship inside–outside that the staff entails is central to any visualisation of madness, and reveals the semantic proximity in iconography of the insane with another particularly disliked category: outsiders, vagabonds and vagrants. While I have thus far focused on the incarnation of insanity in a 'prop' (the staff) and in an 'element' (air) in order to show how the invisibility and immateriality of madness are both overcome and thematised in its visual representation, here I analyse how the visualisation of madness translates into the visualisation of the *insane*; in this case, in relation to the vagrant, the first case we encounter of the *othering* of the insane.

As Laharie (1991, 157) has it, the fool is 'an a-social being, he is not part of any group and his life is that of a vagabond. Or, for that era, to wander alone was a symptom of madness'. Assirelli (1988, 32), in passing, notes that the *insipiens* is often depicted 'walking, carrying the wayfarer's bundle'. Perhaps Foucault's affirmation that 'an itinerant existence was often the lot of the mad' (Foucault 2009, 9) is an overstatement, but the staff of the madman is indeed also a symbol of vagabondage. The iconography of the madman overlaps with 'all the figures associated with any divergence from the society's accepted norms' (Gilman 2014, 2). While Gilman is thinking of 'the maniac, the idiot, the melancholic, the wild man, or the possessed', I would add the vagabond as a central figure in the semantic slippages of key elements of the representation of the outcast. Much has already been written on vagabonds in medieval and early modern times (e.g., Cubero 1998; Geremek 1994; Mazzi 1991; Mollat 1986; Pullan 1978; Riis 1981). As Dani (2018, 15–16) put it: 'The vagabond, like the migrant [...] infringes the founding values of the *civitas* [...]. The vagabond, free from any bond, circumventing these values and thus calling into question the very archetype of *civitas*, ends up incarnating [...] the Other'.

Other social categories share with the vagabond his mobility. In the previous section, in reference to the tonsure of the fool, I have already mentioned vagrant clerics, but we could add 'pilgrims, students, apprentices, merchants and sellers, preachers, healers, knights and soldiers, shepherds, evicted peasants, brigands, nomads and beggars' (Dani 2018, 19). Mobility was considered suspicious and tantamount to vagrancy. As Geremek (1994, 83) says, 'migrating workers were condemned as vagrants, and it became illegal to beg, or to move from one place to another, without special permission [...]. Legislation of this type was enforced with varying degrees of severity in each European country'.

Despite the Christian message of charity, at the apex of medieval development, in the mid-thirteenth century, vagabonds and paupers were increasingly marginalised, probably as their numbers grew: 'from the thirteenth century, the number of *extranei* or *vagantes*, landless paupers trekking here and there in search of work, grew at a sharp pace' (Lis, Coonan and Soly 1979, 16).

The vagabond seems to have a lesser visual presence than the *insipiens*, suggesting that, partly due to the similarities in depiction, the two categories by and large overlapped in medieval iconography, at least until the *insipiens* evolved into the codified image of the jester. The vagabond as a beggar is depicted in the mid-fourteenth-century manuscript *Meditatione de la vita di nostro Signore Ihesu Christo*.[4] Four beggars—a woman, two men and a child—are receiving food from a saint. They receive a loaf of bread, shown as a round white object, similar to the bread of the *insipiens*. The first beggar wears a long fur coat and has a stick (much like the wild man) and wears a straw hat. The beggar in the middle, in contrast, has a monk-like tonsure.

Due to the paucity of visual sources specifically depicting vagabonds, it is interesting to note how much of the representation of the *insipiens* (and also of the cognate wild man) suggests vagrancy; the *insipiens* is dressed in rags, devours bread and his head is often shaven in the guise of vagrant clerics. Most significantly, he carries a staff, that might be a walking stick or the bifurcated pitchfork of peasants/shepherds, which often ends with a bladder or a sack. The bundle of the vagrant, and also of the transhumant shepherd (another 'mobile' category looked at with suspicion for its mobility: see Geremek 2014, para. 28 and 38), is seemingly empty, as is the *follis* in the case of the *insipiens*. In other words, through a varying combination of symbols, he is always depicted as an outcast: a homeless, hungry outsider, a beggar and/or a vagabond.

The insane and the vagabond share in iconography the stick with a bundle and their vagueness, their marginalisation and their condition of being outside society. I believe this condition of outsideness is also represented in the early iconography of the *marotte*. This prop, almost universally used by jesters from the fifteenth century, appears in iconography well before the standardisation of the representation of the court fool, with the earliest occurrences attested in the thirteenth century.[5] While these could certainly be regarded as *ante litteram*

4 Illumination of beggars. *Meditatione de la vita del nostro Signore Ihesu Christo*. Fourteenth century. Siena, Italy. Paris, BNF, Italien 115 f. 8v; see: https://gallica.bnf.fr/ark:/12148/btv1b10527648k/f20.item [accessed 4 Feb. 2025].

5 Arguably, the best-known early example of this is the historiated initial 'D' in Amiens, Bibl. mun., ms. 0124, f. 054v (from around the thirteenth century); see: https://bvmm.irht.cnrs.fr/consult/consult.php?VUE_ID=1388469 [accessed 4 Feb. 2025].

stage props, a symbolic reading, in addition to the representational one, helps us to weave together the semantic slippages of the staff during history. The head at the end of the staff, at least in early depictions of the *insipiens*, seems to represent the condition of folly as being out of oneself. It makes visible the dichotomy inside–outside and its inversion in madness. Early Greek 'psychology' already pointed to a physical seat for the mind, albeit of uncertain location: the *phrenes*. 'One can lose one's hold on [the *phrenes*], be "struck out", ... "no longer in one's *phrenes*"' (Padel 1992, 22). Madness is to be out of oneself—*ekstasis*—not only in negative terms of fury (*mania* from the verb *mainomai*) but also in prophetic terms. Plato had already noted in the *Phaedrus* (244c) that *mantiké*, prophecy, 'the noblest of arts, that [...] foretells the future', and *manike*, madness (which 'men of old [...] thought [...] neither shameful nor disgraceful') are connected. 'Mania, when it comes by gift of the gods, is a noble thing, but nowadays people call prophecy the mantic art, tastelessly inserting a T in the word'.

Etymology might help us to understand this visual overlap and the semantic exchange between vagrancy and folly. Vagabond comes from the Latin *vagus*, rambling, roaming, wandering, thus also unfixed and unsettled, much like animals: 'wandering [*vagi*] through the woods like wild beasts', as Quintilian writes in the *Institutio Oratoria* (VIII, 3, 81). *Vagus* was also used figuratively as unsteady, inconstant, wavering, vague. Catullus, for instance, in verse 4 of *Carmen* 63, describes the state of the enraged Attis as *vagus animi*. Insane, vagabond and wild man converge in the early-thirteenth-century German adaptation of Chrétien de Troyes's Arthurian romance *Yvain*. The author, German poet Hartmann von Aue (1979), tells of Sir Iwein's quests and focuses on his struggle with madness, for which he ends up roaming the forest like a beast, much like Nebuchadnezzar in the Bible (Daniel 4:33).

Vagrancy and madness often overlap in literature. At the turn of the fifteenth century we encounter the first-known first-person description of a mental disorder, by a pivotal figure of fifteenth-century Middle English literature: Thomas Hoccleve. According to Thiher (1999, 47), Hoccleve's work testifies to the fact that 'a poet lives his madness in conformity with the explanatory model that his era offers him', a notion that we could extend to all those living with mental disorders. In the 'Complaint' of his *Series*, Hoccleve (1932, 26) describes his mental disorder:

> Right so, though that my witte were a pilgrim
> and went fer from hom, he cam again.

God me devoided of the grievous venim
that had enfectid and wildid my brain.
See how the cureise leche [doctor] most soverain
unto the seke geveth medicine
In need, and hym releveth of his grevous pine.

Madness for Hoccleve is thus caused by a substance—a 'venim'—a humoral imbalance of sorts. It is also a test sent by God that makes of his madness a pilgrimage, a voyage. While the insane are not described here as vagrants, it is madness itself that is considered tantamount to vagrancy.

One century later, the poet Ludovico Ariosto describes the protagonist of his masterpiece, the chivalric romance titled *Orlando Furioso,* as going mad for love. *Orlando Furioso* is an Italian epic poem first published in complete form in 1532, and is a continuation of Matteo Maria Boiardo's unfinished romance *Orlando Innamorato.* The twenty-third canto of the *Orlando Furioso* is set in a peaceful glade where Orlando seeks shelter for the night. These surroundings trigger Orlando's madness, as they seem to mock him with evidence of his beloved Angelica's betrayal. Consumed by rage and madness, Orlando destroys the elements of nature to silence their voices that speak of this betrayal. A shepherd's story and the sight of a jewel given to Angelica further push Orlando into madness. Two key visual elements emerge in Orlando's descent into madness. The first is that, as part of his fury, Orlando removes his armour and tears his clothes to rags:

At length, impelled by phrensy, the fourth day,
He from his limbs tore plate and mail away.

Here was his helmet, there his shield bestowed;
His arms far off; and, farther than the rest,
His cuirass; through the greenwood wide was strowed
All his good gear, in fine; and next his vest
He rent; and, in his fury, naked showed
His shaggy paunch, and all his back and breast.
And 'gan that phrensy act, so passing dread,
Of stranger folly never shall be said.

(Canto 23: CXXXII–CXXXIII)

Ariosto thus inverts the ritual donning of the knight's armour to visualise Orlando's descent into madness. The undressing of the symbol of knighthood par excellence, the armour, turns into the tearing of clothes into rags, making the proud knight Orlando a figure that resembles the fool of psalters with his appearance like a vagrant.

The second key element to note is that madness is clearly depicted as being 'out of oneself', being outside and being lost like a vagrant in the woods:

> Let him make haste his feet to disengage,
> Nor lime his wings, whom Love has made a prize;
> For love, in fine, is nought but phrensied rage,
> By universal suffrage of the wise:
> And albeit some may show themselves more sage
> Than Roland, they but sin in other guise.
> For, what proves folly more than on this shelf,
> Thus, for another, to destroy oneself?
>
> Various are love's effects; but from one source
> All issue, though they lead a different way.
> He is, as 'twere, a forest, where parforce
> Who enter its recess go astray;
> And here and there pursue their devious course:
> In sum, to you I, for conclusion, say;
> He who grows old in love, besides all pain
> Which waits such passion, well deserves a chain.
>
> (Canto 24: I–II)

Ariosto here tells us that falling in love is tantamount to going mad, that readers should stay away from love and that indeed if someone decides to accept love, despite this warning, they deserve to be chained as insane. Most importantly, he is telling us that the foremost sign of madness is to lose oneself, that it has many visible effects, but there is only one madness that makes them surface, and finally that madness is like a forest in which one can only get lost. The wanderer, the traveller, the vagrant and the insane converge here in the figure of the one who is driven 'out of oneself' by love and madness, whose relationship is a tightly knitted and timeless one in literature and the arts, which goes back to ancient Greek tragedy, at least. For instance, in Euripides' *Hippolytus*, such a link between love and madness is at the heart of the work. Phaedra's forbidden desire for her stepson, Hippolytus, is forced upon her by the goddess Aphrodite as a cruel form of punishment, leaving her tormented and desperate. Eaten up by shame and internal conflict, this love veers out of control, pushing her toward madness and ultimately leading to her tragic death. Similarly, Antonio del Pollaiuolo's painting of 1470, *Hercules and Deianira,* captures the anguish of Deianira, Hercules' wife, who tragically kills him by mistake. In Shakespeare's *Hamlet,* Ophelia's descent into madness is tied to her heartbreak caused by Hamlet's rejection of her and the grief of losing her father, shown through her fragmented speech and sorrowful songs. Tchaikovsky's opera *Eugene Onegin* repeats the love/madness trope through Tatyana, whose heartfelt love letter and Onegin's cold rejection push her into emotional turmoil, echoing a long tradition of love-induced despair in opera. Time and again, love is not just the cause of madness but seems almost indistinguishable from it; a force that consumes, destabilises and transforms. Those madly in love or driven mad by unreciprocated love are often visually depicted with the characteristics of the *insipiens.* Such is the case, for instance, in the illustrations of Tristan madly in love with Isolde. As Zink (2024, 60) has it, 'folly goes hand in hand with love'.

The heroic fury of the warrior or knight could turn into madness and uncontrolled antisocial behaviour, creating in reality, and in the imaginary, 'people without a place in the social hierarchy, who roamed freely abroad and who, like demobilized soldiers, were capable of the invasive violence characteristic of furor' (Kromm 2002, 50). According to Kromm (2002, 54) 'the unpredictability and the violence of these dangerous vagrants, in addition to their bogus association with some of the most frightening incurable illnesses like epilepsy and furor, combined to give observers a clear impression that the vagrants most to be feared were the wandering, violent insane'. A combination of violence, vagrancy and insanity typically converged into the Abram-men and Toms of Bedlam, a famous group of lunatic vagrants who claimed to have been discharged from Bethlem Hospital (Bedlam) without being cured of insanity (Clarke 1975, 237–39). Toms of Bedlam were represented as dishevelled, dressed in rags, having long hair and a beard, and invariably carrying a staff, overlapping their iconography with that of the wild man and the insane. In Shakespeare's *King Lear,* Edgar pretends to be a Tom of Bedlam; this feigning of madness shows us clearly what the expectations were of a madman:

> The country gives me proof and precedent
> of Bedlam beggars, who, with roaring voices,
> strike in their numbed and mortified bare arms
> pins, wooden pricks, nails, sprigs of rosemary;
> and with this horrible object, from low farms,

> pooer pelting villages, sheepcotes, and mills,
> sometimes with lunatic bans, sometimes with prayers,
> enforce their charity. (II, iii, 13ff)

Several ballads narrate the wandering of the Toms of Bedlam, always associating them with rage, furor and insanity. This is the case for instance in *The Mad Man's Morrice* (1637):

> Heard you not lately of a man
> That went beside his wits,
> and naked through the streets he ran
> wrapt in his franticke fits?

As Kromm (2002, 57) has it, 'subsequent efforts to confine the insane were in effect prompted by an interest in containing the danger their vagrancy posed to the social order'. I will return to the representation of insanity by means of confinement, and the breaching of this, in chapter three, but for the purpose of this chapter I will now analyse another semantic overlap connecting madness and outsideness: that between the insane and the traveller.

Ship of Fools: Travellers and Migrants

While it may be true that not all who wander are lost, iconography often tells a different story; travellers are as vague and suspicious as vagrants and the insane. We have seen that blowing air and the wind can cause madness and disease, but it is also that which inflates the sails and sets ships on their journeys. Previously in this chapter, I have shown this semantic overlap at work in the Sanskrit *vāt*. The wind that causes the wind-diseases also inflates the sails; the wind that spins the pinwheel also sets travellers at sea on their journeys. These water-based vagabondages are represented in the numerous images of 'ships of fools' (see Midelfort 1999, 232ff) that follow the publication of Brant's *Narrenschiff* in 1494 and which, according to Gilman (1988, 22), rest on (although I would rather say create) 'the myth of the mad as travelers, an image still with us'.

The motif of the ship of fools originates in Plato's *Republic*. In the sixth book (488a–489a), Plato describes a ship with a shipmaster who is slightly deaf and of impaired vision. His sailors are quarrelling for seizing control of the helm, each claiming they have been taught how to do it, but also incapable of naming the teacher and contradictorily

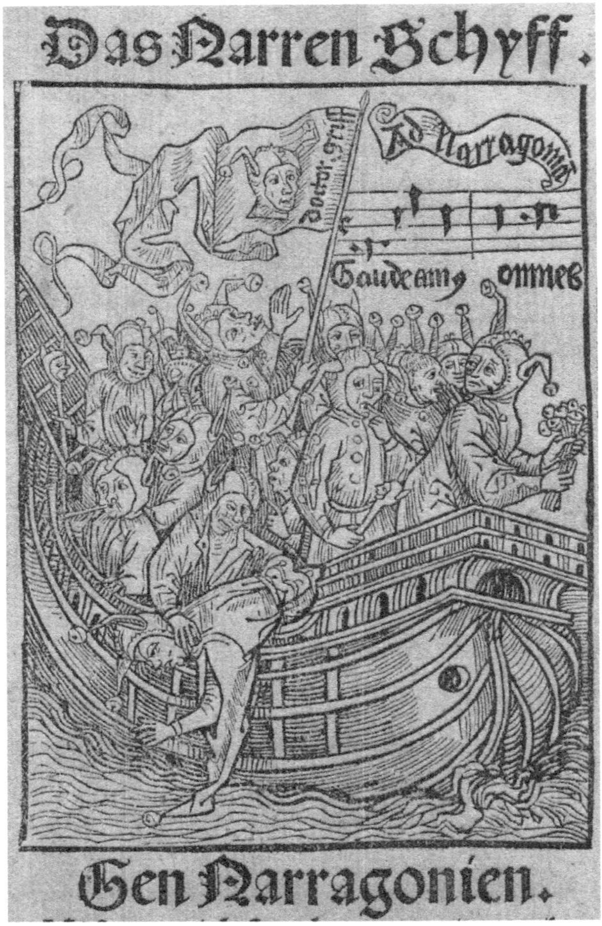

Figure 7: Brant, *Das Narrenschyff*, 1494, [6]–1v.
Public Domain, Courtesy of Staatsbibliothek, Berlin.

affirming that sailing cannot be taught at all. The sailors intoxicate the shipmaster and mount a feast consuming all the stores of the ship. They give the helm of the ship to the most cunning, not to the best sailor. The ship, adrift in the sea, with the sailors feasting rather than piloting it, and naming a cunning rather than competent ruler, is for Plato an allegory of democracy and demagogues: a government that is not led by experts.

It is on this that the trope of the ship of fools emerges, and finds its most notorious (and the first illustrated) incarnation in Brant's *Ship of Fools*, published in 1494 in Switzerland (Fig. 7). The book comprises a prologue, 112 concise satires and an epilogue, adorned with woodcuts. Brant uses the ship of fools to criticise the weaknesses and vices of his contemporaries. In this work, he introduces us to the character of Saint Grobian, whom he envisions as the patron saint of uncultured and indelicate individuals. During the pre-Reformation period, the concept of foolishness served as a widely used concept to justify criticism, as can be seen in the works of Erasmus' *Praise of Folly* and Martin Luther's *Address to the Christian Nobility*. Court fools enjoyed a certain ability to express themselves fairly openly, albeit not entirely freely, so by adopting the voice of the fool in his writing, Brant could effectively legitimise his critique of the Church. However, some, like the Abbot of Sponheim, Johannes Trithemius, lamented Brant's choice of title and preferred to call it the *Divina Satyra*, and likened the work to Dante Alighieri's *Divine Comedy* for their shared usage of local languages. The book was incredibly popular and saw numerous authorised and unauthorised editions, and was published in Reutlingen, Nuremberg, Strasbourg and Augsburg, up until 1512. It was translated into Latin by Jakob Locher in 1497, into French by Pierre Rivière in 1497 and Jean Drouyn in 1498, and into English by Alexander Barclay and Henry Watson in 1509.

The work is known for its elaborate iconographic apparatus made of 103 woodcuts, with approximately two-thirds attributed to the young Albrecht Dürer, while the remainder were created by the artists known as the Haintz-Nar-Meister and the Gnad-her-Meister, and two other anonymous artists. The poem and its illustrations describe the whimsical journey of a group of fools that set sail on a ship, aiming to reach *Narragonien* (the Land of Fools).

During their daring expedition, the fools repeatedly break the Ten Commandments, give in to the Seven Deadly Sins and go on a series of bizarre adventures. The majority of these woodcuts feature at least one fool, which displays the traditional features that I have described above, such as the staff, a bulging cudgel or a marotte. Since we are at the cusp of the transition into the iconography of the court fool and jester, all of the fools feature jester's attire, including the hat with the ass's ears and the bells.

The first woodcut depicts the ship itself in the frontispiece of the book. In the first edition the ship is depicted as being overloaded with fools, all in their jester's attire. Two are fighting, much like in Plato's *Republic*, and at the helm there seems to be a cleric (another vagrant figure associated with the *insipiens*, as I have discussed above), drinking from a round flask reminiscent of the round object associated with *insipientes* in the Middle Ages.

Hieronymus Bosch's *The Ship of Fools* painting (recently dated to 1491) was probably inspired by the frontispiece of Brant's *Narrenschiff* (Fig. 8). Bosch's paintings in general are of great importance for the visualisation of mental disorders in history, and I will return to his work in more detail in the next chapter, but for the purpose of my discussion here, I will focus just on his *The Ship of Fools*. It was probably the upper part of the left panel of a hinged triptych originally, with what is now known as the *Allegory of Intemperance* below it; the other wing contained the painting *Death and the Miser*, with *The Wayfarer* on the rear side, while the central front panel has not been identified yet. In *The Ship of Fools* we see a boat drifting aimlessly in the sea, carrying ten individuals, while two others are overboard. At the centre of the group there is a nun playing a lute in front of a friar or a tonsured cleric. On the left side, a woman seems poised to strike a man who drags a flagon through the water, while on the right side another man appears to be vomiting overboard, while a man dressed as a court fool drinks from a cup above him. One of the boatmen uses a large ladle instead of an oar, and the other has a flagon attached to his oar. Hanging from the mast, there is a round, seemingly edible, object: a pancake or a round loaf of bread, a typical prop of the *insipiens*, which the main group seems to be attempting to eat. Climbing the mast, another character prepares to carve meat from a roasted bird fastened to the mast itself, which resembles a tree adorned with flowers and leaves. While it would indeed not make sense for a mast to be a tree (how could that garner the wind?), it should be noted that in many romance languages (thus not middle Dutch, Bosch's native language), such as Italian, the word for mast and for tree is the same: *albero*. A flag bearing a crescent moon, perhaps symbolising 'lunacy' from the Latin word 'luna', flies from the mast. Perched high in the foliage is an owl, which at first glance appears almost like a skull. In medieval times, much like in modern Greece, the owl symbolises bad luck, whereas in ancient Greece the hoot owl represented *Athena Glaukopis*, the protector of wisdom and philosophy. The painting offers a general portrayal of a group of fools adrift in the sea of life, indulging in excessive eating and drinking. Despite the presence of the Church, represented by the nun and the friar, they lack morals and direction; they seem oblivious to the men overboard, signifying their disregard for consequences.

The motif of the ship of fools rarely appears in the centuries after Brant's *Narrenschiff* outside of its iconographic apparatus, but it was used by Foucault in his *History of Madness* as the opening example of the treatment of the madman in early modern times. In the first

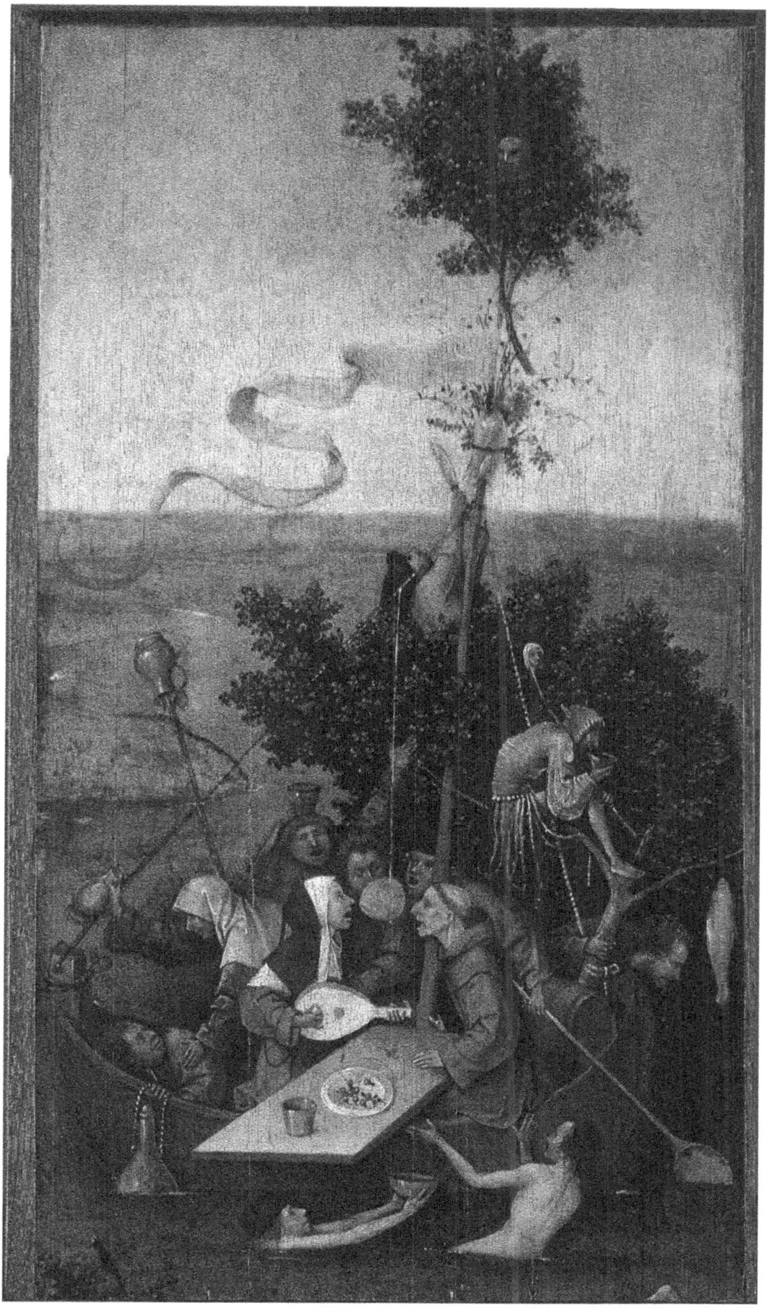

Figure 8: Hieronymous Bosch, *The Ship of Fools*, circa 1494–1510.
2025 © PhotoScala, Florence. Louvre, Paris, RM05947.

chapter, entitled *Stultifera Navis* in fact, Foucault concedes that the ship of fools 'was clearly a literary invention' (Foucault 2009, 6), but continues by remarking that the 'arrival in the great cities of Europe of these ships of fools must have been quite a common sight' (Foucault 2009, 9). Foucault described the custom of handing the mad and the unwanted to boatmen so that they could be exiled, driven away from 'sane' society. According to Foucault (2009, 10), this was a 'constant circulation of the insane', a 'gesture of banishment and enforced embarkation, [that] was not merely aimed at social utility, or the safety of citizens. Its meanings were closer to rituals, and their trace is still discernible'. Maher and Maher (1982) clearly showed that Foucault mis-transposed the literary motif onto a practice that at best might have happened occasionally, and several psychologists took Foucault's statement at face value. What is of interest here is that the ship of fools emerges and returns in the imaginary as a controversial polysemic sign, much like the staff, to reveal the iconographic overlap of madness and travel, the insane and the vagrant. As Foucault (2009, 11) put it, such symbols 'serv[e] to underline in real and imaginary terms the liminal situation of the mad in medieval society'.

Brant's *Narrenschiff* was a very successful publication, translated into several languages, but the trope of the ship of fools recurred only sporadically after Bosch's treatment. Over four centuries later, Katherine Anne Porter revived it in her 1962 novel, *Ship of Fools*. Set aboard a German luxury cruiser crossing the Atlantic in the ominous 1930s, as Hitler's rise began to threaten the fragile Weimar Republic, Porter's ship carries a microcosm of human frailty: proud Jews, disdainful Nazis, restless lovers, broken businessmen, rebellious children and a wise, solitary figure endlessly crisscrossing the ocean in search of a home he cannot find. Drawing on her own experiences from a 1931 sea voyage, Porter allegedly spent 30 years crafting the novel, which became a commercial triumph. In 1965, Stanley Kramer adapted the book into a film with the same name. Much like Brant's *Narrenschiff*, both Porter's novel and its cinematic adaptation were blockbusters in their time but are less widely remembered today. The film captured the metaphor's enduring resonance: the ship as a vessel of human folly and social fragmentation adrift in turbulent waters. A quick, and by no means exhaustive, search on music streaming services returns at least 16 different songs entitled 'The Ship of Fools', by artists such as The Doors, The Scorpions and The Grateful Dead, to name only the three most famous ones.

In contemporary visual culture, the ship of fools makes a striking comeback in the work of American-Nigerian portrait artist Kehinde

Wiley. The iconographic traits of the madman and the fool—those recurring markers of outsiderness we've traced through history—enabled an overlap with other 'undesirable' figures, like vagrants and witches. Wiley's revival of the ship of fools coincides with the rise of political populism and its fixation on a relatively novel target for vilification: migrants and their precarious boats, cast adrift as modern-day symbols of humanity's unwanted. Wiley used the motif of the ship of fools in a series of seascape paintings commissioned for an exhibition at the Stephen Friedman Gallery in 2017. The focus is on the dangers migrants face in search of a better life and, of course, on the legacies of the transatlantic slave trade. In the painting *Ship of Fools* four individuals sail on a boat in stormy seas, their faces reflecting a mix of excitement, determination and uncertainty as they take risks on an old, weathered boat, in the hope for a brighter future.[6] A child stands at the back of the boat looking back at the land left behind, while two women display expressions that could range from excitement to dread. The man standing between the women may represent the challenges and reflections faced by young black individuals in the world; he has a resolute expression, staring ahead towards a potential new life despite the tumultuous sea surrounding them. The single paddle in the boat raises questions about how they will navigate the storm, again perhaps symbolising the additional challenges faced by black men and women. As in Bosch's painting, the mast is replaced by a tree, which does not seem to be fully grown—the green leaves are more prominent on the left side. It is a symbol both of growth and of the land the migrants take with them. Notably, a sailing ship can be seen in the background, representing the transatlantic slave trade, an important but easily overlooked aspect of the painting that impacts the overall context of the scene.

Wiley explicitly engaged with the trope of the ship of fools in the *Narrenschiff* (2017) video installation that accompanied the exhibition. The three simultaneous videos show images of black people swimming and sailing. The videos are accompanied by a cello and a voiceover quoting Foucault and Fanon, among others. The citations describe the shift from what Foucault considered the myth of the *Narrenschiff*—giving safe passage to the multitude of fools—to colonial psychiatry and the use of psychiatry to subjugate the colonised. The images, however, never feature the multitude of the carnivalesque elements that would characterise the motif of the *Narrenschiff*. On the

6 See https://www.rmg.co.uk/queens-house/attractions/ship-fools-kehinde-wiley [accessed 1 Sept. 2025].

contrary,. they are always small groups or individuals swimming and sailing. The carnivalesque journey of fools to their promised land has transformed into the dread and the anguish of real-life migrants journeying towards the promise of a better life.

Inside-Out / Inside–Outside: Conclusions

Vagrants, wild men, *insipientes*, fools, sailors of the *Narrenschiff* and the insane have a long history of being depicted as being 'out of themselves'. At the end of the staff, when there is no bundle, there is often a head (e.g., Amiens, Bibl. mun., ms. 0124, f. 054v), which, as discussed above, does not necessarily represent an *ante litteram* jester's marotte, since it predates its standardisation in iconography. The very head at the end of the stick seems to represent the condition of folly as being out of oneself.

Madness as the condition of being out of oneself, and in particular to be out of one's head, are still common idioms in most European languages: to be out of one's mind, *essere fuori di testa* (to be out of one's head) in Italian; *hors de soi* (out of oneself) in French; *as a meabhair* (out of one's sanity) in Irish; *außer sich sein* (to be out of oneself) in German. Similarly, there are idioms pointing to the idea that to be mad is to be out of one's home, such as: 'the lights are on but nobody's home' in English; *sortir de ses gonds* (to go out of one's hinges) in French; or *eser fora dei copi* (to be outside the roof tiles) in Triestine dialect. These idioms reiterate the permanence of the blurring between insanity and vagrancy (homelessness) in popular culture. In addition to the sense of outsideness, the early *marotte* also incarnates the symbolism of being other from oneself or alien to oneself: *alienatio mentis*, the mind that is alienated, other to itself, a notion which would be frequently used in Western medical jargon well into the 1950s, but which had roots in Roman medicine (first used by Caelius Aurelianus in his *De morbis acutis et cronicis*, from around the fifth century CE; see Coughlin 2018, 114). The insane are, therefore, out of themselves in life as much as in iconography, like the vagabond (and the wild man) who is outside civil society, without a home, constantly travelling.

The overlapping between madness, vagueness, wildness, emptiness and air outlives the iconography of the *insipiens* with his staff. Towards the end of the fifteenth century, the image of the fool has already branched into the codified image of the jester, with his *marotte*, an image that will endure for centuries and is arguably still in use today, such as in carnival costumes, popular culture imagery, or the

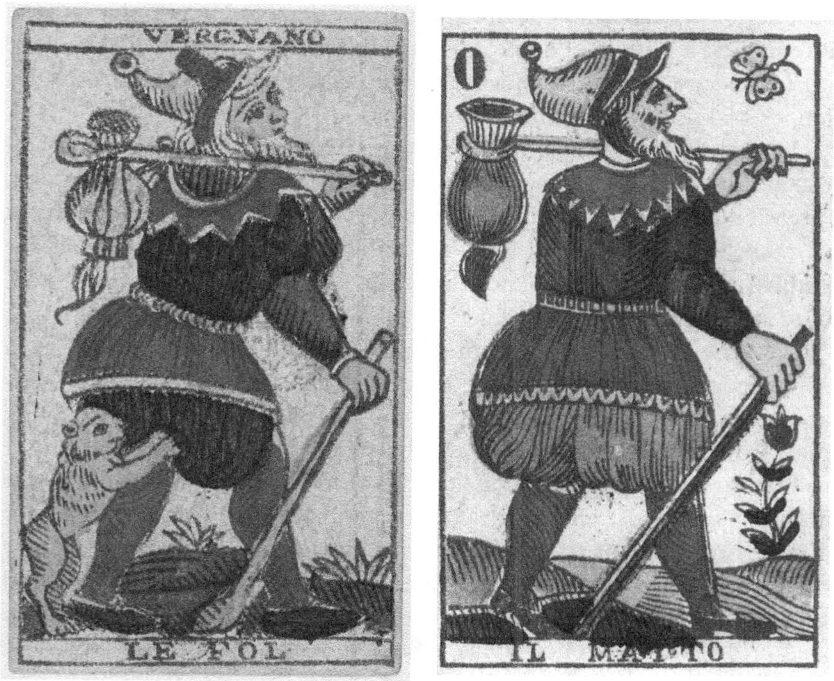

Figure 9: The Fool in two different versions of the Tarot printed in Turin (northern Italy) by Stefano Vergnano: 1827 (left) and around 1830 (right). CC – https://commons.wikimedia.org/wiki/File:The_Fool,_from_Vergnano_Tarot.jpg

jolly or joker card added to the standard 52-card French-suited pack in some games. In the sixteenth century, we see the first images of madmen, as distinguished from court fools and jesters, carrying pinwheels and sometimes also bladders. The image of the *insipiens* carrying a staff with a sack at its end survives almost unchanged, at least in one iconographic repository of the present: tarot cards. In the occult tarot cards (as well as in the *Tarocco Piemontese* gaming cards) *le mat, le fou, le fol, il matto* or the fool on the first (0) or the last (XXII) of the major arcana is invariably depicted as carrying a bundle at the end of a stick (Fig. 9). This bundle resembles the post-Depression bindle of American hoboes, and is now recognised as the universal icon of vagabondage, possibly thanks to its use in comics and cartoons (from Donald Duck to the Smurfs). Of course, I am not suggesting that Disney intentionally depicts its characters with a bindle to recall the iconography of the *insipiens*, but simply that both madmen and vagabonds are traditionally and enduringly depicted in popular culture as carrying a bundle of some sort, a symbolic reminder that they have no home, are outsiders and travel with few possessions (or even an empty sack in the case of the madman).

In this first chapter, I have analysed many instances of the use of the staff as a symbol of madness, especially in connection to the fool, intended not only as the court jester but as the *insipiens* who is devoid of reason. I have shown that several characteristics of the insane revolve around the staff, including different iterations of 'unwanted' outcasts, such as the witch and the outsider, the vagrant.

Are the insane driven out of society to become outcasts as a consequence of insanity or are they regarded as insane because they are outcasts already? Do they become outsiders as a result of being marginalised because of their odd behaviour (and is this tantamount to 'madness') or is their behaviour regarded as mad because they are already vagabonds? Do the insane turn feral because of their insanity or are they regarded as mad because they live in the forest? Legal history might help us distinguish these categories, for example insanity could be used to plead innocence of a crime (insanity defence), but vagrancy was criminalised. Iconography, however, blurs the answers to these questions, showing clearly that wild men, outcasts, vagabonds and *insipientes* (whether they were born as fools or driven mad) are very intimately related in terms of their representation. This, in turn, shows that in the common perception, popular culture and in the imagination, there is an element of vagrancy and vagueness in mental disorder, just as there is something insane in being a vagabond. The fool, the vagabond and the wild man unsettle the status quo, for good or for ill, just with their presence and existence. Outsiders trouble boundaries: the boundaries of reason, of the nation, of civilisation. There is therefore something witch-like, evil and threatening in everyone who is marked as other, as different; almost invariably, the other comes from the outside, whether this outside is populated by vagabonds coming from foreign lands, mental ailments coming from the outside of the head or madness chasing someone out of themselves.

I started this historical overview with the staff of the madman as a pivotal and polysemic iconic element that encompasses numerous references, including the *follis*, air, emptiness, and lightness, the dialectics inside–outside and inside-out, vagrancy and vagueness. I have thus unravelled the overlap in the representation of different outcasts, in particular the insane, showing that it pivots on dichotomic/binary 'root metaphors' (Pepper 1942, 92), such as visible–invisible, empty–full, inside–outside, that recur in history. These indeed emerge in iconography through specific elements (such as the bladder or the pinwheel) representing, both realistically and metaphorically, a condition of emptiness (also absence or lack?), vagueness, changeability, that is incarnated in the insubstantial element par excellence: air. This element is by and large invisible, but not in its effects (e.g., inflating a bladder, moving the pinwheel), much like insanity. Using air to represent the unrepresentable does not bring madness closer to being made visible though, and in the next chapter, by focusing on the actual procedures for literally extracting madness, we might uncover more effective and concrete incarnations of an invisible malady (Gilman 2014, 36–42). Yet, the images I have analysed in this chapter, by foregrounding air, show us the struggle to deal with mental disorder; something so historically and culturally mutable, so ephemeral and invisible, yet deeply impactful on individuals, communities and societies.

The next chapter will focus on a rather different way of visualising madness: through the procedures for extracting it—medical or otherwise. When pictured as being extracted, madness is embodied in a variety of materials. From the ephemeral vapours or spirits that need to be distilled, evaporated or let out, to much more solid metaphors such as stones that need to be extracted, to metaphysical entities such as demons that have to be exorcised.

CHAPTER TWO

The Extraction of Madness

As I HAVE SHOWN, by discussing air and its invisibility, over the course of history numerous semantic slippages blurred the representation of madmen, vagabonds and other 'unwanted' human types, implying that the struggle to deal with mental disorder corresponds more generally to the struggle of dealing with difference and otherness. Here I move to a different trope of the visualisation and othering of madness: how it is seen as an extractable entity. The concept of extraction is an interesting one, and in medical practice, as much as in iconography, as we shall soon see, there are several instances of extraction involving mental disorder. Whether it is Galenic medicine prescribing purges and emetics to let melancholia out, Rogerius recommending a cross incision in the head to let the vapours of melancholia evaporate, the numerous depictions of exorcisms illustrating a demon exiting the body of the possessed through their mouth (which I will examine later in this chapter), Bosch representing charlatans in the process of extracting the stone of madness from the head of the gullible, Cheyne and contemporaries debating the difference between hypochondria and the 'vapours' or Henry Cotton extracting teeth to uproot mental disorders, all extractions of madness have one thing in common. In order to depict the extraction of madness they *presuppose* a certain materiality of mental disorders; the possibility of their incarnation as a tangible entity. It is in the representation of the process of extraction that madness assumes a material form, which does not seem to pre-exist it, nor are there many clues as to how these materials made their way into the body. While iconography is rife with images of exorcisms and demons, there are very few indicating the way in which such demons entered in the first place. In the same way, the vapours that circulate in the body of the mad and need to be evaporated are rarely seen getting in, at least not in iconography nor in medical writings (the misericord of Great Malvern Priory of Figure 6 above being a notable exception).

The extraction of mental disorder thus presupposes that madness has some sort of materiality (visible, invisible or ephemeral as it may be) that has to be identified in order for it to be extracted. This process of recognition, I claim in this chapter, underpins the second leading narrative in the discourse on madness and visibility: if the first is that madness is invisible and has to be made visible (either in the arts to represent it or in medical practice to treat it), the second is that madness is *other*. Madness represented as a foreign body thus presupposes that madness is other to the person affected by it, which also itself contributes to the 'othering' of madness. This is not an exclusively iconographical process; the visual 'othering' of mental disorders proceeds in parallel with, and continuously overlaps, the arts, culture, religion and medicine. Yet, it does not necessarily mark, as one might assume, a passage to the medical treatment of a condition that has found a material substratum. Some extractable incarnations of madness certainly call for medical intervention, but others, for instance demons, require exorcisms.

If in the Middle Ages and early modern eras the most prominent visual symbol of madness is, as discussed above, the staff of madness with its symbolic references (including air, invisibility, vagrancy and otherness, to mention only the main ones), in the modern era another symbol for this condition emerges and becomes prevalent, especially in the Netherlands. This is the 'stone of madness', an approximately golf-ball-sized stone that is depicted as being extracted from the head of the mad person.

The most famous depiction of this operation (and the first) is certainly Bosch's *Cutting the Stone* or *The Cure of Folly*, a *c.*1494 painting that features a surgeon cutting something that looks like a tulip out of a patient's head, under the supervision of a monk and possibly a nun (Fig. 10). Bosch's *Cutting the Stone* gives rise to a wealth of paintings and prints with the similar theme of the extraction of the stone of madness, especially in the Netherlandish regions (Scull 2016, 21). This trope survives for at least two centuries in the fine arts, and has even re-emerged in contemporary paintings, such as Giovanni Gasparro's 2012 *L'estrazione della pietra della follia. After Jan Sanders Van Hemessen*. What does this trope represent? Was it an allegory of madness and its potential treatment? Was it the representation of a real surgical operation? And if this were the case, was the operation depicted a *bona fide* operation done by surgeons or was it quackery practised by charlatans?

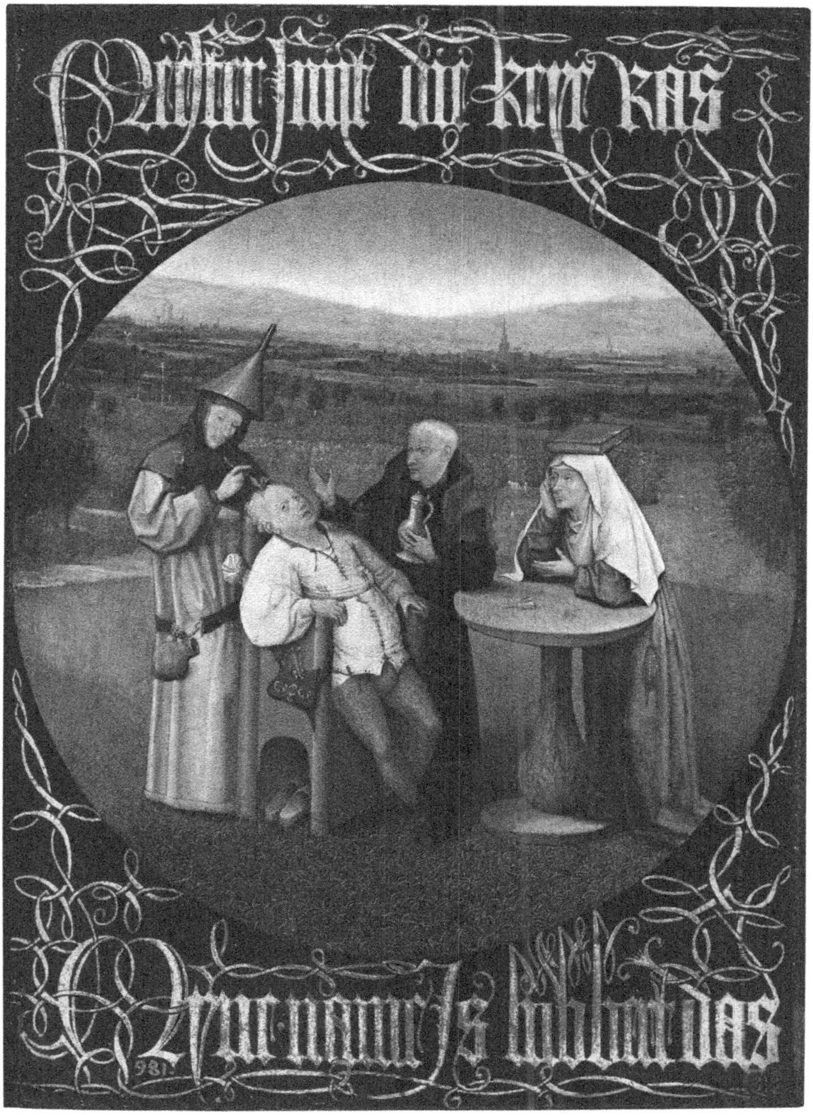

Figure 10: Hieronymous Bosch, *Cutting of the Stone*. 1501–1505. Oil on Wood, 48.5 x 34.5cm (P002056). Madrid, Museo Nacional del Prado.

Bosch's painting might be a satirical reference to charlatans; however, the vast corpus of later images depicting the extraction of the stone of madness suggests it was a commonplace metaphorical depiction for the curing of mental disorders. Other materials were also extracted to depict the curing of madness in iconography, including a wealth of different fumes or vapours that could be distilled (e.g., Theodor de Bry's sixteenth-century engraving) or baked (e.g., Greuter's sixteenth-century broadside in Figure 12). Crazy thoughts were depicted as leaving the head, carried out by the smoke.

In order to better understand this materialisation of madness in the form of extractable entities (stones, etc.) and the representations showing its potential extraction, we need to reconstruct the history of possible surgical procedures for the extraction of madness, whether real or quackery. For this reason, I will start the chapter by analysing the practice of trephination and its connection to the extraction of madness. After discussing the extraction of different real or metaphorical entities from the head as a possible cure of madness, I conclude the chapter with an analysis of the iconography of exorcisms and its overlap with the extraction of mental disorders.

Trephination and Extractions

As Horsley (1888, 105) put it,

> No cases afforded the savage mind more striking proof of demoniacal influence or the efficacy of magical cure than epilepsy. It seemed, therefore, highly probable that the process of trephining had been employed by primitive man in order to expel the demon who possessed the patient, especially in cases of epilepsy.

Whether it is a demonic, gaseous, liquid or solid entity, madness seems to need a hole to be let out. Trepanned crania are relatively common archaeological finds, and indeed trephinations are the most common type of surgical procedure encountered in the archaeological record (Ortner 2003, 169). To date more than 1,500 specimens of trepanned skulls have been excavated, more than 450 of these dating back to the Stone Age. The oldest were found in the Dnieper Rapids cemeteries, in particular in Vasilyevka II, whose crania date back to 7300–6220 BCE (Lillie 1998, 854). Trephination—which consisted of opening a hole in the cranium either by scraping, boring, sawing, drilling or gouging—was practised all over the world, including Australia (Webb 1988), the

Pacific, the Middle East, North Africa and pre-Columbian Latin America (Stewart 1958; Stone and Miles 1990). Trephination was performed on the living and there is evidence that (most) patients survived: no signs of violence appear on the bones, the hole is regular (thus it was not a traumatic injury) and the bone healed after the procedure (thus it was neither performed on a corpse nor was it lethal) (Ortner 2003, 171).

While research on prehistoric trephination is extensive (Arnott, Finger and Smith 2003, ix), there is no consensus as to why humans bored holes in the skulls of the living. There is certainly good evidence that some of these trephinations were of a medical nature, for example, to treat complications from skull fractures. Others, however, were performed on perfectly healthy skulls, suggesting a possible ritual or magical purpose. Paul Broca (1876, 572), one of the fathers of cerebral localisation theory, after whom the area of the brain most involved with speech production is named, suggested that in such cases trephination could have been used to treat mental disorders. We will probably never know with certainty.

In the fourth century BCE, in *On Injuries of the Head*, Hippocrates recommended, with caution, the use of trephination to treat skull fractures, although it was never made clear why; for instance, there is no mention of draining a hematoma (Missios 2007, 4). Hippocrates is clear though that care should be taken to preserve the meninges, the dura mater in particular, the first meninge under the bone of the skull, to avoid infections. Galen also recommends protecting the dura mater in trephination, describes in detail how to use trephination to treat skull injuries and is also clear on the purpose of trepanning to drain hematomas and what he calls 'phlegmatous' lesions of the head. Galen also extensively studied hydrocephalus and recommended trepanning to drain the fluid, unless this is located between the meninges and the brain, in which case it is untreatable (Rocca 2003, 253–71).

The first mention of using trephination to treat anything other than a skull injury comes from Aretaeus the Cappadocian (*c.*150 CE) who lists it as a possible cure for epilepsy. He recommends trephination to reach the diploe first, while wax and plasters should be applied to cauterise the dura mater underneath. Trephination should then be repeated to expose the cauterised dura mater, which should be suppurated and healed (Aretaeus 1923, 469). Caelius Aurelianus, however, mentions that the methodist Themison used a *terebra* (trephine) as a therapeutic aid to treat epilepsy and paralysis (Tardae passiones, I.iv.118, 127, 143; II.i.59) but he disapproves of the method (Temkin 1971, 235).

Trephination was thus primarily recommended to treat head injuries. When it was recommended to treat epilepsy, nothing was extracted.

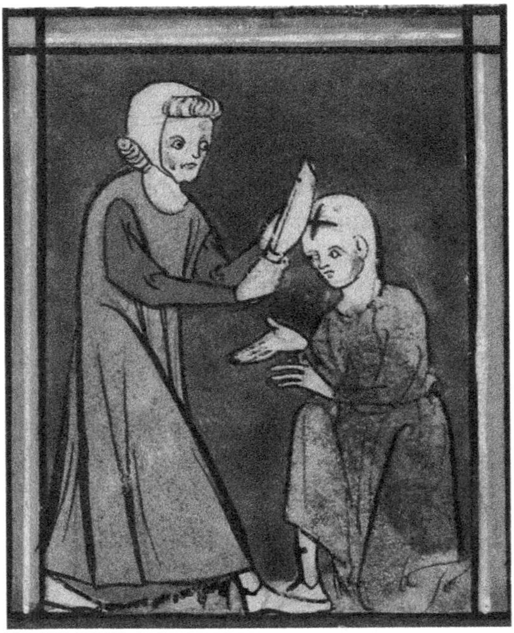

Figure 11: Detail of a page from Rogerius Salernitanus's *Chirurgia*. France (near Amiens), 1300–1310. Sloane 1977, f.2v. Courtesy of British Library.

If anything it was mostly carried out so as to be able to cauterise the brain directly. The first to mention the extraction of something related to mental illness—epilepsy—was the Persian physician al-Rāzī, also known as Rhazes (854–925 CE), who, in his *Liber Nonus ad Almansorem*, denounced 'the quacks who wanted to cure epilepsy making an incision in the front and pretending to draw something that was hidden in their hands' (al-Rāzī 1490). This is the first document detailing the charlatan practice of 'palming' to pretend something that causes mental disorders is extracted from the skull. No trephination was involved, only a cut in the scalp.

Medieval surgeon Rogerius Frugardi, in his twelfth-century treatise on surgery, describes trephination on several occasions, in particular in reference to head injuries (chapter I) (Fig. 11). Section XXVI, however, is of particular interest to us because it describes a procedure to cure mania and melancholia:

> I, XXVI: De cauteriis que fiunt contra maniam vel melancoliam: Ad maniam vel melancoliam in summitate capitis incidatur cutis in

> Modum crucis et craneum perforetur ut materia exhalet ad exteriora. Patiens autem in vinculis teneatur et vulnus curetur, sicut in curis Vulneum superius diximus

> [On Cauterisations Performed Against Mania or Melancholy:
> For mania or melancholy, the skin at the top of the head should be incised in the shape of a cross, and the skull should be perforated so that the matter may exhale outward. The patient, however, should be restrained in bonds, and the wound should be treated as we have previously described in the care of wounds.]

A cross-shaped incision is made on the top of the head and the skull is 'perforated' so that 'matter' can be let out. While we do not know exactly what the matter that is let out is, 'exhalare' refers exclusively to gaseous elements, such as breath and vapours.

The translation into Old French (BL Sloane 1977 at F.186ra) renders the sentence as: 'fore le test, que la matere de la maladie s'en isse fors'. The 'matter' is qualified only as being the 'matter of the illness'. Rosenman's translation of Rogerius's Latin Venetian edition of 1546 is clearer:

> In cases of mania and melancholia we make a cruciate incision at the crown of the scalp and we perforate the cranium to allow the escape of the offensive matter (i.e. vapors) while the patient is restrained by bonds. Then we treat the wound with our usual methods. (Frugard 2002, 53)

The matter that is extracted—or, rather, let out—is a vapour. The thirteenth-century *Tractatus de egritudinum curatione* (a collection of texts by different physicians of the Salernitan School) recommends to trephine the skull to let humours and spirits exit and exhale:

> Item melancolici et epileptici incenduntur sic: in summitate capitis fit incisio usque ad craneum; hoc facto inscidatur craneum ad modum dictum ut inde humores et spiritus possint exire et exalare, et teneatur apertum per XL dies. Multi enim melancolici et epileptici, frenetici, vertiginosi, maniaci, cephalargici hoc opere perfecte curati sunt; et etiam appoplectici, stothomici et multe alie passiones capitis. (Renzi 1853, 698)

> [Melancholics and epileptics are treated in the following way: an incision is made at the top of the head down to the skull; once this is done, the skull is cut open in the prescribed manner so that the humours

> and spirits may exit and evaporate, and it is kept open for forty days. Indeed, many melancholics and epileptics, as well as the frantic, those with vertigo, maniacs, and sufferers of cephalalgia have been perfectly cured by this procedure; and also apoplectics, those with stammering, and many other afflictions of the head.]

As Arnott, Finger and Smith (2003, 32) remark, 'during the European Renaissance, craniotomies continued to be performed for epilepsy, especially of traumatic origin, although the purpose of the operation was still to remove broken bone or a buildup of fluid or "evil" air—not to remove diseased brain tissue'.

Holes could also be needed to cool the blood. In *The Diseases That Deprive Man of His Reason*, Renaissance alchemist and physician Paracelsus maintains that mania is caused by heat. This is why 'it often happens that by opening fingers and toes mania can be made to disappear' (Paracelsus 1979, 150). This was not, however, to let mania out, but to let air in, in order to cool the humours. Heat can distil the humours 'which rise in the heat of the other limbs [...] and cause insanity on touching the particles of the brain' (Paracelsus 1979, 149). There mania can make 'worms grow' (Paracelsus 1979, 150). There is no mention of the extraction of mania or said worms. Later in the text, however, Paracelsus returns to the possible cure for mania and mentions a surgical procedure, which should be attempted only by the best trained surgeons. It consists of making 'an aperture at the place from which mania rises; but if you are in doubt, open all extremities—at the toes, fingers and the head—in a circle which must be as wide as possible' (Paracelsus 1979, 173). 'If the disease is strong and intense, the first opening of the skin is not sufficient to give an *outlet* to the origin of mania, but the second opening can, because it leaves more holes; each separate hole has the capacity to serve as an *outlet*' (Paracelsus 1979, 173, my emphasis). According to Paracelsus, therefore, cuts in the fingers and in the head were outlets, from which the origin of mania could be let out. His preferred approach to curing mania was, however, pharmacological (Hartman et al. 1976, 273).

Burton, in his *Anatomy of Melancholy* (1621), recommended trephination, following Galenic physicians Salvianus and Gordonius, as one of the possible cures for this ailment, precisely to let the vapours out:

> 'Tis not amiss to bore the skull with an instrument, to let out the fuliginous vapours, because this humour hardly yields to other physic [...] for that it much avails to the exhalation of the vapours; 'I saw' (saith he) 'a melancholy man at Rome, that by no remedies could be healed,

> but when by chance he was wounded in the head, and the skull broken, he was excellently cured.' Gordonius would have these cauteries tried last, when no other physic will serve. 'The head to be shaved and bored to let out fumes, which without doubt will do much good.' But Alexander Messaria a professor in Padua, lib. 1. pract. med. cap. 21. de melanchol. will allow no cauteries at all, 'tis too stiff a humour and too thick as he holds, to be so evaporated.
>
> Guianerius c. 8. Tract. 15. cured a nobleman in Savoy, by boring alone, [4294] 'leaving the hole open a month together,' by means of which, after two years' melancholy and madness, he was delivered. All approve of this remedy in the suture of the crown; but Arculanus would have the cautery to be made with gold. In many other parts, these cauteries are prescribed for melancholy men, as in the thighs, (Mercurialis consil. 86.) arms, legs. Idem consil. 6. & 19. & 25. Montanus 86. Rodericus a Fonseca tom. 2. cousult. 84. pro hypochond. coxa dextra, &c., but most in the head, 'if other physic will do no good'. (Burton 2004, Pt. 2, Sect. V, Memb. I, Susect. IV, para. 5)

Much like Paracelsus, Riverius, in his 1655 book *The Practice of Physick*, also concedes that trephination could be used to treat epilepsy but only if all else fails:

> If all means fail the last remedy is to open the fore part of the Skul with a Trepan, at distance from the sutures, *that the evil air may breath out*. By this means many desperate Epilepsies have been cured, and it may be safely done if the Chyrurgeon be skilful. (Riverius 1655)

The Oxford neuroanatomist and physician Thomas Willis (1621–75) believed that 'threatening, bonds or strokes' were 'Curatory' for madmen but noted that 'Specifick Remedies such as St. Johns-wort as well as Chirurgial Remedies such as Trephining or opening the skull' have been recommended (Willis 1683, 192–93), though he does not specify why that was the case.

As I have shown in the previous chapter, madness and mental disorders have been visualised, across history and cultures, as the invisible element *par excellence*: air. The visualisation of madness as air thus seems to prompt the trepanation or trephination of the skull, in order for the vapours, the air, the spirits, that have swollen, obfuscated or even rotted the brain, to be let out. As I have shown in this section, in the majority of sources, if not all of them, trephination of the skull, other than for the treatment of head injuries, was carried out to let mental disorders out in a gaseous form (Fig. 12). We can also find cases

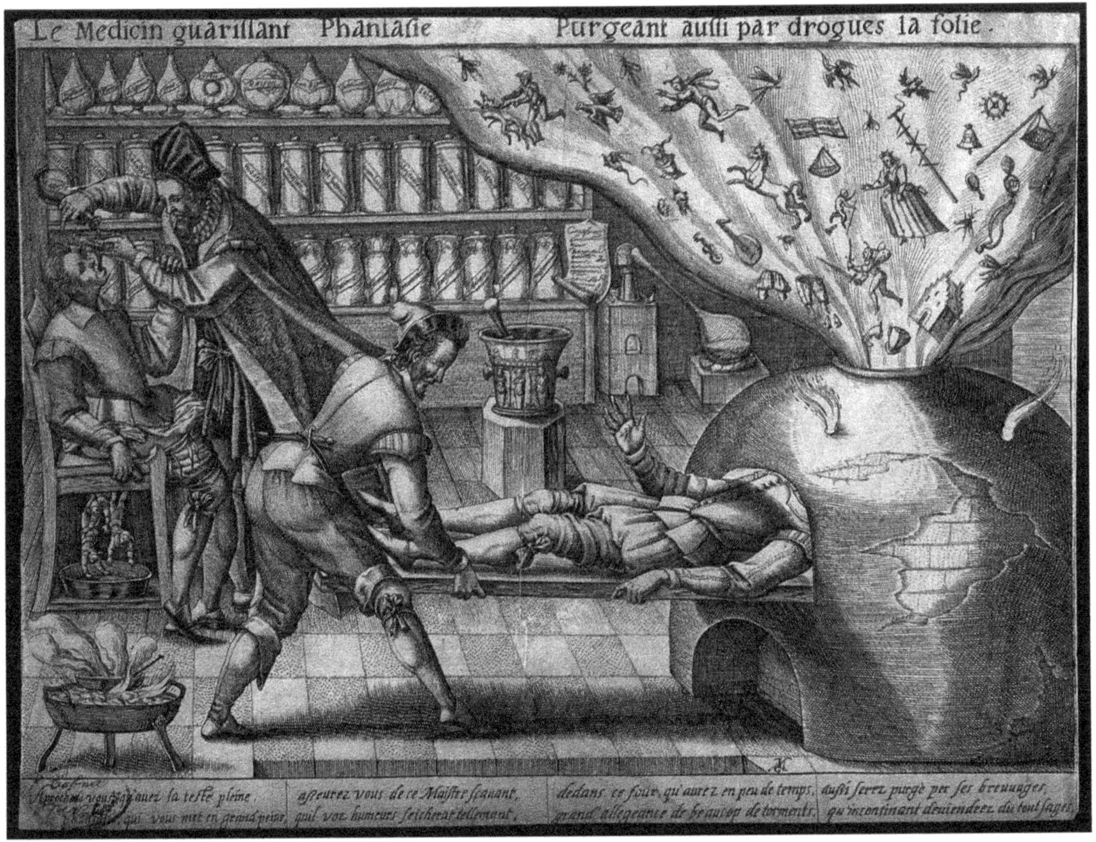
Le Medicin guarissant Phantasie Purgeant aussi par drogues la folie.
la teste pleine,
qui vous met en grand peine,
asseurez vous de ce Maistre scauant,
quil voz humeurs seichera tellement,
dedans ce four qu'aurez en peu de temps,
grand allegeance de beaucop de torments.
aussi serez purgè per ses breuuages,
qu'incontinant deuiendrez du tout sages.

Figure 12: A surgery where all fantasy and follies are purged and good qualities are prescribed. Line engraving by M. Greuter, c. 1600. Source: Wellcome Collection.

of extractions of liquids or solids taking place that materialise mental disorders; these, however, deserve a separate section, since the majority revolve around the extraction of the 'stone of madness', a procedure whose existence beyond the allegorical is debatable, to say the least.

Removal of Diseased (Solid) Matter

Famously, around 1494, Hieronymus Bosch painted *The Cure of Folly,* also known as *Cutting the Stone* or *The Extraction of the Stone of Madness* (Fig. 10). The painting depicts a 'surgeon' with a funnel on his head ('far more insane than the patient he is attempting to cure' remarks Foucault (2009, 25)), cutting through the scalp of a 'patient', with the assistance of a monk and a nun. The golden inscription around the painting reads, in middle Dutch: 'Master, cut the stone out fast. My name is Lubbert Das', a classic fool character in Dutch comedy. Despite the protagonist of the painting requesting the cutting out of the stone of madness, and the painting indeed declaredly depicting a *keisnijden* (stone cutting), the object that is shown to be extracted is actually a flower, possibly a tulip. This painting gave rise to a tradition of paintings and prints in the Netherlands (the Flemish and Dutch areas especially) portraying either the extraction of this stone of madness or a stone (strapped to the head, bulging out of the head or even simply carried around) as a symbol of madness, akin to the staff. Examples of the former are very numerous, such as Pieter Huys's *c.*1561 painting *A Surgeon Extracting the Stone of Folly* (Fig. 13), in which the surgeon cuts the stone out of a patient strapped in a chair, with the assistance of a nurse and in front of a small audience. Jan Sanders van Hemessen's *c.*1563 painting *An Operation for Stone in the Head* is very similar, whereas Pieter Jansz's slightly later (early-seventeenth-century) wood painting *An Operator Extracting 'pierres de tête' from Behind a Man's Ear with Four Other People in Attendance* shows the stone being extracted from behind the ear rather than the front.

There are no signs in these images that these might be allegories of quackery, such as strange dresses or funnels on the head; all the people depicted are serious and focused on the task at hand. Stones employed as symbols of madness but without an accompanying image of an extraction can also be found, though less frequently. Flemish painter Quentin Matsys (1466–1530), in his early-sixteenth-century painting *An Allegory of Folly,* depicts the fool with a staff/marotte, bells around the waist, a hood with ass's ears and a lump on the forehead containing the stone of madness. Around the same time, Pieter Bruegel the Elder

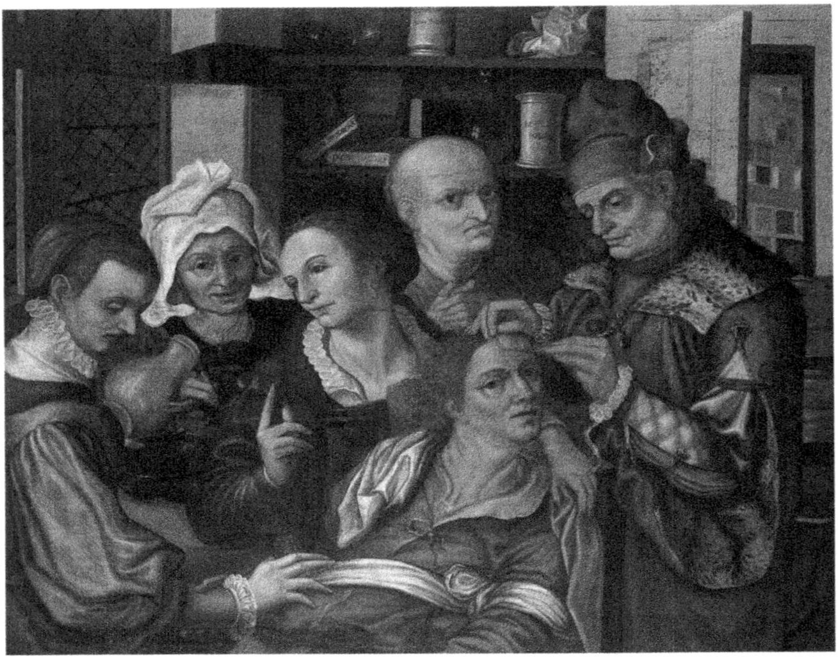

Figure 13: A surgeon extracting the stone of folly.
Oil painting by Pieter Huys, ca. 1561. Source: Wellcome Collection.

(*c.*1525–69) also employed the stone as a symbol of madness, but in his undated painting *The Feast of Fools*—better known through Pieter van der Heyden's 1559 reproduction in print—Bruegel shows the square of a city being 'invaded' by fools (a visual motif on which we will return in chapter three). Fools carry their marotte, have an eared hood and are generally dressed like jesters. Many bring large orbs that they seem to offer to others, and several of these orbs are scattered on the pavement, in the foreground. This is very similar to his other collective depiction of madness, also printed by van der Heyden (published 1559, painting now lost), commonly referred to as *The Witches of Malleghem* or *The Stone Operation of the Witches of Malleghem*. This title appeared only 40 years after the original painting was created, but it should be *The Extractor of Stones of Madness* (Fig. 14). According to Weemans (2024, 413) it depicts a charlatan arriving at Malleghem, claiming to be able to free everyone from their stones of madness, while, in fact, his accomplices free the 'insane' from their coins.

The focus in these depictions is the material being extracted, not the operation itself. A variety of tools are depicted: scalpels, razors,

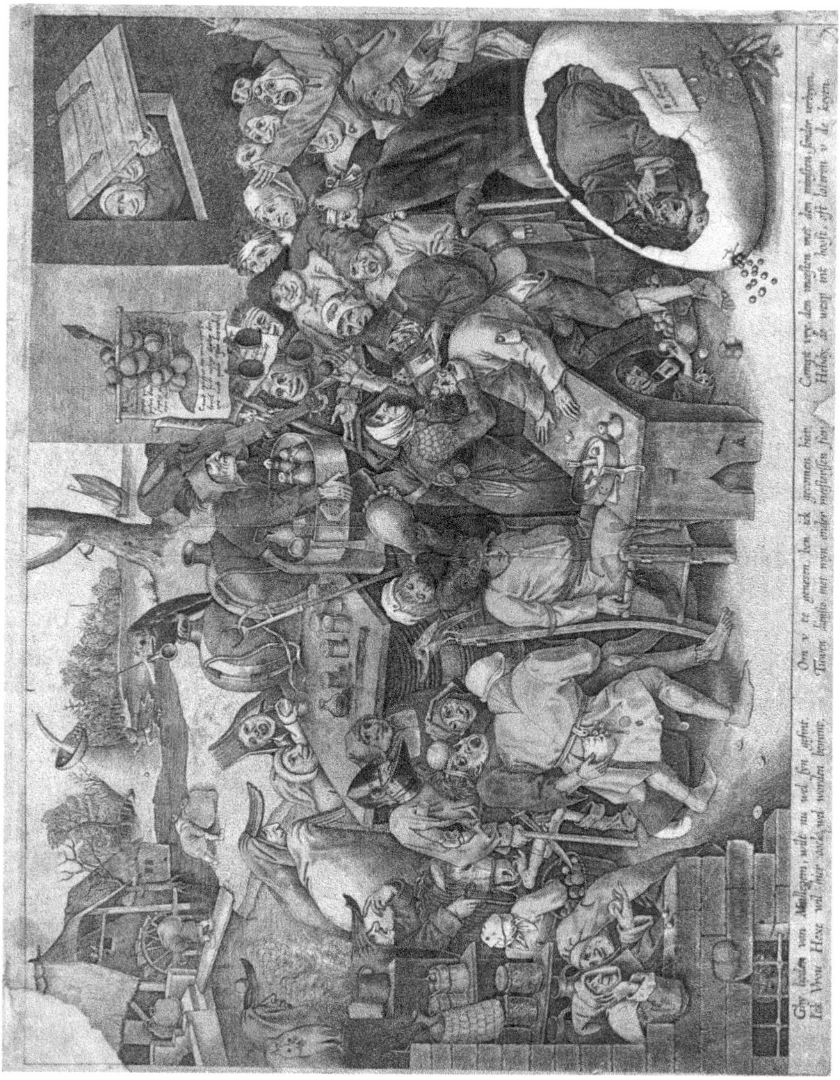

Figure 14: Pieter van der Heyden after Pieter Bruegel the Elder. *The Witch of Mallegem*. Circa 1595–1633. RP-P-1924-700. Courtesty of Rijksmuseum, Amsterdam.

tweezers and forceps but never the trephine or drill that would have invariably been used to cut through the bone of the cranium. As Wauters remarks, there is a

> significant discrepancy between the surgical materials used. The method recommended by the Roman author Aulus Cornelius Celsus, with a bow or a drill rotated by hand becomes the norm during the Middle Ages, but these tools do not recur in any preserved depiction of the *keisnijding*. What has been frequently depicted in these scenes are a (flat) scalpel, scissors and tweezers. (Wauters 2018, 12)

The extraction of the stone of madness therefore does not seem to be a representational depiction of trephination.

Given the above discussion on trephination, it is highly improbable that these depicted real surgical operations done in good faith. As we have seen, any attempt at accessing the brain would have needed a trephine and the matter to be extracted was almost invariably gaseous. Some 600 years before Bosch, Rhazes referred to 'palming', the technique of concealing something, even a small stone, in one's palm and pretending to extract it from someone's body, specifically the head. Bosch's seminal painting on the cutting of the stone clearly depicts the 'surgeon' as a quack, most notably by his donning of a funnel as a head ornament. While the majority of Bosch's successors depicted the surgeons extracting stones from the head of their patients as serious physicians performing a delicate operation, it would then stand to reason to regard the cutting of the stone as a representational depiction of 'palming' or quackery, in reference to fraudulent practices that promised miracle cures for mental ailments. This, however, is not the case. As Schupbach (1978, 271) has it, 'since charlatans travelled all over Europe, it is not surprising that the descriptions of quackery left by Netherlandish, French, English, German, Italian, and Spanish writers of the Renaissance are almost interchangeable, but all alike omit to attribute to Netherlandish quacks the operation for *pierre de tête*'. Indeed, as Schupbach noted, there is no documentary evidence to support the idea that charlatans in early modern Europe actually practised palming or pretended to extract stones to cure madness. This has not stopped scholars from continuing to believe that the extraction of the stone of madness was indeed a representation of quackery, for example Babiloni and colleagues (2003, 1775) note (referring to Bosch's painting) that, 'in fact in that age head surgery for the extraction of "stones" from the brain in the psychiatric disorders was relatively widespread'. However, in Gilman's words, it might well have been neither a representation of quackery nor of 'Renaissance trepanning, but rather the mocking of those who needed to see madness as rooted in some sort of objective physical cause' (Gilman 1988, 20).

Given the examples mentioned above of the depictions of feasts of fools—real carnivalesque events, to which I will return in chapter three—which often used the stone as a symbol of madness, it is possible that paintings of the extraction of the stone of madness in fact referred to allegorical scenes staged by actors in popular theatre, especially comedies (Schupbach 1978, 277). I might not subscribe to this theory with the same certainty as Wauters, according to whom 'it was demonstrated that the roots of the *keisnijding* should mainly be searched for within the textual tradition' (Wauters 2018, 30), but I do agree that a likely explanation for the boom of depictions of the extraction of the stone of madness can be found in linguistic equivalences. According to Wauters, this would be

> in line with what is known about the development of Bosch's visual language. This artist actually derived numerous elements from the Dutch language, which beforehand only had a textual existence. In this respect Bosch leans on an age-old tradition. The custom to play with language symbolism in a cryptical way occurs as early as the 13th and 14th century coats of arms. In this context the stone *kei* is a frequently occurring symbol of foolishnes [...] Bax remarked that 'van iets zoveel weten als de domme stenen' ['to know as much about anything as the stupid stones'] is used as an allegory for stupidity. Stones are after all symbols of rudeness and dullness. (Wauters 2018, 31)

Similarly, Schupbach had already pointed out that such paintings might be illustrations of 'popular phrases "to have a stone in one's head" (to be imbecile), "to have a stone cut out of one's head" (to be cured of imbecility or [...] to be deceived)' (Schupbach 1978, 269). Cornelis Kiel's 1599 *Etymologicum teutonicae linguae* mentions *keye* (*cerebri morbus*) and *Keyaerd* (*homo insanus*) as two words that come from *key* (stone) and relate to madness. Such expressions find equivalents in other European languages, for instance in north-eastern Italian languages ('astu glerje tal çurviel?' / 'Do you have gravel in your head?' in Friulano) and dialects ('te ga piere in testa?' / 'do you have stones in the head?' in Triestine). Curiously, neither in Danish nor in Norwegian does this reference survive, it being replaced by dirt or soil as the matter that causes stupidity and insanity ('have jord i hovedet' / 'to have dirt in your head').

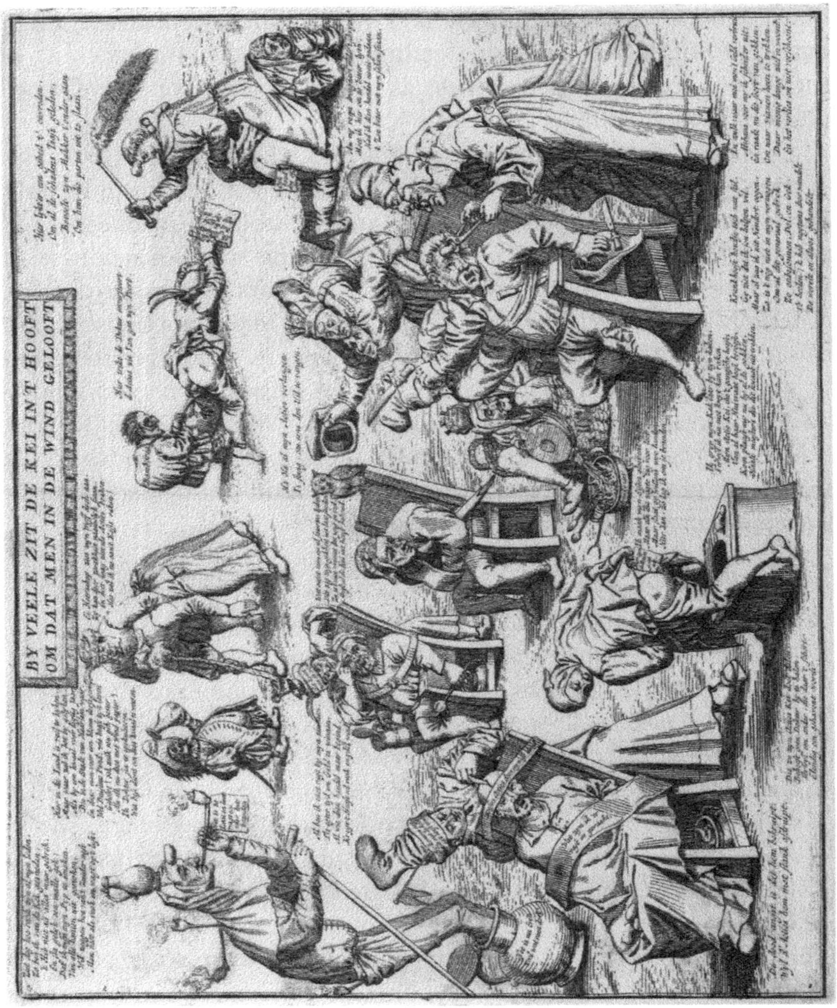

Figure 15: Carolus Allard, *By veele zit de kei in't Hooft om dat men in de Wind gelooft*. 1720. Courtesy of Library of Congress – https://www.loc.gov/item/2006677592/.

According to Wauters (2018, 21), the extraction of the stone of madness would fit in 'with the tradition of removing a negative object—such as a wasp, a worm, or a parasite—from the head'. The negative object par excellence would of course be excrement, and the stone might in fact be a 'symbolic fecal equivalent' (Hartman et al. 1976, 288); after all, purges and emetics were common cures for all kinds of mental disorders and the coexistence of the extraction of stones and the purge of excrement can be found in Allard's engraving on the cures of madness (Fig. 15). Several expressions in English connect excrement and mental disorder, stupidity or foolishness, namely 'being full of shit' or a 'shithead', or their opposite, 'putting one's shit together', for instance. Stones and excrement are also linked in some of the expressions mentioned above, in which the negative object is not a stone but rather soil/dirt/gravel. There are also numerous examples involving insects and parasites. We have seen above that Paracelsus, for instance, theorised that the sublimation and coagulation of mania might make worms grow in the head (Paracelsus 1979, 150), even though the surgical intervention he recommends is not to extract the worms, but to let the mania evaporate from cuts (Paracelsus 1979, 173). Under one of the most popular versions of Bruegel's *Witches of Malleghem* engraving there is an inscription in middle Dutch that invites the good people of Malleghem to love the 'Hexe' (the witch) and go to her without hesitation if they have a wasp in the head ('wesp int hooft') or are troubled by stones ('oft loteren v de keyen'). Similarly, in Pieter Huys's painting *A Surgeon Extracting the Stone of Folly*, while the scene is definitely a surgeon extracting a stone from a patient's head, in the background there is a jar of 'conserva van Wespen' (conserve of wasps) (Fig. 13). The connection between madness and insects (or spiders) in the head also surfaces at a linguistic level with expressions such as 'bee in one's bonnet' in English, 'qualcosa ronza in testa' (something buzzes in the head) in Italian, and 'hanneton dans la cervelle' (beetle in the brain) and 'araignée dans la cervelle' (spider in the brain) in French to indicate an obsession or madness; we even see this in the etymology of *estrus*—the scientific term for animal heat—which derives from 'οἶστρος [oîstros]' in ancient Greek (gad-fly, wasp, sting, frenzy). Shakespeare in *Henry IV Part I* (I.iii.236) refers to a 'wasp-stung and impatient fool'. As Hartman and colleagues (1976, 285–86) note, insects are common hallucinations in schizophrenia and drug-induced altered states of consciousness, and several flying insects lay their eggs under animals' skins creating lumps such as those depicted in stone extraction scenes.

'Like exorcism', continue Hartman and colleagues (1976, 292), 'the Stone operation is meant to remove the foreign matter of inner badness and evil'; we should add that it might mean to *represent metaphorically* the removal of a foreign matter of inner badness. There are two major advantages of attributing madness to a foreign object, according to Hartman and colleagues (1976, 293). The first is 'to make the unknown knowable, the intangible concrete', the leitmotif of this book. 'Another purpose', they continue, 'is the externalisation of unwanted badness. This well-known mechanism protects the person from having to own up to badness and weakness, which is attributed to outside agencies. This is essentially the paranoid position described by Melanie Klein'. In other words, the stone serves, like the staff, the dual purpose of making madness visible and of othering it.

Real Stones in the Head and Medical Extractions

Metaphorical, psychoanalytical or symbolic interpretations notwithstanding, real 'stones' can form inside the cranium and the brain. As Saade and colleagues (2019) note, 'intercranial calcifications are frequently encountered in non-contrast computed tomography scans in both adult and pediatric age groups', with a prevalence ranging from 1 per cent in young individuals to 20 per cent in the elderly population. Additionally, up to 72 per cent of autopsies worldwide report brain calcifications, the majority of which at a microscopic level, that cannot be picked up by the CT scan. Some of these calcifications have rock-like, conglomerate, mass-like and dot appearances that could make them appear, on dissection, as stones. Several such calcifications are physiological and age related, most notably those found in the pineal gland (on which I will return shortly), the choroid plexus, the habenula, the falx and the tentorium. Other calcifications are pathologic and can indicate a variety of illnesses, including: vascular (e.g., atherosclerosis), genetic (e.g., primary familiar brain calcification), infectious (e.g., HIV), neoplastic (e.g., meningiomas), metabolic (e.g., hypothyroidism), inflammatory (e.g., sarcoidosis) or even lead and CO poisoning. Some of the pathological causes of brain calcification might present with a symptomatology that could have been regarded as tantamount to melancholia or mania (e.g., seizures, clumsiness) but also neuropsychiatric manifestations, such as dementia and psychosis. Schenck, in his monumental treatise of 1608, *De Lithogenesia*, had already noted that *calculi* can be found everywhere in the body, including in the brain, where they could cause 'cephalgia, phrenesis, mania, vesania' (Schenck 1608, n.p.). But in the history of medicine, there are no other notable mentions of *calculi* in the brain, and Schenck does not mention any possible cure or form of extraction for any of them. Given the variable position of these stones and the impossibility of ascertaining their existence *in vivo* without imaging techniques such as the CT scan, it is very unlikely that extraction operations for such calcifications were performed at all in the past; and if they happened—and we have no record of them—survival would have been almost certainly impossible.

In his memoirs, neurosurgeon Daniel Cardinali remarks that the pineal gland calcifies in two adults out of three, a phenomenon which is clearly visible via X-ray. Cardinali, however, believes that 'since it had been known since ancient times that such stones (or calculi) were associated with urinary or biliary diseases, it seems reasonable to conclude that someone would have associated mental illness with the presence of a cerebral stone' (Cardinali 2016, 1). He continues his introductory argument by presenting cases of trephination as evidence of attempts to access the calcified pineal gland, and indeed concludes that 'considering the unique petrous nature of the pineal gland, the stone of madness was undoubtedly simply the pineal gland!' (Cardinali 2016, 2). The key issue is that prehistoric and historic evidence of trephination clearly shows the patient surviving it, which would not have been the case had the pineal gland, which is located very deeply and centrally in the brain, been accessed or extracted. The first successful pinealectomy on a human was performed only in 1915, and before this brain calcification and calcification of the pineal gland could have been ascertained in postmortem dissections only. According to Wauters (2018, 14), at the time of Bosch's paintings 'there was a revival of the notion (although refuted by Galen) that the pineal gland worked as a valve-like structure regulating the flow of animal spirits'. For this reason, she claims, 'this led to the concept that the pineal gland is connected with the "stone of madness", with the assumption that stones develop in the brain which by generating pressure result in brain damage and mental disorders'. It is unclear whether Wauters is here referring to Cardinali's stance or not, but she also dismisses the possibility that scenes showing the extraction of a 'stone of madness' might be reconstructions of actual operations of removing cerebral or pineal calcifications, or good faith attempts thereof. The same conclusion is reached by Ladino, Hunter and Téllez-Zenteno (2013, 87).

Overall, while it is certainly interesting to note that, with the pineal gland, we see the return of the motif of animal spirits, vapours and air moving in and out of the body—and potentially causing mental disorders—this does not add much to explaining the origins of the motif of the extraction of the stone of madness. While there are cases of intracranial calcifications, including the common and physiological calcification of the pineal gland, it is highly unlikely, and, in fact, almost inconceivable, that the extraction of the stone of madness might have represented the removal of one such stone.

Over time, however, there have been medical attempts purposefully aimed at extracting diseased matter that was believed to have caused a form of mental disorder, although such solid matter was not intracranial calcification. As Finger and Clower (2003, 32) note, the physician of Charles IX of France, Louis Duret, cured a boy of his epilepsy 'by removing some broken bone pressing on his brain'. In 1886, the surgeon Victor Horsley operated on his first patients with epilepsy by means of trephination, with the intention of removing diseased brain tissue. He was successful in removing a vascularised scar on the superior frontal sulcus and a tuberculoma, and in both cases the epilepsy did not return.

Even the infamous lobotomy, a procedure vastly popularised in horror and thriller films and novels (e.g., Ken Kesey's 1962 novel *One Flew Over the Cuckoo's Nest*, adapted for the big screen in 1975 by Miloš Forman, and Brad Anderson's 2001 film *Session 9*) originated in medical attempts at extracting diseased matter. Lobotomies notoriously involved severing the neural connection between lobes in the brain. Certainly the most portrayed (and widely used) procedure was the transorbital lobotomy (a.k.a. the 'icepick' lobotomy due to the shape of the tool used), which involved accessing the brain from the eye socket of the patient and severing, rather imprecisely, the connection between lobes, presumably between the prefrontal cortex and the thalamus. In spite of its permanent and devastating side effects, in the 1940s and 1950s it is estimated that more than 60,000 lobotomies were performed in the United States alone (Faria 2013). Lobotomy was first performed under the name leucotomy by Nobel Prize winner Egas Moniz in 1935. His procedure involved drilling small holes in the front of the skull and injecting pure ethyl alcohol to destroy the relevant tissues. While none of these procedures involved extracting supposedly diseased tissue, they did, however, originate in the late 1880s experiments of Swiss physician Gottlieb Brukhardt. Brukhardt carried out brain ablation (removal of tissue) on six of his patients, removing parts of the brain cortex that he believed were involved in their schizophrenia. One of the patients died some days after the operation, the other five all committed suicide at a later date; a gruesome procedure that had equally gruesome origins, grounded on the notion that madness can be extracted.

The most bizarre—and fortunately also the last—medical theory involving extraction in relation to mental disorders dates back to the first three decades of the twentieth century, at the hands of Henry Andrews Cotton, the superintendent of Trenton State Hospital in New Jersey. Inspired by advancements in the study of neurosyphilis and the demonstration that the spirochaete of syphilis causes brain damage (and symptoms that might look like mental disorders), Cotton extended this notion to all mental disorders. He developed what he called the 'bacteriological model of madness', postulating that all forms of mental disorder are caused by an infection. In parallel to this, he also subscribed to the theory of focal infection or focal sepsis, according to which several diseases could be explained by an infection in a specific part of the body (the 'focus' of the infection). By overlapping the two theories, Cotton postulated that mental disorders are caused by infections, which are in turn localised in different foci. Cotton started with teeth in 1913, extracting them from patients suffering from a variety of mental disorders. He soon identified different foci of infection, and exodontia evolved into evisceration, ablation of the gall bladder, tonsils, uterus, ovaries and testicles. Even though Cotton was not a surgeon he performed many of these operations himself, the majority of them without the consent of the patient. Several of these operations were fatal, in fact about 30 per cent to 40 per cent of colectomy patients died. Cotton claimed a success rate of 80 per cent and his methods became very popular. Several eminent physicians and scholars visited Trenton to study his outcomes, and he also opened a private clinic to treat his wealthiest patients. In 1925, the *New York Times* praised Cotton's hospital as the most progressive mental institution. By the time the mortality rates due to his interventions (perhaps as high as 45 per cent) became patent, Cotton had already retired from the state hospital, even though he continued to practise in the private sector until his death in 1933 (Scull 2007).

Possession and Exorcism

Cotton extracted teeth, gall bladders and bits of the intestine to remove, according to his theory, the bacteria that festered there and caused mental illness. The medical reasons behind this were no more scientific than the reasoning behind the need to extract demons from the possessed. If anything, regardless of one's personal beliefs, possessions and exorcisms have much more tangible manifestations than Cotton's 'focal infections'.

Much has already been written on mental disorders and demonic possession in history (see, e.g., Levack 2013). In this section, it will suffice to note that the trope of the extraction of madness relates to the iconography of possession and exorcism. In this, the demon is often depicted exiting the possessed from their open mouth, sometimes simply ascending from their body. Several representations of possession in history depict the demon leaving the body of the possessed after an exorcism, much like the *materia* causing mania was supposed to exhale from the cut in the head according to Rogerius (see above). This is the case for instance in the illumination of Jesus exorcising the Gerasene demoniac in the eleventh-century Hitda codex, Spinello Aretino's frescos in San Miniato (Florence), Girolamo di Benvenuto's painting of Saint Catherine exorcising the possessed (Fig. 16), woodcuts from the early-seventeenth-century *Compendium Maleficarum* and Rubens's famous *c.*1618 painting *The Miracles of St Ignatius*.

Of course, when considering possession in relation to mental disorders we are facing a double bind. On the one hand we can argue that, especially in medieval and early modern times, certain conditions which today we would consider mental disorders were ascribed to demonic possession. On the other, we must remember that demonic possession itself has been, and is still, regarded as a psychiatric condition (see Oesterreich 1966).

> Possession [...] is rarely encountered today by psychiatrists [...] though cases are occasionally reported [...] Some of the symptoms occur somewhat more frequently in other disorders, for example, belief that one is possessed is sometimes found in schizophrenics. The disorder sharing the most common symptoms is probably Gilles de la Tourette's syndrome, which is also rare and is characterized by involuntary tics and compulsive utterance of obscenities [...] A key factor in producing a case of possession syndrome is a culture or subculture which believes in the reality of possession. (Kemp and Williams 1987)

In contemporary terms, 'a possession state can be defined as the presence of a belief, delusional or otherwise, held by an individual (and sometimes by others) that their symptoms, experiences and behaviour are under the influence or control of supernatural forces, often of diabolical origin' (Enoch, Puri and Ball 2020, 224). Possession is therefore always a matter of interpretation. It is about someone interpreting their own symptoms as deriving from possession. In other

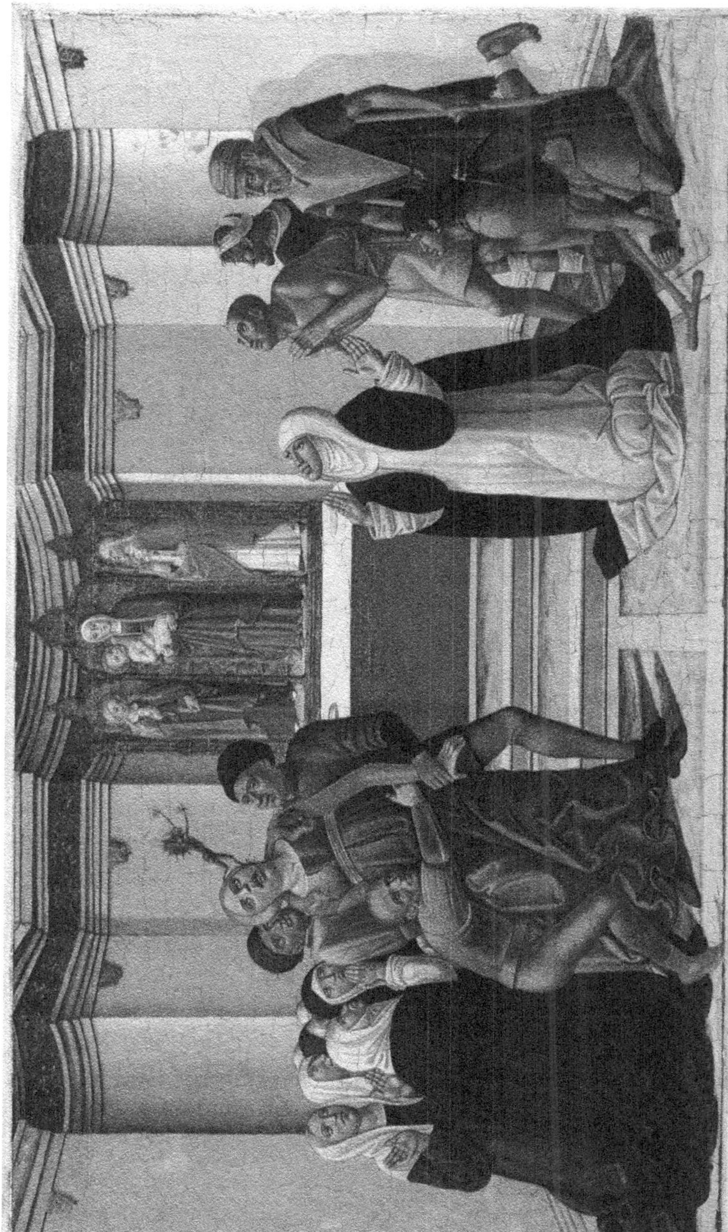

Figure 16: Girolamo di Benvenuto, St. Catherine of Siena Exorcising a Possessed Woman, about 1505. Denver Art Museum: Gift of the Samuel H. Kress Foundation, 1961.171. Photography courtesy of Denver Art Museum.

words, it is considered 'pathoplastic colouring [that] can be understood in the context of the patient's cultural background' (Enoch, Puri and Ball 2020, 231) in that 'the patient's belief structure and cultural background influences and is represented in the content of the symptoms exhibited' (Enoch, Puri and Ball 2020, 234).

When we cast our gaze to the history of possession, we are thus inevitably looking at it as an interpretation of a mental disorder: possession itself is a way to represent mental disorders. We must also bear in mind that this double bind was already present in the first descriptions of possession. In the New Testament for instance, Matthew tells us that from the whole country of Syria people were brought to Jesus: 'all those who were sick, suffering from all kinds of diseases or disorders: people with demons, and epileptics, and paralytics—and Jesus healed them all' (Matt 4:24).

Possession, which we could define as a state in which one's body and mind are taken over by an entity (spirit, demon, etc.), is a cross-cultural and trans-religious phenomenon. It occurs in Buddhism, Christianity, Haitian Vodou, Hinduism, Islam, Wicca and Native American traditions. It may, depending on the context, be voluntary or involuntary, beneficial or injurious, and may or may not require exorcism. Bourguignon's 1968 study (Bourguignon 1968) found that 'belief in spirit possession' was claimed to exist in 74 per cent of the 488 societies under consideration. She noted that possession-believing states were more prevalent among the cultures of the Pacific than among Native Americans. Religions such as Christianity, Islam and Judaism tend to attribute this phenomenon to malevolent spirits, or demons, using exorcism as a way to purge an evil spirit from the individual. Catholicism views it as one of the rarest forms of possession, whereas Islam recognises *jinn* and other spirits, which, depending on their context, cause a positive or negative possession. Similarly, Jewish mysticism refers to the *dybbuk*, a restless soul that seeks resolution through its host.

African traditions are replete with variant meanings for possession. For instance, in the Democratic Republic of the Congo, a therapeutic framing for possession can be seen in the Zebola dance ritual. Such a belief extends across Kenya and Mozambique to the African diaspora, where Haitian Vodou, Umbanda and Hoodoo include spirit possession in their rituals of healing and wisdom.

China also has a deep-rooted belief in spirit possession. Shamans (*Jitong*) invoke possession for protection, seen with the Boxers during the Boxer Rebellion of 1899–1901. In India, particularly in the Himalayan regions, belief in possession is widespread, while the

Veddas of Sri Lanka enter trances during religious festivals, where they are believed to be possessed by spirits. In south-east Asia, Indonesia practises *sanghyang*, a form of voluntary possession where such a trance-like state is used for cleansing and restoring spiritual balance.

Exorcism is a reaction to ideas of spirit possession across cultures. Such a religious practice includes recitation in Buddhism, Hindu mantras, Islamic verses from the Quran, Jewish Kabbalistic ritual, and prayers and other rituals in Christianity to keep away the evil spirits from the possessed person. Christian exorcisms are characterised by prayers and rituals designed to expel malevolent forces; however, the specific methods vary depending on the denomination. The Chinese also have their version of exorcism, wherein the ceremony is performed by a Taoist priest who uses talismans for warding off the spirits.

These are just some of the most prominent examples of possession and exorcism across cultures, testifying to the widespread nature of this belief. The main focus of this section, however, is of course to analyse the visualisation of possession and exorcism as a scene of extraction; to present them as an alternative and enduring iconography of mental disorder represented as an entity that can be extracted. To this extent it is important to note that 'the most prominent features of demonic possession do not exist before the exorcism ritual but are its products' (Zempléni 2022, 26). While it is the possessed who we can equate, in iconography, to the insane and the fool, it is in the exorcism, and thus in the action of extraction of the demon/mental disorder, that their characteristics are defined.

As Zempléni (2022, 3) reminds us, it must be borne in mind that 'most anthropological studies on spirit possession have been—and still are—infused with Western concepts of self and personhood and Western notions of body–soul dualism, and they convey a whole set of presuppositions inherited from Christian models of "good" and "bad" possession once prevalent in Europe'. It is undeniable that possession and exorcism are phenomena present in the vast majority of cultures and historical periods, but in many cultures, possession is sought by people, craved and seen as a positive contact with deities. In this section, therefore, where I focus on representations of exorcism as extraction, I will necessarily focus on cultures that see possession as a negative, and thus exorcism as a necessary remedy. This is in line with my approach, whereby I discuss possession only inasmuch as it is considered either a mental disorder or an illness/disease that has to be eradicated. Being aware that this limits the scope of my analysis, I refer the reader to Pócs and Zempléni's edited volume on possession across cultures for a comprehensive study of the phenomenon (Pócs and Zempléni 2022). As Zempléni (2022, 5) put it, I will be inevitably focusing on the

> dualistic ethics and way of thinking of the religions of the Book which emphasize the opposition between good and evil, pure and impure, faithful and unfaithful, believer and pagan [...] religious dualism is at the origin of a whole series of oppositions that shaped how the adepts understood and judged possession.

Exorcism is visualised as the extraction of demons in particular, if not exclusively, in the Christian tradition. In these, which are mostly depictions of either Christ or saints expelling demons, taken from either the Gospels or hagiographies respectively, there are several recurrent characteristics, most notably that the demon exits the possessed from the mouth after having been expelled by the exorcist. One of the most frequently depicted scenes of exorcism is that of the Gerasene demoniac, known as the Miracle of the (Gadarene) Swine and the exorcism of Legion, recounted in the synoptic Gospels (Matt 8:28–34; Mark 5:1–20; Luke 8:26–39). The story depicts Jesus casting out one or more demons from a possessed man, who then enter a herd of swine. The swine rush down a hill and drown in a lake. In all the three accounts in the canonical Gospels, Jesus is seen performing the exorcisms. In Mark 5:1–20, Jesus crosses the sea and arrives in the 'region of the Gerasenes', where he meets a man possessed by a demon. This man had been living in caves and tombs, and despite several attempts to restrain him with chains, he kept breaking free and harming himself with stones. When Jesus confronts the demon, it addresses him as 'Jesus, Son of the Most High God' and pleads not to be tormented. Jesus then asks for the demon's name, to which it responds, 'My name is Legion, for we are many'. The demon(s) ask not to be sent away, but instead ask to be sent into a group of pigs nearby. Jesus grants their request, after which the pigs rush down a steep bank into the sea, drowning in the process. The formerly possessed man is now restored to sanity and is fully clothed, and expresses a desire to follow Jesus, but Jesus tells him to stay in the Decapolis region and tell others the great things the Lord has done for him. In the Gospel of Matthew (Matt 8:28–34), the story is considerably condensed, but involves two possessed men rather than one. Interestingly, in this version, Jesus does not inquire about the demon's name, which is usually an essential part of exorcism practice. Additionally, the location given for the exorcism is not the Decapolis but rather the region of the 'Gadarenes' (Gadara) in most Bible translations. The King James Version mentions 'Gergesenes', which is likely to be modern Kursi (Kheras), the most plausible location for the Gospel event. Luke's version (Luke 8:26–39) is shorter than Mark's, but largely agrees with its core details. One unique aspect of it though is the mention of the demoniac's nakedness and subsequent clothing after the exorcism. Initially, the man is depicted as naked, symbolising his animal-like state due to his possession, but after the exorcism, he is fully restored as a human being and portrayed as being 'clothed and in his right mind'. In these depictions we see again the association between nakedness and outsideness/madness (or possession in this case), and clothing as the return of civilisation/sanity.

One of the many depictions of this event can be found on an ivory panel by the Milanese workshop dating to *c.*968 CE, and donated by Emperor Otto the Great to Magdeburg Cathedral. Jesus and the apostles stand on the left, whereas the demoniac stands on the right, being restrained; three swine are at the bottom right of the panel and the demon is depicted as exiting the mouth of the demoniac. The Hidta Codex (University State Library of Darmstadt, Hs. 1640), an evangeliary commissioned by Hidta, Abbess of Meschede in 1020, depicts the same scene in fol. 76r (Fig. 17). In this depiction, Jesus and the demoniac are on their own and there are no swine.

The demoniac stands in a lower position than Christ with his arms spread in front of him, in a position of submission. The demon is exiting from the mouth, but instead of ascending like in the ivory panel, it seems to fall to the ground, as if the demoniac were vomiting it. The celebrated Armenian illuminator Toros Roslin illustrated the Gospels in 1262 under the commission of a priest also named Toros, the nephew of the Emperor Constantine. At fol. 40r Toros depicts the 'sick and the possessed', an illustration for the verse 'When evening came, many who were demon-possessed were brought to him, and he drove out the spirits with a word and healed all the sick' (Matt 8:16). Two of the six people queueing to be healed by Jesus feature a demon exiting their mouths, although no exorcism is being performed in the illumination.

A very similar iconographical model is used to depict the miracle of the numerous saints who are said to have healed demoniacs, that is to say, performed exorcisms. One of the bronze panels on the right door of the twelfth-century Basilica di Zeno Maggiore in Verona (Italy) depicts St. Zeno performing an exorcism on the daughter of the Emperor Gallienus. While she is held by a third person, the demon exits from her mouth. The same happens to the demons being exorcised by St. Egidius and St. Donatus in the 1320–40 *Acta Sanctorum pictis imaginaribus adornata*, an illuminated version of the *Acts of the Saints* that

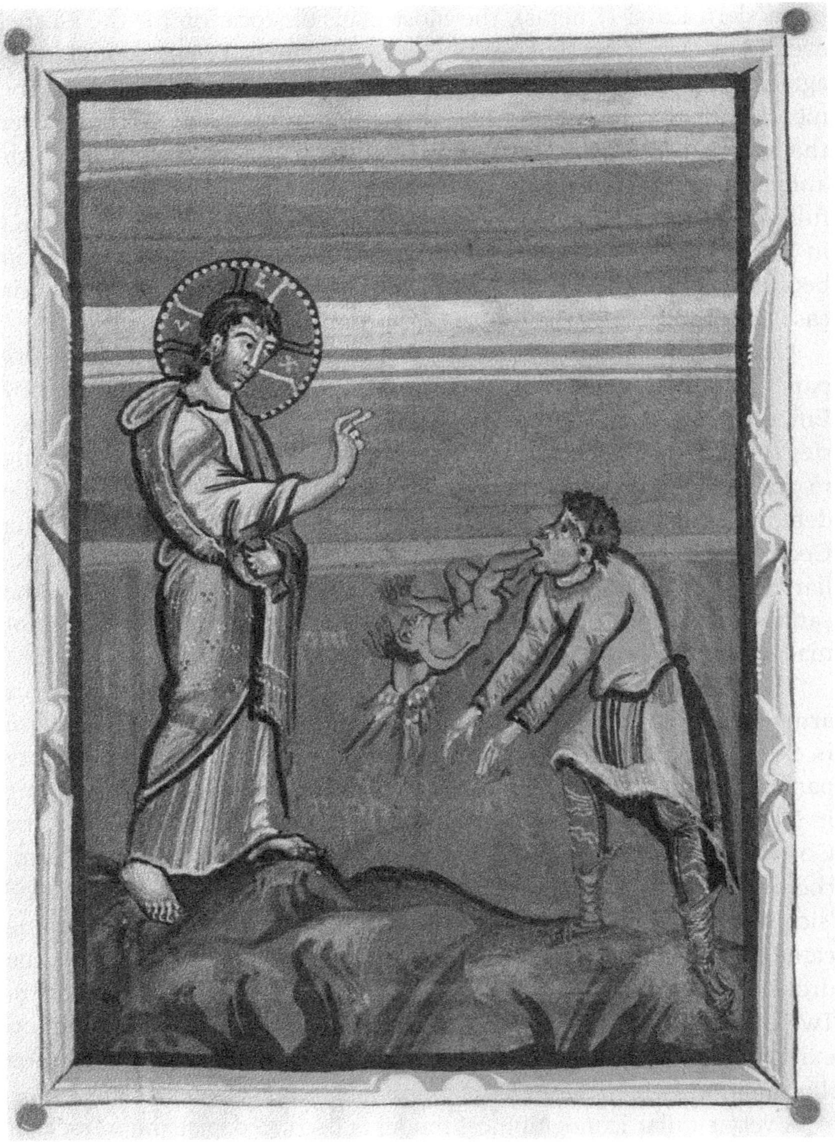

Figure 17: Jesus exorcising the Gerasene Demoniac.
Hidta Codex, Hs. 1640, fol 76r. Courtesy of Universitäts- und landesbibliothek Darmstadt.

is now split between the Vatican Apostolic Library, the Hermitage Museum and the Morgan Library. Three demons leave the possessed from the mouth in the mid-thirteenth-century altarpiece of the Master of Bardi Chapel in Santa Croce (Florence) that depicts one of the many exorcisms of St. Francis. Some early modern paintings also repeat the same trope: Antonio Vivarini's *c.*1450 depiction of St. Peter exorcising a possessed woman, for instance, and the *c.*1500 painting by Girolamo di Benvenuto that depicts St. Caterina exorcising a woman—she is being held by several helpers and, while St. Caterina prays at a certain distance, the demon exits from the mouth of the possessed (Fig. 16). While in this chapter I am focusing on the expulsion or extraction of demons, it is worth noting also that the posture of the possessed is very significant and overlaps with postures historically associated with mental disorders. Postures of convulsions and rigidity—such as the opisthotonos—recur in the iconography of mental disorders and we will encounter them again in the next chapter.

The expulsion of matter from the mouth is not only a motif in the visualisation of exorcisms. Human vomiting of unlikely matter, such as hairballs—in medical jargon known today as trichobezoars—was considered to be a possible sign of possession. Enoch, Puri and Ball (2020, 229–31) describe a case in which a woman, claiming to be possessed, lamented vomiting 'pieces of fat covered with hairs'. They note that the vomiting of trichobezoars was rather common in medieval and early modern demonological writings. Guazzo, in his *Compendium Maleficarum*, quotes Cornelias Gemma's account of a 15-year-old girl who, in 1571, vomited (and defecated) several different objects including 'hairs [...] like those which fall from old dogs' (Guazzo 1988). By the same token, emetics and purges were often used as a treatment for mental disorders, whether these were prescribed to rebalance the humours in the body (in Galenic medicine) or to expel the obnoxious matter, as discussed above in reference to Allard's engraving on the cures of madness.

Spirit possession and exorcism are beliefs and practices that are very widespread across cultures and historical periods. Yet, the visualisation of exorcisms as the extraction/expulsion of demons, most often from the mouth of the possessed, is a very Christian iconographical trope that presupposes that it is an evil entity that possesses the demoniac, and that its expulsion is much needed. To this extent the iconography of possession and exorcism reveals telling parallels with that of the extraction of madness: mental disorder is incarnated into an unwanted substance or object that needs to be extracted/let out to cure the person.

Conclusions

As in the previous chapter, here I have focused on different aspects of the othering of madness, and how this translates into the othering of the insane. The visualisation of mental disorders as solid or gaseous entities that can be extracted takes many forms and it is impossible to give a definitive interpretation of these. Trephination, the practice of boring holes in the skulls of the living, has been practised since time immemorial, and there is evidence in medical treatises from all eras that it was also practised to extract madness or let it evaporate. The medical procedure of attempting to extract madness does not stop with the advent of modern medicine; we have seen some fine and gruesome examples of twentieth-century extractions. However, artistic depictions of madness as a material object, such as a stone, and their extraction are almost certainly allegorical representations. They depict neither real operations nor charlatan practices, such as palming, but there is no definitive answer as to what they could be allegorising. Perhaps they are an allegory of charlatanry or the gullibility of humankind, or perhaps they represent the vain hope of finding a cure for madness, or the insanity of considering madness as something that can, or should, be cured by physicians. What is most surprising, perhaps, is that calculi and calcifications can indeed form inside the skull, but none of the procedures of extraction depicted could relate to their extraction, something which would have been impossible. This is another example of the continuous exchange and parallels between medical practices and iconography that testifies to the complexity of this relationship, especially in reference to the invisible ailments of the mind.

'Is it mad to imagine a cure for madness?' (Hartman et al. 1976, 266) ask the authors of one of the seminal articles on the study of trephination and extraction of the stone of madness, a question that we could legitimately ask of several of the depicted practices I discuss in this book. As we will continue to see in the following chapters, as we unravel the visual othering of madness as much as the visual othering of the insane, the history of the visualisation of mental disorders is laden with semantic slippages and borrowings. In visual representations there is something mad about being an outsider, as much as there is something alien in being mad. By the same token, as much as we have identified madness and mental disorders as ailments to be cured, there is something mad, in visual representation at least, in imagining a cure for madness. But madness and genius often touch, something we will return to towards the end of the book, and even if it is not an act of genius to visualise a mad cure for madness, there is something profoundly human in giving a visual shape to something otherwise invisible and unknown, the leitmotif of this monograph. Making madness visible—in stones and in other materials that can be extracted, even if they are just vapours—enables us not only to visualise the invisible and make the unknown known, but also to picture a potential cure for madness, be it via extraction, evaporation or ablation. The visualisation of madness as an entity that can be extracted has led to concrete medical practices for such extraction, some of which still took place until quite recently and all of them rather gruesome. The potential extraction of mental disorder has led us to another practice that is closely related to the extraction of an unwanted, evil, entity: exorcism, in particular the Christian version. The study of the visualisation of madness in the prop of the staff has unravelled the depiction of madness as air and, with it, the othering of the insane as fools, witches, wild men, outsiders and vagrants. The study of the visualisation of madness in the form of an entity to be extracted, be it gaseous or rocky, leads us to conclude that, in visual cultural history at the very least, another category of 'undesirables' overlaps with that of the insane: the possessed and the demoniacs. We will return to this in later chapters, when we will look more closely at how the stigma of madness etches itself onto the very bodies of the insane, by means of seizures, dances, postures, expressions and even subtle differences in the shape of skulls. For the time being though, as a partial conclusion, we should note how in visual culture, numerous categories of unwanted individuals are marked as 'other' by means of recurrent and exchangeable visual characteristics.

PART TWO

The Body of the Insane

CHAPTER THREE

Madness Troubles Borders: Externalising and Containing Mass Madness

OVER THE PREVIOUS CHAPTERS, we have seen how madness is visually articulated in the individual, often coming into being through props, objects or direct representation of the body of the mentally ill. However, madness is not solely an individual affliction; it emerges as spectacle in the social body, whereby it reveals deeper anxieties about the boundaries of sanity and the communal fear of disorder. In its visual and cultural presence, madness is not just that of an isolated madman; instead, it poses the possibility of spillover into society. These depictions of insanity in association with crowds (dancing, overflowing, invading, etc.) reflect new dimensions in the ways in which one conceives mental illness—themes of contagion and overflow, for instance—and the urgent social need to contain them. Much like with individuals, as we have seen in the previous chapters, so also in multitudes, insanity borders with other states of marginality: vagrancy, poverty, social outcasts, migrants. This chapter approaches the visualisation of madness as a diffuse, social one that, if left uncurbed, might shake the very foundations of society.

One of the most enduring motifs in the visual representation of madness is its performative aspect, a notion that becomes even more pronounced when addressing the phenomenon of collective insanity. Unlike the isolated madman, who can be 'othered' through marginalisation or exclusion, the mad multitude brings to mind images of widespread disorder, hinting at madness as a potential epidemic that may afflict the masses. This collective dimension of madness, as we shall see, reveals how precarious societal boundaries are, and is a reflection of the anxieties around the contagious nature of mental illness. This fear of madness infiltrating the 'sane' social body often leads to visual representations that stress the necessity for containment, both physical and metaphorical. Whether through the walls of an asylum, the isolation of the mad in cages or visual metaphors that emphasise their difference, such depictions demonstrate the lengths to which societies will go to control and restrain madness, at least in terms of iconography.

The iconography of collective madness often employs the motif of the 'fool'. These depictions of mass folly, such as those seen in the 'Feast of Fools' engravings and paintings, often feature court jesters, *insipientes* and participants wearing fool's caps and bells or distributing them to the crowd. Yet, despite the festive overtones, these visualisations contain a variety of deeper meanings. The collective madness portrayed in these works is not only a carnival or festive inversion of social norms, but also a commentary on the anxiety that the thin line separating reason from madness provokes. These images represent the porous nature of the boundary between sanity and insanity, depicting groups of fools spilling into the streets, public squares and even sacred places. The world itself becomes a stage for this madness. The sane and the insane are constantly at risk of swapping places.

A good example of the visualisation of mass madness are those images depicting dancing mania, a phenomenon that swept across Europe from the fourteenth to seventeenth centuries. These events, in which large groups of people engaged in uncontrollable dancing, were often seen as a form of collective insanity and were linked to spiritual or supernatural causes. The historical sources that describe dancing mania reveal that such episodes were viewed as disturbing by contemporaries, especially as entire towns or villages were sometimes affected. The fear that madness could erupt either spontaneously or recurrently, without any clear cause, and spread across the entire population further muddied the boundary between sanity and insanity, and reinforced the anxiety to control and contain madness. Such a fear is evident in the visual representations of manic dancing, such as Pieter Bruegel's *The Dancing Pilgrims at Muelebeek* (1564) (Fig. 18), where the bodies of the 'afflicted' appear contorted and chaotic, showing madness to be something that invades and overwhelms the human body and society alike.

Yet, despite its chaotic and invasive nature, dancing mania also blurred the lines between madness and its cure. Some historical accounts suggest that the uncontrollable movements were the madness, whereas the dance itself was its therapy, a form of cathartic release that might help those afflicted to purge the madness from their bodies. This ambiguity—whether the dance was a symptom or a

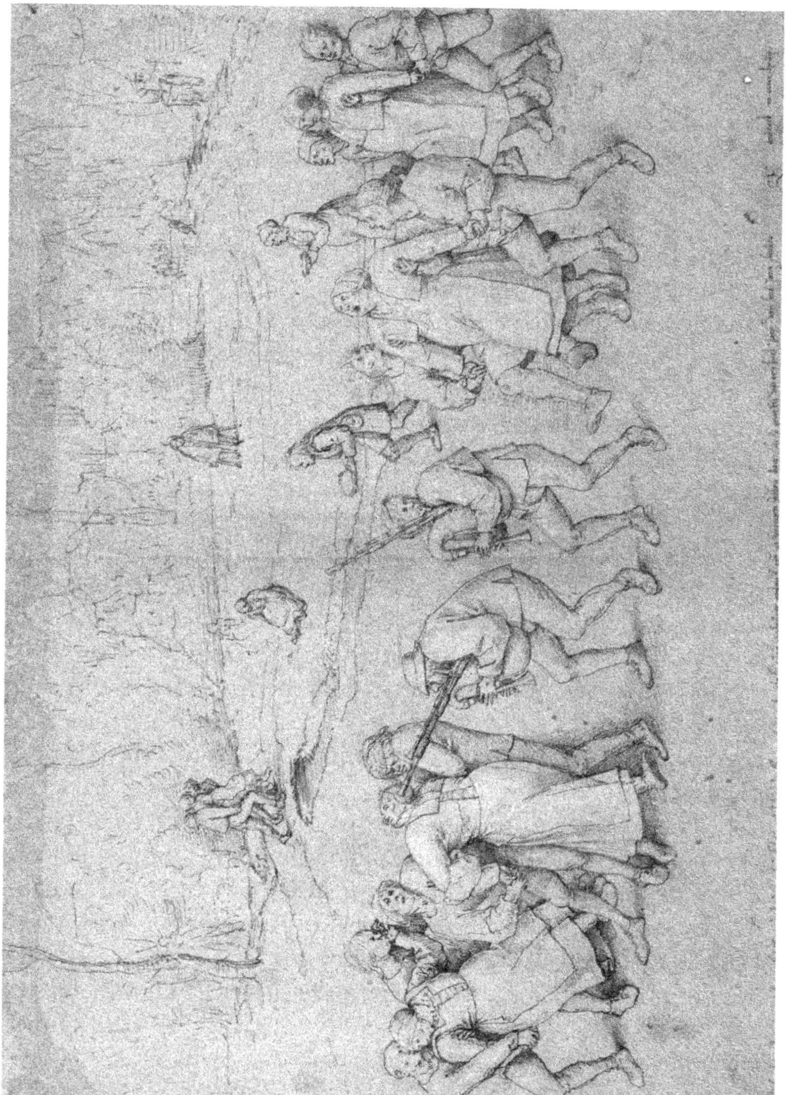

Figure 18: Pieter Bruegel, the Elder. The Dancing Mania. Pilgrimage of the Epileptics to the Church at Molenbeek. Drawing 1564. Courtesy of the Albertina Museum (Vienna).

cure—demonstrates how deeply intertwined madness and its visualisation are with notions of performance. Madness, in these contexts, is not only something that is seen but something that is enacted, often in public spaces, where the mad become unwilling performers in a spectacle of disorder. In performing the dance, the insane also become agents of their own madness and its cure. They are no longer only represented, talked about, construed as mad by others; they also move, dance, invade—that is to say, they have some level of agency and opportunity for self-representation.

Such collective forms of madness—whether depicted as dancing mania, feasts of fools, or multitudes of the insane—foreground the tension between externalisation and containment. Madness, in these visual tropes, is something that overflows, something that cannot easily be kept at bay. But it is precisely this uncontrollable nature that necessitates the creation of boundaries—both physical and symbolic—around the mad. The visualisation of madness frequently returns to the motif of cages, walls and other forms of restraint to represent this containment. We have already seen the *Narrenschiff*, for example, on which the insane become the travellers. The ship of fools serves as a metaphor for the way in which societies seek to distance themselves from the madness that threatens to engulf them, setting the insane adrift.

In the visualisations we will explore in this chapter, the containment of madness becomes a visual and cultural necessity: an act of both protection and exclusion. At the same time, however, these visual representations also end up depicting the permeability of these boundaries. The walls of the asylum, the cages that hold the mad and the ships that carry them away cannot conceal that madness *is everywhere*, always capable of resurfacing and troubling the borders that societies erect to contain it. Not only this: the necessity of containment, we shall see, foregrounds also its impossibility. The cage of fools cannot contain madness because it is the world itself that is mad.

Within–Without: Dances and Convulsions

Choreomania

In this section it will become clear that the otherness of madness is often represented as the surfacing of the inside on the outside of the body, whether it is in physiognomic characteristics, as I will show in chapter four, or bodily movement. In this section I focus on bodily movements, especially the extent to which they are portrayed in relation to multitudes of the insane. Additionally, because madness becomes visible by it seizing control of the body—influencing facial traits, expressions, posture and movement—numerous 'treatments' leverage parallel principles: for example, raving maniacs must be contained; idle melancholics must be made active. Here I thus analyse the most iconic performances of madness, such as the collective and relatively common phenomenon of 'dancing mania', which seized groups of up to hundreds of people in medieval and early modern Europe, and even Charcot's hysterics, that inspired Freud in giving birth to psychoanalysis.

Even though 'dancing mania' is not often depicted in visual culture—most images are variants of Bruegel's sixteenth-century drawing *The Dancing Pilgrims at Muelebeek*—the fact that collective mental distress appears in the form of uncontrollable movement is, I claim in this section, a way to make madness visible. Interestingly, dancing mania also allows us to blur the line between mental disorder and its cure, as it is often impossible to distinguish whether the dance is symptomatic, therapeutic, cathartic or even iatrogenic. This ambivalent relationship between inner and outer disorder resides also in the therapeutic approach that is still used today, namely convulsive therapy (i.e., inducing a grand-mal seizure to treat mental disorder, now practised in the form of electroconvulsive therapy (ECT)). Whether contemporary convulsive therapy was erroneously inspired by the myth of the dance cure—as catharsis of inner troubles—or the dance cure was effective precisely because it leveraged the same biology as convulsive therapy, iconography and medicine display a continuity across history in relating convulsive movements to mental disorders and their cure.

Dancing mania was a peculiar phenomenon, and is often also referred to as the dancing plague, choreomania, or St. John's or St. Vitus' dance. It was a social phenomenon that appeared primarily across mainland Europe between the fourteenth and seventeenth centuries, and involved groups of people engaging in erratic dancing, sometimes involving hundreds of participants at once. The term 'dancing mania' originated from the Greek 'choreomania', a combination of *'choros'* (dance) and *'mania'* (madness). Paracelsus coined the term in his 1532 treatise *The Diseases That Deprive Man of His Reason*, and the condition was initially attributed to the influence of saints, particularly St. John the Baptist or St. Vitus, thus the names St. John's dance or St. Vitus' dance for the phenomenon (Paracelsus 1979).

Throughout history, outbreaks of dancing mania occurred at irregular intervals with varying characteristics, and were often triggered by difficult circumstances; such episodes involved large groups of people dancing for extended periods, from hours to sometimes months on end. Musicians occasionally accompanied the dancers in the belief that their music would alleviate the mania, although this approach sometimes simply led to more people joining the dance. While it is thought that women participated more in these events than men, the historical sources actually indicate a broader spectrum of participants, which included both adults and children who danced until they became exhausted or sustained injuries. Whether the dancing was spontaneous or organised is not known, but the participants typically seemed to be in an altered state and lacked control over their actions (Bartholomew and Goode 2001, 132–36).

The earliest known outbreak seems to come from the seventh century (Backman 1952, 171), although Waller (2009, 16) claims the first event took place in the Saxon town of Kölbigk in 1070. In 1237, a notable outbreak is recorded as having taken place during a journey involving a large group of children travelling from Erfurt to Arnstadt (about 20 km apart). Throughout the journey, the children engaged in continuous jumping and dancing, a striking resemblance to the famed story of the Pied Piper of Hamelin, which emerged around the same period (McAlister 1977). Later, in 1278, approximately 200 individuals are recorded as having danced on a bridge spanning the River Meuse, causing the bridge's unfortunate collapse, with many survivors finding refuge at a nearby chapel devoted to St. Vitus (Bartholomew and Goode 2001, 194). On 24 June 1374, a major outbreak began in Aachen, then spread to Cologne, Flanders, Franconia, Hainaut, Metz, Strasbourg, Tongeren, Utrecht, as well as to Italy and Luxembourg (Midelfort 1999, 138). More incidents followed in 1375 and 1376, across France, Germany and the Netherlands. In 1381, another dancing mania event occurred in Augsburg, and more are recorded in Strasbourg in 1418, possibly due to exhaustion from fasting, and in Schaffhausen in 1428, where a monk danced to death. At the same time, some women in Zürich featured in a dancing frenzy (Bartholomew and Goode 2001, 138). Another extensive outbreak took place in July 1518 in Strasbourg, where a woman initiated the dancing and was then joined by between 50 and 400 people. Further occurrences took place during the sixteenth century: in 1536 in Basel involving children, and in 1551 in Anhalt when a lone man was involved (Midelfort 1999, 38). Although there are numerous reports of dancing mania up until the seventeenth century, the 1374 and 1518 incidents are the best documented (Waller 2009, 625).

There is no agreement among scholars as to the exact cause or nature of this dancing mania. Various theories have been proposed, ranging from religious cults orchestrating them (Bartholomew and Goode 2001, 134–37) to people dancing to cope with mass stress events in order to momentarily escape the hardships of their era (Hetherington and Munro 1997, 92). Some theories suggest it might have been a form of mass psychogenic illness, where physical symptoms without apparent physical causes spread through a group due to social influence (Hetherington and Munro 1997, 73; Bartholomew and Goode 2001, 135; Midelfort 1999, 73). Physical causes behind dancing mania have also been advanced, with hypotheses including ergot poisoning, encephalitis, epilepsy or murine typhus (Blom 2010, 126). St. Vitus' dance in individuals may also have been caused by Sydenham chorea (an autoimmune reaction to streptococcal infection, primarily seen in children), so episodes of dancing mania have thus been referred to as 'epidemic chorea'. Additionally, phenomena like tarantism are similar to dancing mania, with victims dancing to counteract perceived venomous bites. Tarantism is a Southern Italian phenomenon, which is often accompanied by specific music and elaborate rituals to 'cure' the victims. Given the group nature of the documented episodes of dancing mania though, the most plausible explanation is that it represented a collective reaction to periods of enormous stress, as Waller (2009) has convincingly argued.

Having noted that episodes of dancing mania are far from isolated oddities, and that they have, much like possession, cross-cultural manifestations, what is interesting for the purpose of the present study is to discuss how such episodes were visually depicted, but also to consider these episodes as visualisations of madness in their own right. That is, the otherwise invisible mental distress surfaces in the bodies of the affected and, much like the staff or the stone, makes madness visible.

Despite its prevalence, to date only two visual representations of these dancing mania events exist: an anonymous seventeenth-century etching of the dancing plague of Strasbourg, as well as several engravings and paintings all based on Bruegel's drawing *The Dancing Pilgrims at Muelebeek* (1564) (Fig. 18).

The 1564 drawing shows a procession of four women each being carried by two men. The women are seemingly in the grip of fits and seizures, their bodies are contorted and one features an expression of stupor; she is also being carried and constrained by the two men in a position that is very similar to that of the possessed. Other 'dancers' and companions are featured in the background, and the procession in the foreground is accompanied by two pipers. The inscription by Bruegel at the bottom reads, in Middle Dutch: 'On this Saint John's Day, outside Brussels, in Molenbeek, they must dance, and when they have danced or jumped over a bridge, then they are cured for a whole year from the sickness of Saint John'. In the sixteenth century, a small spring existed at Muelebeek with healing properties that was dedicated to St. Gertrude. Bruegel's accompanying description indicates that the dancers would be 'healed', thus implying that they were seen as unwell in their current state (and their dancing was consequently undesirable), and that the healing effects would endure for a full year. This suggests that the pilgrimage depicted in the illustration had to be repeated on a yearly basis. From this, one can infer that certain individuals experienced recurring, undesirable symptoms each year around the time of St. John's day, and likely embarked on an annual pilgrimage to Muelebeek during that period to seek healing for the upcoming year (McAlister 1977). Waller (2009, 139), in contrast, considers that the image represents an embryonic folkloric possession cult, as 'these people wanted to suffer from the dance frenzy for a day, apparently believing that for doing so St John would relieve them of the curse for the remainder of the year. By implication, they repeated the performance year after year'. According to Waller, Bruegel did not depict dancing mania, but rather people ritually dancing to *prevent* falling prey to dancing mania for the rest of the year.

Bruegel's drawing was subsequently turned into a painting (undated) by his son (Brueghel the Younger) and as part of a booklet of etchings by Hendrick Hondius (1642) (Fig. 19). This booklet opens with a 'Presentation' in Middle Dutch that is very similar to Bruegel's original caption:

> How the Pilgrims, on St. John's Day, outside Brussels, must proceed to Meulebeke; and as they have crossed over this Bridge, or are compelled in the following manner, then they seem to be cured of the falling Sickness.
>
> First, these Players or Minstrels, playing on Bagpipes, go ahead; after that, the Pilgrims follow, who are seized by strong Villagers, very unwillingly (as is shown in the second and third following Figure), crying and shouting; but upon reaching the Bridge, they turn around and put up a great resistance; but being captured, they are lifted and carried over the Bridge; having crossed, they sit down as if exhausted; and then the Villagers from that place come, offering them something to drink, and giving them something warm; and thus this work is completed.

Some of Hondius's etchings are interpretations and expansions of Bruegel's drawing: the first is a detail of the bagpipers, followed by a

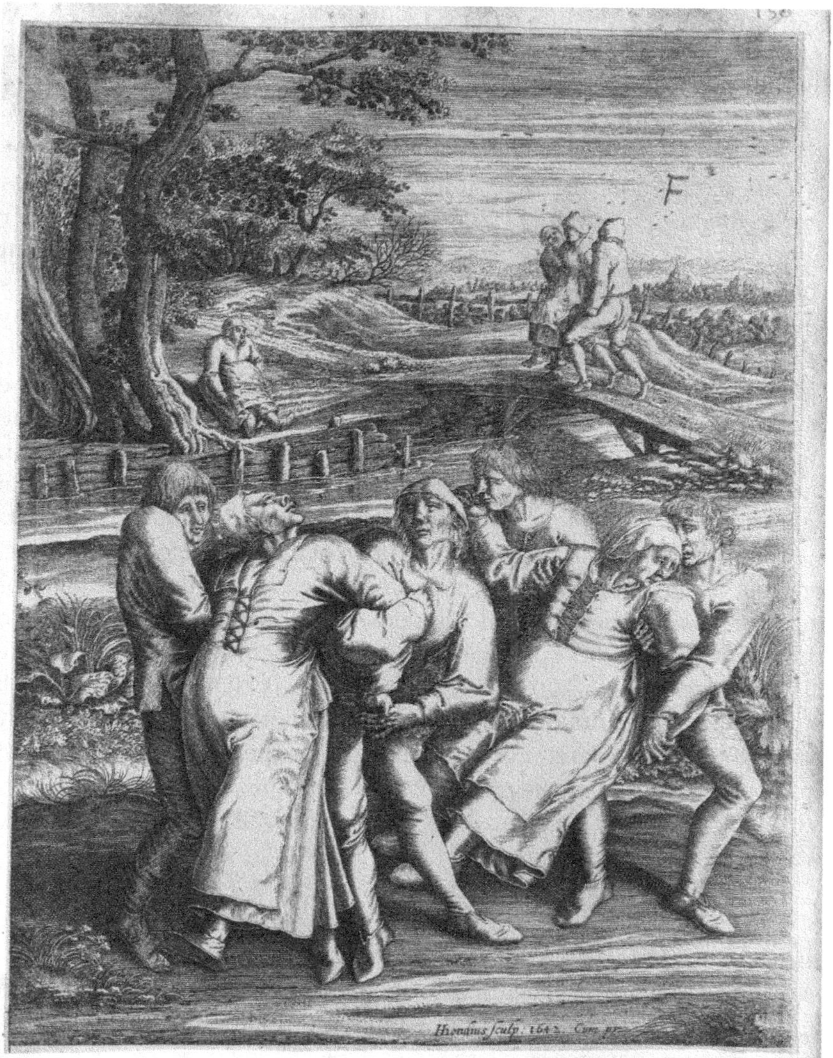

Figure 19: Hendrik Hondius, After Peter Bruegel's Drawing. Engraving 1642. Collection Museum Boijmans Van Beuningen, Rotterdam. Purchased with the support of Lucas van Leyden Foundation / Photography: Studio Tromp.

court fool playing the lute to lead a dancer. These are followed by etchings after Bruegel's drawing that capture some of the details, including the dancers being forcefully dragged over the bridge. The disease for which the pilgrims are seeking a cure is the 'falling sickness' (*vallende Sieckte*), which would normally indicate epilepsy.

One of the noteworthy details is that in all of these the dancers are accompanied by pipers and musicians, who guide them in their pilgrimage. These seem to have been often hired by the authorities in the belief, as we shall soon see, that the dancing was the disease as much as it was the cure (Burton has already noted this in the *Anatomy of Melancholy* (Burton 2004, I.I.IV)). Despite the noticeable similarities, this distinguishes these epidemics of dancing mania (and the preventive practices such as the ones depicted by Bruegel) from the Italian *tarantismo*. This involved those who believed they were bitten by a tarantula dancing for days on end to sweat out the venom; in the case of *tarantismo*, the dance was the cure for melancholic symptoms.

Whether in a ritual pilgrimage to prevent a recurrence of the mania, or whether affected by the dancing mania itself, the dance of choreomaniacs makes their mental distress surface and become visible, to the point where the epidemic nature of dancing itself rests in the visual field. Waller (2009, 114–15) reminds us that, during the 1518 epidemic, the regents of Strasburg realised dancing mania was highly contagious, and ordered not only the dancers themselves to be hidden from public view before and whilst being sent to the church of St. Vitus, but also that no dance was to be performed until the epidemic was over.

Dancing fools in jester's attire also appear in two distinct corpora of images, unrelated to the feast of fools. First, it is worth mentioning that jesters are recurrent characters in *danse macabre* scenes, as part of *memento mori* warnings: death also catches up with those who ignore it and foolishly dedicate their lives to lust and material pleasures. Such is the case for instance in a late Swiss copy of the *Danse macabre de Bâle* by Johann Rudolf Feyerabend (1806) (Antoine-König 2024) (Fig. 20). Additionally, between 1560 and 1570, Frans Hogenberg produced a diptych whose prints are entitled *Stultorum Chorea* (Fig. 21) and *Stultarum Chorea*. They, respectively, depict male and female forms of foolishness (not mental disorder) and are comparable with each other, in that in both the fools dance in circles within a walled square, and are overlooked from arched windows by two people of the relevant gender, who exemplify a wise demeanour (they are old, with long beards and are well dressed). Hogenberg's dances are a mix of tropes: the dancers are dressed in fool's/jester's attire, they dance in a circle

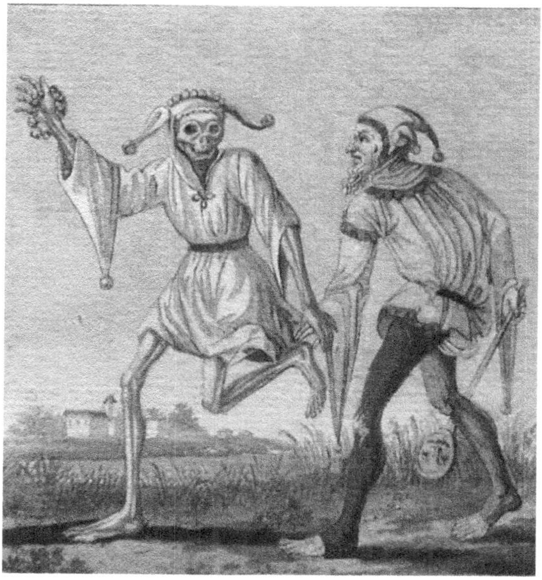

Figure 20: Detail of *Danse Macabre* of Basel, watercolour copy by Johann Rudolf Feyerabend, 1806. Historisches Museum Basel. The (destroyed) original was a mural of Predigerkloster (Basel), first half of 15th century.

around a trumpet player and they do so in a square, all similar to feast of fools depictions. These are not feasts of fools though. Each of the dancers is captioned with a form of foolishness/sin: either they are the greedy and the lustful, the gluttons and prodigal sons and daughters, or the curious and the idle. So, these are worth mentioning in their connection with dance, but they are visualisations of mental disorders, and in both cases the iconography of the fool is used allegorically to depict foolishness and stupidity.

Dancing mania offers a compelling perspective for understanding the visualisation of mental disorders, regardless of its relatively scant manifestation in visual culture. Dance serves as a medium for lunacy to manifest, to emerge and to be externalised, and as such this perplexing manic phenomenon may be a sign of underlying psychological disorder. Although less prominent in visual culture than the image of the *insipiens*, the collective phenomenon of dancing mania, evidenced by several well-documented examples, might be interpreted as a collective unconscious reaction to psychological anguish. Such mania events vividly and dramatically symbolise the concealed 'chaos of crazy', externalising internal conflicts into a visible and public display. Similar to the images of the staff or the extraction of the stone in the brain, the representation of dancing mania illustrates the human desire to render the intangible facets of mental disorders tangible, albeit through metaphorical and symbolic motifs.

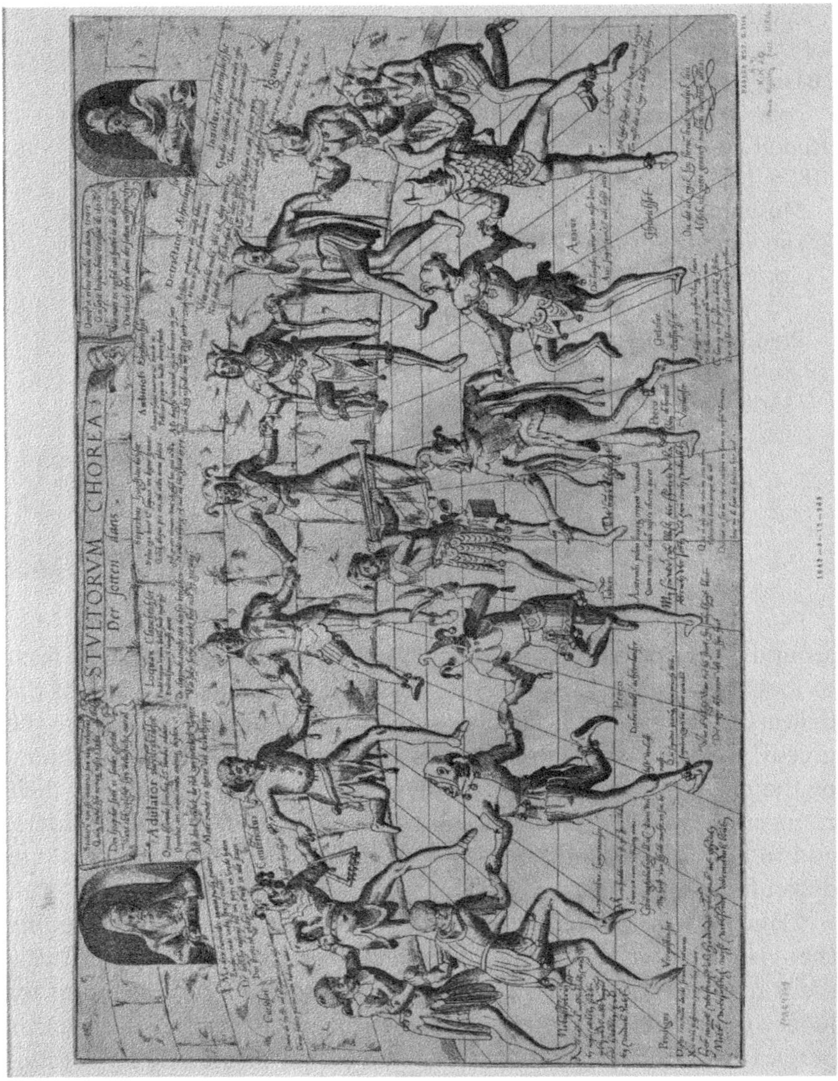

Figure 21: Frans Hogenberg. Stultorum Chorea. Engraving 1550–1600. © The Trustees of the British Museum.

Charcot's Hysterics

Dancing mania not only represents mental distress and disorder becoming visible, but also its *performativity*: to make madness visible, choreomaniacs perform it and make a spectacle out of it. While digressing into the theatricality of manifestations of madness would take us away from the topic of this monograph, it is important to note, as eloquently surmised by Waller (2008, 155) that dancing mania epidemics 'highlight the remarkable fact that even when we lose control, we often do so in culturally prescribed ways'. This does not mean that the manifestations of mental disorder and distress are 'just' psychological; on the contrary, it means that very real and very impactful disorders and pains often surface into visibility through channels that are defined by the dominant surrounding culture. To this extent, dancing epidemics present us with more than just a hint of what is currently called 'conversion disorder' (also known as 'psychosomatic disorder', 'hypochondria', but also 'hysteria'): a series of potential physical symptoms (including paralysis, deafness, blindness or fits) that have no organic cause and no established neurological pathway, but seem to be triggered by psychological states or external stressors. Hysteria in particular has been at the centre of the visualisation of mental disorders as performance.

Neurologist and mentor of Freud, Jean-Martin Charcot is best remembered for his descriptions of ALS (amyotrophic lateral sclerosis or Charcot's disease) and MS (multiple sclerosis). One of his most remarkable publications, however, is one that, despite being well intentioned, had little scientific basis: the *Iconographie Photographique de la Salpêtrière*, a major collection of photographic 'evidence' detailing the stages, gestures and poses of the hysteric attack. While ever present in history, hysteria was a disorder regarded with suspicion by medical doctors, 'the wastebin of medicine where one throws otherwise unemployed symptoms' (Lasègue quoted in Goldstein 2001, 324). On the contrary, Charcot believed that 'hysteria was a genuinely organic disorder, a disease rooted firmly in the higher nervous system, and in these respects part of the broader spectrum of neurological disorders' (Scull 2011, 108). According to him, hysteria, along with choreas and epilepsy, are 'morbid states, evidently having their seat in the nervous system, which leave in the dead body no material trace' (Charcot 1889, 14). While they left no lesions on the brain, they 'displayed the next best thing: physical stigmata revelatory of the underlying inherited physical inferiority that gave birth to their symptoms' (Scull 2011, 110). Charcot's *Iconographie* was a work of visual documentation of these

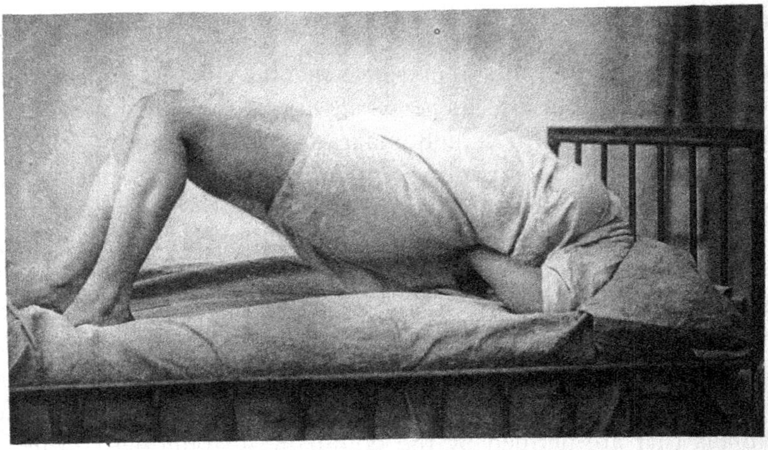

Planche III.

ATTAQUE HYSTÉRO-ÉPILEPTIQUE

ARC DE CERCLE

Figure 22: Page from Charcot's Iconographie (Volume III, Plate III). 1878. Courtesy of Wellcome Trust.

transient physical stigmata. According to him, a complete hysteric attack presents in four stages 'with mechanical regularity': '1st epileptoid; 2nd great movements (struggling, purposeless); 3rd, passionate attitudes (purposive); 4th terminal delirium' (Charcot 1889, 13) (Fig. 22). During the first period, the patient suffered fits and seizures similar to *grand-mal* epileptic episodes, including typical postures such as the locking of the arms in the tetanic position. In the second period, patients performed dramatic gestures, often shouting and crying and ending in the typical position of the *arc-de-cercle* or opisthotonus, something also used in the iconography of possession. Charcot also referred to this as the period of clownism. He considered the third phase typical of female hysteric patients: it consisted of erotic poses, feigning orgasms, or religious attitudes including mimicking crucifixion. Finally, the physical expressions would give way to hallucinations and delirium in the fourth phase. While he conceded that simulation was certainly possible, he also devised numerous methods of measurement to discern the phases of real hysteric episodes from simulations, such as the oscillations of outstretched arms, and 'a hundred other examples' (Charcot 1889, 18).

According to Didi-Huberman, with the *Iconographie*, Charcot addresses 'the *figurative problem* that obsessed every medical clinic, the problem of the link—the phantasmatic link—between seeing and knowing, seeing and suffering' (Didi-Huberman 2004, 8, emphasis in original) since 'one truly cannot get under the skin of a nervous patient to see how the illness works' (Didi-Huberman 2004, 20). Charcot created a symptomatology of an invented disorder, choreographing it and fixating it on photographic paper. So it is appropriate that his contribution is called an 'iconography', since this is his creation: the iconography of what he considered to be a mental disorder. Most importantly, however, what he invented was

> an ethics of seeing. This is called, in the first place, the glance [*coup d'oeil*], which also implicates the 'fine sensibility' with which the clinical gaze identifies. It is an 'exercise of the senses'—an exercise, the acting-out of seeing: glance, diagnosis, cure, prognosis. The clinical glance is already *contact*, simultaneously ideal and percussive. It is a stroke [*trait*] that goes directly to the body of the patient, almost palpating it. Charcot went 'further' in percussion in a straight line, in ideal contact and the instantaneity of the stroke [*trait*]; he armed his gaze for a more subtle, less tactile percussion, for he was disputing with neurosis, an intimate, specific intertwining of ground and surface. And he armed himself with photography. (Didi-Huberman 2004, 8)

While Charcot did consider male hysterics (Micale 1990), the iconography portrays exclusively women, in particular one: Augustine. Charcot's iconography is a prime example of a visual othering not only because it is a visual othering of a mental disorder. It is so also because it deploys in its fullness a male gaze, redoubling the otherness of the subject portrayed. It thus confirms once again how in iconography the process of othering enables the blurring of different categories of those who deviate from the norm or are just different from the normative gaze: the insane, the vagrant, the witch and, in this case, women tout court.

Through photography, Charcot brought to life what Paracelsus called *chorea lasciva*: the dance of lechery. Mental disorder is not only made visible in the bodies of patients, it is spectacularised and performed. The visible manifestations are borrowed from other iconographic repositories (such as demonic possession) or other (real) disorders (such as epilepsy or tetanic paralysis), creating a catalogue of visual expressions of suffering, and its storyboard. Despite its 'extreme visibility', however, hysteria 'retained a secret in its possession, an invisibility and a changeability, the freedom of absolutely untreatable manifestations: an irreducible unpredictability' (Didi-Huberman 2004, 74). Rather than manifesting itself in full visibility, dramatic and patent as its manifestations were, hysteria still brought to visible representation its own invisibility, much like the staff of madness and its attachments visibly representing the invisibility of insanity. As Harpin and Foster (2014, 4) put it, the 'history of madness is intertwined with performance', which creates a 'bonding of madness and sensational visual imagery', of which we are exploring both still and performative iterations. Like other visible props of mental disorder, performance too 'sustains a diagnostic gaze towards individuals and offers up superficial surface behaviours as decipherable clues to inner enigmas' (Harpin and Foster 2014, 4).

In relation to madness and mental disorders, there is a fine line between convulsions and dance; both are aspects of a certain performativity and theatricality of the disorder itself. Both convulsions and dance had a dual valence as possible symptoms of the disorder and its cure. As we have seen earlier, even the episodes of dancing mania displayed this ambiguity, with pipers accompanying those who suffered from St. Vitus' disease. This was either a therapeutic dance to cure dancing mania or to prevent it—*similia similibus curentur* (like cures like)—one of the two principles of Galenic medicine. In a similar vein, Paracelsus recommended administering camphor by mouth to those suffering from mania, so as to cause convulsions and thus treat the manic state. To add to the complexity, dance and convulsions can also incarnate the opposite principle of Galenic medicine: *contraria contrariis curentur* (opposite cures opposite). The frenetic *tarantella* dance, for instance, was initiated so that the dancers could sweat out the poison of the tarantula, whose symptoms were similar to melancholia. During the 1800s, mental institutions frequently used dance to foster patients' abilities to cultivate self-discipline, self-esteem, endurance and productivity (Showalter 1980, 166–68). Dance was thus regarded as a highly regulated form of movement that could, by virtue of the *contraria contrariis curentur* principle, bridle the irrationality of the insane.

Even the still-used electroconvulsive therapy (ECT) is rooted in similar considerations. While Paracelsus applied an *ante litteram* convulsive therapy to treat mania, with others following in his footsteps, the first 'modern' use of convulsive therapy, the grandfather of contemporary ECT, was practised by Ladislas Meduna in 1934. Meduna treated patients with catatonic stupor with injections of camphor oil at first, and then pentylenetetrazol (Metrazol or Cardiazol) to induce convulsions. His use of convulsive therapy was exclusively based on his (mistaken) belief that schizophrenia and epilepsy are antagonistic disorders, thus inducing the latter would cure the former.

In this section, the visual has expanded into considerations of performativity and spectacularisation, which I had already touched on when discussing possession. I have explored one of the ways in which madness manifests itself in the public sphere, whether through the choreographed movements of groups afflicted by dancing mania or the pseudo-documented stages of hysterical attacks staged and captured by Jean-Martin Charcot. I have also, and perhaps most importantly, unravelled the dual valence of convulsions and dance as both symptoms of mental disorder and potential cures. From therapeutic dances to the modern practice of electroconvulsive therapy, these interventions show madness being treated both with similar and opposite actions, echoing the principles of Galenic medicine.

My Name is Legion: For We Are Many—The Multitude of the Insane

'My name is legion: for we are many' says the Gerasene demon(s) before Jesus exorcises them from a man into a drove of pigs (Mark 5:9). The dancing maniacs, much like the Gerasene demon(s), are many, and contort their bodies in an uncontrolled and lascivious way. The visualisation of madness as externalisation, by means of dancing or convulsive movements, brings us to another recurrent trope that often shares several characteristics with representations of *chorea lasciva*: the multitude of the insane, its potential overflow and the contamination of the 'sane' world, the necessity to contain and marginalise it, but also the permeability of any membrane that is placed between the 'sane' and the 'insane'.

The Multitude of the Insane

According to an Italian proverb, 'La madre degli imbecilli/idioti/cretini è sempre incinta' (The mother of fools is always pregnant). The notion that the world is crowded with fools, in addition to everyday experience, seems to date back to an incorrect translation of Ecclesiastes 1:15: 'numerus stultorum infinitus est' (the number of fools is infinite), which is more accurately rendered in the New International Version of the Bible as 'what is crooked cannot be straightened; what is lacking cannot be counted'. As discussed in the previous chapters, we could certainly try to narrow down the notion of fool and foolishness, for instance to what we might today consider foolish behaviour, thus regarding this iconographic trope as relating to stupidity rather than mental disorder and madness. This would not, however, do justice to the complexity of the iconography I am looking at here, which in turn shows us that we should not extend contemporary definitions to a historical study of madness. The visual trope of the fool was often employed as a catch-all symbol for fools, court jesters, madmen and wild men alike.

In this context, an illustration of Thomas Murner's *Schelmenzunft* (1513) depicts a fool planting (or harvesting) fools in a field, while Wolfgang Strauch (active 1554–72) illustrates Hans Sach's *Narrenbad* (*Bath of Fools*) verses as a pool overflowing with fools. In his drawing 'The Tree of Fools', Hans Weiditz depicts a well-dressed noble woman shaking a tree, from which, like overripe fruits, fools fall in great numbers. In an anonymous Flemish print of *c.*1570 we can see a 'family of fools' where fools are hatched from a basket, perhaps by the very mother of fools of the Italian saying. We also see the hatching of fools in an anonymous painting of the same decade, the *Chicken Hatching Fools*, whereas in Theódor de Bry's *Quale granum talis est farina* print of 1580 fools, like grain, are milled in great quantities to produce fool's flour. In all of these images, fools are recognisable by their characteristic jester attire (in particular the ass's ears and the hat with bells), even though it is evident that in this case they are not court fools but *insipientes*, of which the world is full. Bruegel's *Witches of Malleghem* (Fig. 14) situates the multitude of the insane in an ambiguous position, as it declaredly depicts those suffering from 'wasps' or 'stones' in the head flocking to a 'witch' to excise insanity from their heads (see chapter two). So in Bruegel's illustration the world is indeed full of fools, but at least they do want to be 'healed' from foolishness as they flock to a 'witch' to cure them.

Derived from one of Bruegel's sketches, Pieter van der Heyden's 'Festival of Fools' print (after 1570) (Fig. 23) depicts a multitude of fools adorned in typical jester attire, many wielding marottes and some carrying featureless orbs, possibly symbolising the stones of madness (or the bread of the *insipiens*), either to be eradicated or introduced into the town. The scene unfolds with a multitude of fools spilling into the town square from the doors of the buildings around it. They engage in music, dance and revelry, ensnaring the townsmen in their antics. Bruegel's drawing and van der Heyden's print illustrate the tradition of the feast of fools, known by various names such as *asinaria festa, libertates decembris, festum stultorum, festum fatuorum, fete*

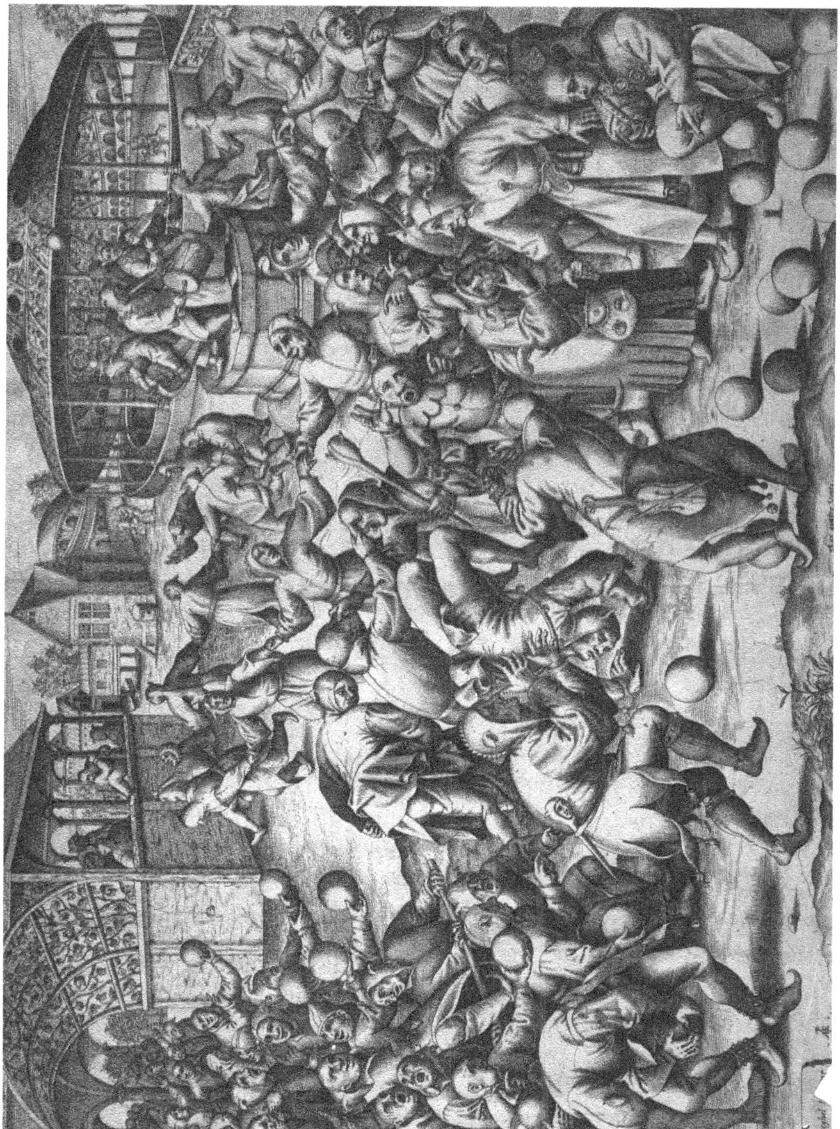

Figure 23: Pieter van der Heyden. Feast of Fools, after Pieter Bruegel the Elder. Engraving after 1570. Courtesy of MET Museum (New York).

des fous and *festum baculi*. Note that the last one means the feast of the staff; the king of fools was given a staff of madness as a sceptre. This subversive event, generally observed between Christmas and Epiphany, satirised Christian rituals through carnivalesque activities, including the election of mock abbots, priests or kings—sometimes even an ass—leading the irreverent festivities. Originating around the late twelfth century, likely as an homage to the biblical verse 'God chose what is foolish in the world to shame the wise' (1 Cor. 1:27), the feast of fools initially appeared in France *c.*1160. Despite early disapproval from the Church, official condemnation only came from the Ecumenical Council of Basel in 1435, signalling the demise of the tradition. It was eventually conflated with the still-continuing festivities of Carnival and April Fool's Day. Contrary to popular belief and scholarly assertions, the feasts of fools may not have been as pervasive as we think: many of the descriptions of it were likely exaggerated by Church officials to underscore its disruptive nature to ensure its condemnation. Indeed, the feast of fools often coincided with festivals for subdeacons or the Feast of the Innocents and, until its outlawing, it was often supported by the local chapter (Harris 2014). Bruegel's depiction therefore, created over a century after the censure at Basel, was produced without any firsthand knowledge of such celebrations, and instead likely draws from embellished accounts propagated by Church ministers keen on emphasising the festivity's problematic nature. Thus, the feast of fools is depicted as an invasive motif: fools overtake city squares, crown their king, infiltrate churches and infect the populace with their revelry-induced madness.

Such a multitude of madmen, threatening the social order and its norms with a potential invasion, is, perhaps unsurprisingly, also depicted in reference to means of containment and marginalisation. The *Narrenschiff*, discussed above, could, for instance, be regarded as one of the possible ways the 'multitude of the insane' was represented as being contained—on a ship—and marginalised, to the extent that the ship is set adrift in the sea. The relationship between Dürer's engraving and the text by Sebastian Brant it illustrates of course complicates this visual metaphor (see chapter one).

In a more literal sense, madness is also depicted as being contained within cages, as is the case in Erhard Schön's woodcut *Narrenkäfig* (1530) (cage of fools). At the centre of the woodcut a large cage stands out. In it there are several fools locked up, and three well-dressed women stand outside of the cage. The one on the left tells the fools that since they burn with love/lust they have to sing while they, the women, whistle and dance. The woman in the middle asks the woman on the right to let them out, since they are listening to gentle music and they already know how to sing. The third woman obliges and opens the door to the cage, urging the fools to get out and telling them 'we need to have our satchels full'. At the top left a fool is carried in a cart and at the top right three men in plain clothes discuss: 'the heat is over, the money is gone, we are now dressed'. Reading the image left to right it seems to be the narrative arc of the insane, in particular those driven insane by lust. They are carried into the cage where they are tamed with gentle music, and from which they can get out only when they have shed their foolish attire, but their money is gone, possibly spent in lascivious entertainment or given to the women to 'fill their satchel', perhaps to pay them for their services in 'curing' their lust.

The cage of fools has a twofold meaning that gives rise to two different, albeit related, tropes of the representation of madness. The first is a representational strand, where the cage is a real tool used to contain the insane, either individually or as a group, and represents all the related methods of constraint used in 'treating' the insane. The second is a metaphorical one, where the cage is the *locus* of madness in its many possible meanings, for example the cage is the place to contain the insane and from which the insane can overflow; the world is a cage of fools, and madness is that which cages the insane individual's head/rationality.

Real Cages and Asylums

A diverse array of implements, including literal cages, have historically been employed, and regrettably are still utilised in some cases today, to confine individuals afflicted with mental disorders. As early as the initial version of *Orlando Furioso* (1516), Ludovico Ariosto, in cautioning readers against the perils of love, equates those consumed by passion to the insane, who warrant being fettered: 'a chi in amor s'invecchia, oltr'ogni pena // si convengono i ceppi e la catena' (XXIV.2). This does not suggest that chaining the lovesick was considered the norm, but rather that it was a readily acceptable fate for the mad. The Italian language preserves this notion in the commonly used expression 'matto da legare' (so mad he needs to be tied up). In the early seventeenth century, Cervantes also portrays cages for the insane in the madhouse of Seville in the first chapter of the second book of Don Quixote, a section of the novel that is a cautionary tale by a barber who doubts Don Quixote's recovery from his madness (II.2, para. 19). Isolation cages and cage beds were commonly seen fixtures in psychiatric institutions throughout the nineteenth and twentieth

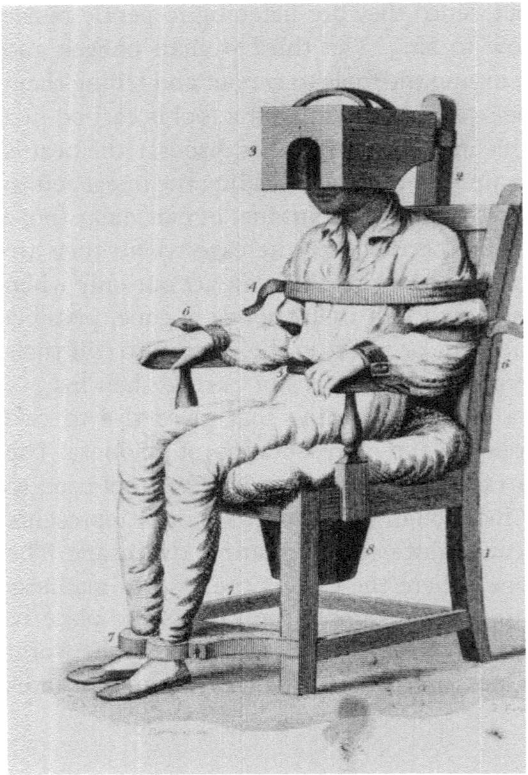

Figure 24: Benjamin Rush. Tranquillizer chair. Engraving ca 1800. Courtesy of National Library of Medicine.

centuries. Some countries, such as Czechia, only banned them in 2020. Moreover, an assortment of handcuffs, manacles and wrist restraints were commonly employed alongside the cages. Benjamin Rush (1979, 179), one of the founding fathers of the United States of America, perfected the 'composing chair' into what he termed the 'tranquillizer': a commode on which inpatients were strapped, often for entire days, which also had a helmet to muffle sound and to cover the eyes to reduce any source of stimulation (Fig. 24). Of course, readers will also be familiar with the straitjacket of Quaker invention, still used today (Colaizzi 2005), and all of these methods of restraint famously and prominently emerge in visual culture: from Rush's own illustration of the 'tranquillizer', all the way to the numerous films that depict the contemporary use of the straitjacket, most notably Forman's 1975 cinematic adaptation of Kesey's abovementioned *One Flew Over the Cuckoo's Nest*. What is most important, however, is not that such means of restraint were visually depicted (of course they were), but that these means of constraint themselves were a visual remedy to a

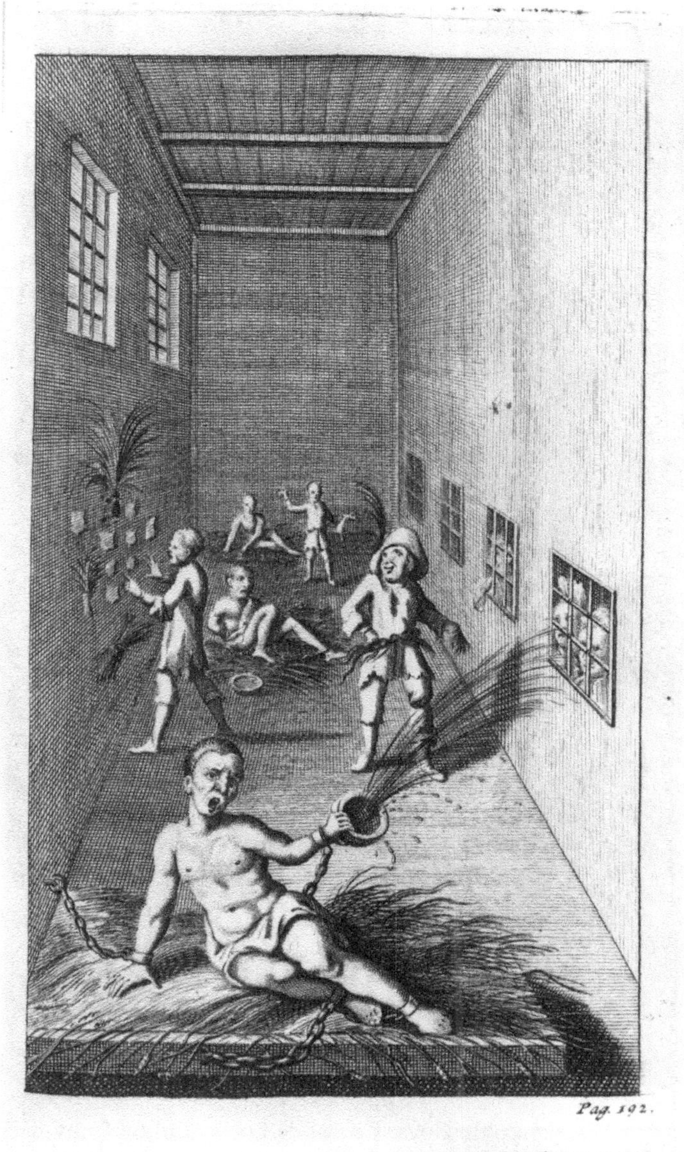

Figure 25: Bernard Lens, Illustration of Bedlam from 'A Tale of a Tub' by Jonathan Swift. Engraving 1710. Division of Rare and Manuscript Collections, Cornell University Library.

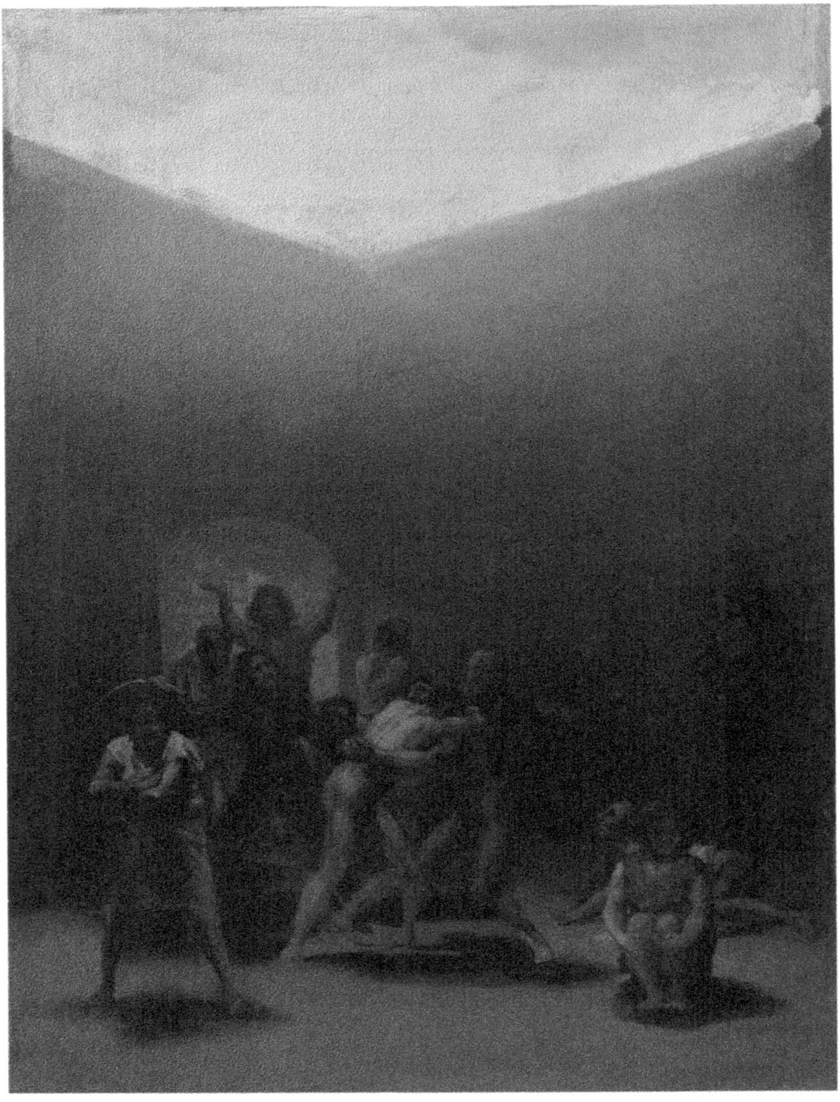

Figure 26: Francisco de Goya. Corral de Locos. Oil on Canvas 1794.
Photo by Robert LaPrelle. Courtesy of Meadows Museum, SMU, Dallas.

visual issue. Madness surfaced into visibility by means of uncontrolled, disorganised, violent, badly behaved gestures—sometimes resembling seizures and convulsions—a visual expression that troubled decency, composure and reason. The response was to limit and restrict such gestures, shrinking the space within which the insane could express their madness through movement. Some, like Rush's tranquilliser, went as far as limiting the movements of the insane while at the same time preventing them from seeing.

Just as the individual madman is contained by straps and handcuffs in real life and in visual culture, so the multitude of the insane is contained within the walls of the lunatic asylum. Bernard Lens and John Strut's print in the fifth edition of Jonathan Swift's *A Tale of a Tub* (1710) is a classic and very telling example (Fig. 25). It represents Bedlam—London's Bethlem Hospital—to illustrate Section IX of the book, entitled 'A Digression Concerning the Original, the Use, and Improvement of Madness in the Commonwealth'. In this passage, Swift puts forward a satirical solution to address the issue of madness in society by appointing commissioners to inspect institutions like Bedlam, and identify individuals whose talents could be used in various professions. He then describes the differing types of madness shown by the individuals in these institutions, and suggests that with proper guidance and employment, they could make a significant contribution to society. In Lens and Strut's print, the insane are all locked up in a long, narrow room, the walls of which are disproportionately tall. The madman in the foreground is chained and throws the contents of his chamber pot onto the onlookers. These could have been the inspectors Swift proposed to create or general visitors, who could, famously, pay a shilling to watch the insane as if they were animals in a zoo. I will return to this print in chapter eight as it also contains one of the first depictions of the insane producing art.

When picturing the containment of the insane, the idea of the asylum is possibly the most familiar. The asylum becomes the space in which to place those who must be removed from the social body, much like the way the stone is extracted from the individual body. The insane are thus made invisible and marginalised in the asylum, where the unruly mass is depicted in relation to insurmountable walls, as we see in the engraving of Bedlam by Lens and Strut described above. We also see this in Goya's 1794 painting *Corral de locos*, which depicts, in deep chiaroscuro tones, a group of the insane in the courtyard of Saragoza's asylum (Fig. 26). As Gilman (2014, 129) notes, each individual represents a different kind of madness, from mania to melancholia, and the figures are all placed in the bottom third of the

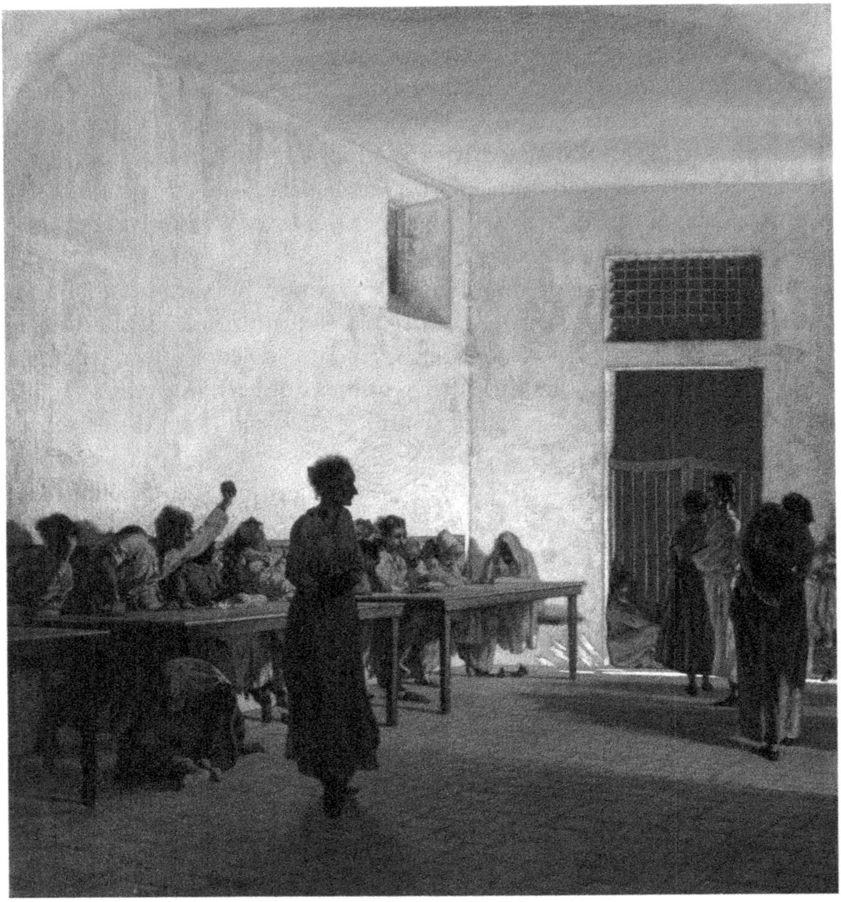

Figure 27: Telemaco Signorini. La sala delle agitate al Bonifacio di Firenze. Oil on Canvas 1865. © Archivio Fotografico – Fondazione Musei Civici di Venezia.

canvas, in the shade. The middle third of the canvas is filled by the featureless wall that separates the insane from the light (either the sky or a very bright ceiling). Similarly, in the 1810 painting *Casa de locos,* half of the frame is filled by the wall and the barred window, with the group of the insane relegated to the darkest bottom of the canvas. Even without a chiaroscuro effect, the orderly and imposing walls of the asylum tower over the belittled group of inpatients in Thomas Rowlandson's print of St. Luke's hospital from 1809. The bright walls here feature a repetitive and orderly geometry that seems to symbolise the dominance of reason over the small figures of the raging mad, who appear in the bottom third of the composition.

In 1865, when Telemaco Signorini paints the agitated female inpatients room of the San Bonifazio hospital in Florence, the majority of the canvas continues to be occupied by a bright featureless wall, containing, rather than towering over, the patients in this instance (Fig. 27). The protagonist of these paintings is neither the group of the insane nor madness, it is the walls and structures that contain it, the asylum itself in its function of segregating the insane and separating them from the sane. While the illustration of Swift's *A Tale of a Tub* suggests a minimal communication between the exterior and the interior, with a few onlookers on the outside, no such idea is featured in other depictions of the asylum. The separation between the sane and the insane is a physical and mechanical one as much as it is a visual one: the population of the insane is removed from the view of the sane, to hide the 'unsettling picture [...] of a violent insanity apparently on the increase generally as a threat to public welfare' (Kromm 2002, 147) and to avoid offence to public decorum.

Metaphorical Cages, the World as a Cage of Fools, Permeability

Despite their height, their grates and their lack of features, the walls of the asylum are not insurmountable and, at least in visual culture, they cannot keep madness at bay. In the eighth plate of *A Rake's Progress* (1763), Hogarth portrays Rake finally being admitted to Bedlam. In the corridor and among the usual catalogue of different types of madness, slightly in the shade but still quite visible drawn on the wall, is the personification of the British Empire, Britannia: Bedlam not only houses the mad, it houses the whole world (Fig. 53). Similarly, Peter Dutsman's 1781 print portrays the melancholic George III signing the declaration of war against Holland, spurred on by his raging mad ministers. The print is entitled *Bedlam of the World*: the world itself is a lunatic asylum. The walls of the asylum and other means of containment of madness are thus metaphors of permeable membranes. The world itself is an asylum, much like the world itself is a 'cage of fools', 'una gabbia di matti', as the saying goes in Italian.

The first appearance in Italian iconography of the 'gabbia di matti' comes a little after the *Cage of Fools* print discussed above. It is a popular print by Sebastiano di Re, dated between 1557 and 1563 (Fig. 28). The print uses the trope of the cage of fools as an expedient to catalogue all the mad behaviours and stances that human beings display, hence it is not *only* an inventory of mental disorders.

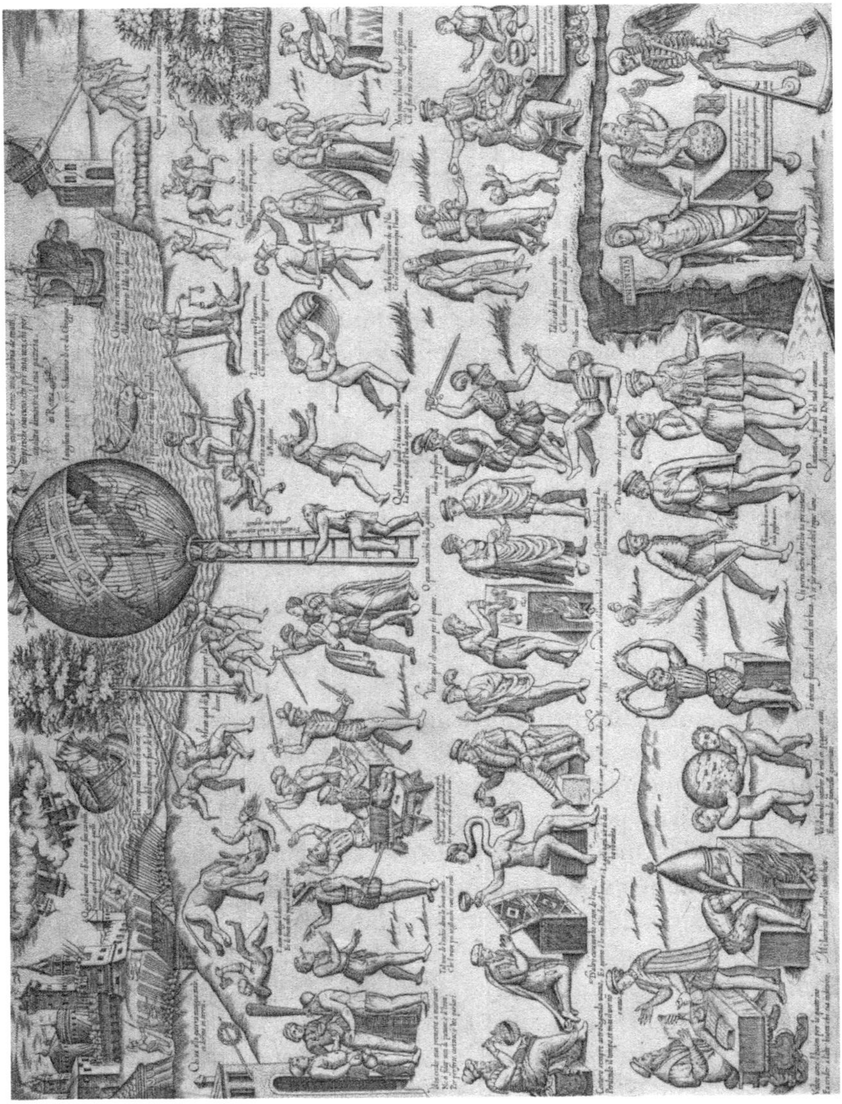

Figure 28: Sebastiano di Re. La gabbia de' matti. Engraving 1557–1563. Courtesy of MET Museum (New York).

The spherical cage features at the top centre of the print, filled with fools dancing, but from the bottom of the spherical cage a ladder allows the mad to climb in and out. 'O quanti sciocchi nella gabbia vanno' (Oh! How many fools go into the cage) reads the caption at the bottom of the ladder. The rest of the print is a series of scenes that depict either daily and mundane forms of foolishness—such as scenes of force prevailing over reason (*La Forza vince et caca adosso la Ragione*) or people being idle (*Io niente faccio, et il cervel mi becco*)—or proverbs and common sense, such as not to trust the ill doctor nor those who brag (*Non ti curar per medico ammalato, ne creder troppo à chi da se si vanta*). No person in the print, not even the fools in the spherical cage, seem to be wearing any traditional uniform of the fool, save for the personification of 'ignorance' in the vignette that illustrates 'La giustizia sta sopra l'Ignoranza, Che sempre hebbe di lei maggior posanza' (Justice sits above Ignorance, since it is heavier), in which ignorance is naked with ass's ears. Bottom right the catalogue of daily follies and words of wisdom concludes with a *memento mori*: 'Studisi ogniun far ben mentre che puote, Che'l Tempo da à la Morte il bollettino, Et ella con sua falce ognihuom percuote' (Everyone should strive to do good, because time keeps Death up to date and she hits everyone with her scythe). Like with the *Narrenschiff*, and even with the walls of the asylum at times, the cage of fools serves in this case as a container for the catalogue of forms of madness.

The expression 'gabbia di matti' is also picked up by Tommaso Campanella in the second madrigal of the third song to the *Primo intelletto* (Campanella 2011, 89–92):

> A stupendous thing Eternal Intellect has wrought,
> that every being, though vile, does not want to trade places
> with others; so it guards itself
> against death, which would change it;
> but it would like to be and believes it is blessed
> only in itself because it is ignorant of the good of others.
> Oh highest Wisdom,
> Who takes advantage of our ignorance
> to make each happy and glad,
> and to advance the universe.
> The world is a cage of fools; and if it ever
> were without madness, everyone
> would kill himself to become greater.

Campanella explains these verses in the following way. Each being

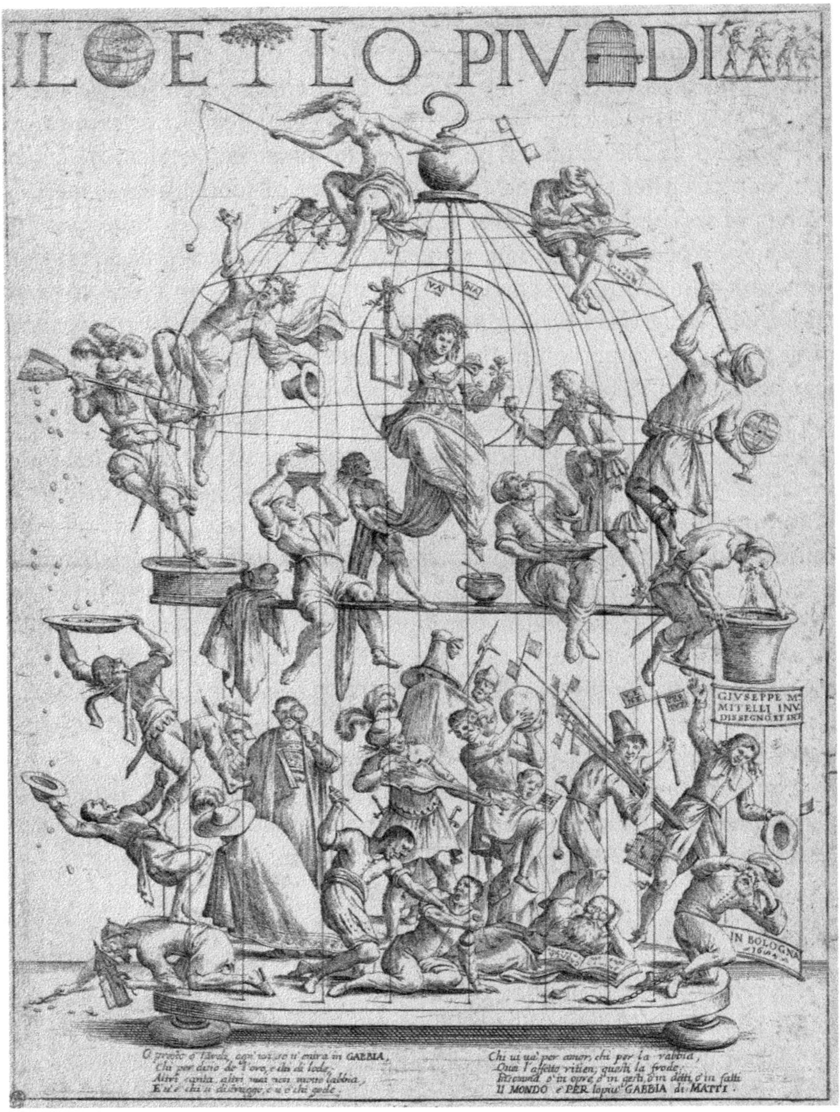
IL
E
LO PIV
DI
VA
NI
GIVSEPPE M.
MITELLI INV.
IN BOLOGNA
Chi ui uà per amor, chi per la rabbia,
Quei l'affetto ritien, questi la frode;
Il MONDO è PER lo più GABBIA di MATTI.

Figure 29: Giuseppe Maria Mitelli, Gabbia di Matti, Engraving 1684.
 – Raccolta delle Stampe "Achille Bertarelli", Castello Sforzesco, Milano.

has an innate sense of self-awareness and takes pleasure in their own existence, which is a participation in divine matters, thus it never wants to die and only seeks enjoyment in its own being. Therefore, it is evident that God, to ensure our happiness, uses our ignorance for as long as they see fit to preserve each entity. Thus, the world can be seen as a madhouse; if it were not, everyone would strive for improvement to the point of self-destruction. At the same time, however, being all mad, we still believe ourselves to be gods. Madness therefore preserves human beings in a state of blissful ignorance, making them content with being what they are, caging them within the confines of what they are supposed to be. Even so, we think ourselves as gods.

An excellent depiction of the cage of fools comes from Giuseppe Maria Mitelli in his popular 1684 print entitled 'Il Mondo è per lo più gabbia di matti' (Fig. 29). The title towers over the top of the page. It is not spelled out but rather is laid out in the form of a rebus. 'World' is represented by the globe; 'per' in 'per lo più' (by and large) is rendered as a pear tree (*pero*, poetically truncated into *per*); 'cage' is represented by the drawing of a bird cage; and 'matti', which translates as the insane rather than 'fools', is represented by a group of fools in classic jester attire, handling pinwheels (see chapter one) instead of marottes/staffs. The bottom of the print reads:

> Ò presto ò tardi, ogn'un se n'entra in GABBIA,
> Chi per disio de l'oro, e chi di lode;
> Altri canta, altri mai non move labbia,
> È v'è chi si distrugge, e v'è chi gode;
> Chi vi và per amor, chi per la rabbia,
> Quei l'affetto vi tien, questi la frode.
> Insomma ò in opre ò in gesti ò in detti ò in fatti
> Il MONDO è PER lo più GABBIA di MATTI.

[Sooner or later everyone enters the cage. Some for gold lust, some for lust of praise; Some others sing, some don't move their lips, and there are those who destroy and those who enjoy; some go in it for love, others for rage, some stay in it for affection, others for fraud. All in all, either in deeds, gestures, words or facts, the world is by and large a cage of fools.]

The cage is populated with drunkards and gold diggers, musicians and fortune tellers, prostitutes and artists, to name but a few. At the bottom right of the cage a street seller carries numerous pinwheels on his shoulder. In his left hand he carries a pinwheel, which is also the

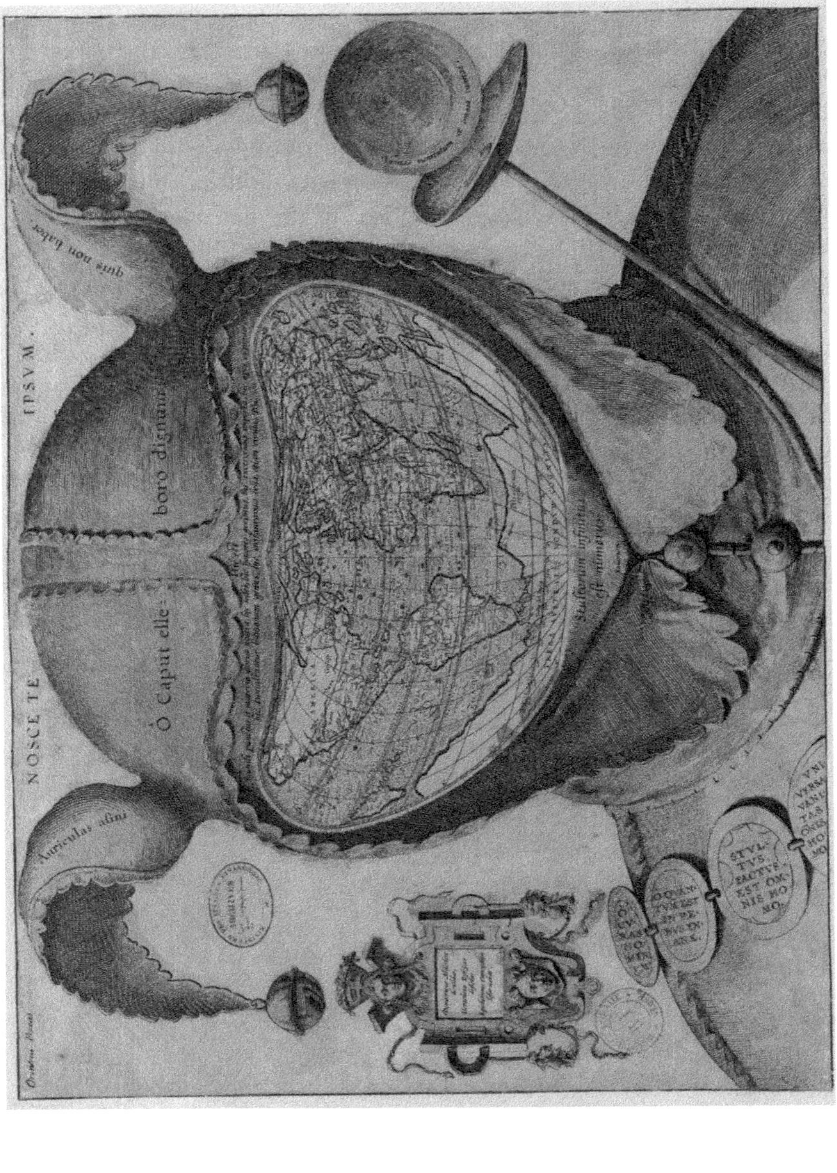

Figure 30: Epichtonius Cosmopolites (Pseudonym of Jean de Gourmont). O caput Elleboro Dignum. Engraving ca 1580. Courtesy of BNF– *Bibliothèque nationale de France*, ID/Cote :GE DD-2987 (64 RES).

sign to his business, that reads 've n'è per tuti' (there's enough for all), suggesting that everyone is welcome in the cage; everyone is welcome to their own folly.

Conclusions

In this chapter, I have explored how the visualisation of madness troubles borders and, *mutatis mutandis*, how madness troubles visual borders. This exploration reveals the permeability of the membrane that is created/visualised to contain madness and the mad. Across centuries, the iconographic trope of the insane troubling borders has blurred the lines between folly, mental disorder and societal norms. The feast of fools captures not only a tradition of subversion but also a certain fluidity of social norms and the porous nature of boundaries. Alongside the invasive celebration of folly, a need for containment and marginalisation emerges in the visual. This is a literal containment (cages, straitjackets and lunatic asylums) as much as it is a metaphorical one: madness needs to be contained, restrained and concealed. However, even the confines of cages and walls seem to represent, at least metaphorically, permeable membranes, troubled borders between sanity and insanity. Rather than a representation or metaphor of containment, the motif of the cage of fools is much more a reminder that it is the world itself that has gone mad. The world becomes a metaphorical asylum, where individuals are both captives and creators of their own folly, trapped within the paradox of their own existence. The watercoloured print after a drawing by Jean de Gourmont entitled *O Caput elleboro dignum* (dated *c.*1590) reproduces a map of the world inside the jester's cap, and seems to be the best image on which to conclude this chapter: the whole world is mad (Fig. 30). The plant hellebore was considered one of the possible remedies to mania, and *Nosce te ipsum* (know yourself) is the first sentence that we encounter at the top of this watercoloured print: know yourself, world, you are worthy of hellebore!

CHAPTER FOUR

Looking Madness in the Face: Physiognomics

IN THIS CHAPTER, I move more clearly in focus the body of the insane, and the (pseudo)science that developed to study it: physiognomics. This marks a milestone in terms of the relationship between medicine and visual representation. As Fraser (1998, 140) put it, in fact, 'the move from artistic representation of madness to the science of physiognomy employed in the service of medical illustration constitutes a significant shift in both established modes of perception as well as in the motivation behind the production of such images'. In this chapter, I therefore start with a historical overview of physiognomics, with the aim of studying how it has shaped our visual understanding (or lack thereof) of mental disorders. I thus study the portraitures of those suffering from a mental disorder, focusing on the pseudoscience of physiognomics, which I introduce as the study of facial appearance in relation to one's personality. I discuss in brief the history of physiognomics, and I draw on some case studies from notable psychiatric treatises that used such illustrations and descriptions, including Philippe Pinel's *Traité medico-philosophique sur l'aliénation mentale ou la manie* (1801), Jean-Etienne-Dominique Esquirol's *Des maladies mentales* (1838) and Alexander Morison's *The Physiognomy of Mental Diseases* (1840). I conclude this chapter with considerations that move beyond the study of the face of the insane, and will elaborate on the discussion started in chapter three by analysing how posture, beyond Charcot's portraiture of hysterics, became an indication of mental disorders. In the next part, as bodies in general become the domain of medicine, I will shift the focus to the evolution of the tools employed to capture medically meaningful images of the bodies of the insane: first photography and then brain and neuroimaging.

The Roots of Physiognomy

French and Italian, among other languages, distinguish between *physionomie/fisionomia* and *physiognomonie/fisiognomica* to distinguish between physical appearance (the former) and the, very loosely put, pseudoscience of the alleged association between the appearance of the body, especially of the head and the face, with behavioural and personality traits (the latter). English does not have this distinction and employs the term *physiognomy* for both. This section is about physiognomy understood as the pseudoscience of physical appearance, a pseudoscience that is 'by definition essentialist and deterministic, [in which] the body always serv[es] as an index to some fundamental, innate truth which orders and explains an individual' (Rivers 1994, 9).

The origins of physiognomy as a discipline date as far back as writing itself and cut across cultures, even though, as Rivers (1994, 18) has it, 'physiognomical practice is obscure and disjointed even in treatises on the subject [...]. Physiognomical skill, it is implied, is the fruit of some unspecified form of innate "genius"'. We can for instance retrieve associations of bodily appearance and divinatory significance in cuneiform clay tablets from the first Babylonian dynasty (Rivers 1994, 18), and Chinese face reading (*mianxiang*) is referred to in texts of the Zhou dynasty (Hinrichs and Barnes 2013, 374). The Sanskrit term 'Samudrika Shastra' refers to the 'knowledge of features of the body' and is an integral part of Indian astrology. The term itself, 'physiognomonia', appears for the first time in the fifth-century BCE Hippocratic treatise *Epidemics* (II.5.1), and the nascent foundations of a developed physiognomic theory begin to manifest in fifth-century BCE Athens, as glimpsed through the writings attributed to Zopyrus and recounted in dialogues attributed to Phaedo of Elis. In the fourth century BCE, Aristotle repeatedly alluded to theories and literary works exploring the nexus between external appearance and internal disposition.

The earliest systematic treatise on physiognomy is a short work titled *Physiognomonica* traditionally attributed to Aristotle but likely stemming simply from his philosophical tradition rather than directly authored by him. This treatise is comprised of two sections, believed to have initially circulated independently of each other. The first section examines arguments derived from observations of nature, discusses various non-Greek ethnicities and focuses on human behavioural patterns. The second section looks at animal behaviour, dividing the animal kingdom into distinct male and female prototypes, and drawing parallels between human physical morphology and character attributes. The main tenet of the text, which echoes later interpretations of physiognomy, was that animals held essential qualities (the fox is cunning, the lion is strong, for instance) which, because of their simple structure, was reflected in their appearance. Specific animal facial characteristics in humans would therefore indicate, by analogy, these essential qualities: a human with a beard and the hair of a lion is strong; one with tiny eyes and a pointy chin is cunning, like a fox, etc. This reveals 'a fundamental basis of physiognomical thought: the relation between the particular and the general' (Rivers 1994, 20). The logic that underpins the origins of physiognomy is that 'the grounding of particular judgements about a particular object (a human body) [is based] on observations about a group in which the particular object can (supposedly) be classified' (Rivers 1994, 20). The rhetoric of this argument is a syllogism: if a person looks like a lion and if the lion is strong, then it follows that the person is also strong. In addition to this 'zoological' method, pseudo-Aristotle proposes an ethnological method—according to which certain bodily and behavioural characteristics are specific to a race or a nationality—and a pathognomical one, which is more concerned with volatile expressions rather than permanent characteristics. Cicero and numerous other Roman authors, such as Tacitus, Suetonius and Seneca, referred at least in passing to physiognomy, which, also thanks to Arabic treatises, continued to be read in medieval Europe. In thirteenth- and fourteenth-century Europe, thanks to the work of Michael Scot, Petrus Hispanus, St. Albert the Great and Giovanni Buridano, physiognomy was located at the crossing of natural philosophy, moral philosophy, medicine and astrology (Agrimi 1997). Notable works of Renaissance physiognomy include Magnus Hundt's *Antropologium de hominis dignitate* (Hundt 1501), Cocles's *Physionomiae et chiromantiae compendium* (Cocles 1536) and Girolamo Cardano's *Metoposcopia* of 1558 (Cardano 2003), in which the physical traits of humans are associated with the essential qualities of the stars and constellations. In medieval and early modern times physiognomy sits astride medicine and divination.

In 1586, Giovan Battista Della Porta (Della Porta 1586) published the work *De humana physiognomonia* in four volumes, and would later (Della Porta 1599) expand it to six volumes on the occasion of the second edition. Della Porta's treatise of physiognomy was arguably one of the most influential, in that he abandoned astrological considerations and founded physiognomy entirely on Pseudo-Aristotle's zoomorphic approach. Della Porta's work marks the departure of physiognomy from divination, consolidating its position in the realm of medicine. 'Many divinatory sciences are vain, false and pretentious',

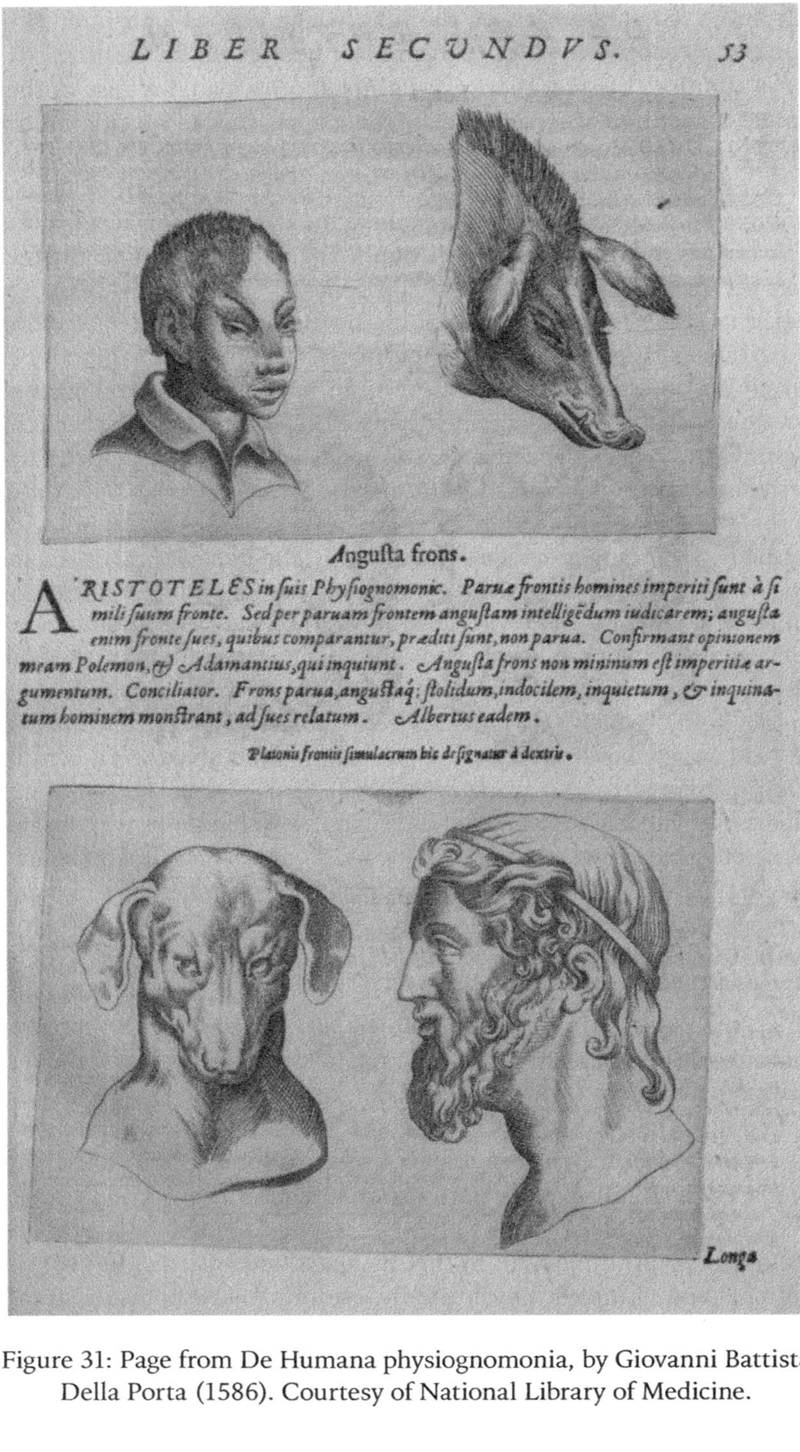

LIBER SECVNDVS. 53

Angusta frons.

ARISTOTELES in suis Physiognomonic. Paruæ frontis homines imperiti sunt à simili suum fronte. Sed per paruam frontem angustam intelligẽdum iudicarem; angusta enim fronte sues, quibus comparantur, præditi sunt, non parua. Confirmant opinionem meam Polemon, & Adamantius, qui inquiunt. Angusta frons non minimum est imperitiæ argumentum. Conciliator. Frons parua, angustaq; stolidum, indocilem, inquietum, & inquinatum hominem monstrant, ad sues relatum. Albertus eadem.

Platonis frontis simulacrum hic designatur à dextris.

Longa

Figure 31: Page from De Humana physiognomonia, by Giovanni Battista Della Porta (1586). Courtesy of National Library of Medicine.

Della Porta (1610, 1) writes, 'whereas grand is the excellence of physiognomics, borne out of natural principles' (Fig. 31).

Modern Physiognomy

In the seventeenth century, Descartes played a significant, but often overlooked, role in the development of physiognomy, despite not being commonly recognised as a physiognomist himself. Rivers (1994, 25) notes that Descartes' contribution to the discipline was both indirect and direct. Indirectly, in his *Discours de la méthode* (1637) (Descartes 1995), Descartes defined the principles of 'rationality' and 'method', creating an intellectual milieu which corresponded to the revival of physiognomical thought. The most direct impact of Descartes on physiognomy can be found in his last work, *Les Passions de l'âme* (1649), where he presented his thoughts about the relationship between the body and soul, in particular the 'passions' as both physiological and affective phenomena. Locating the centre of these passions in the pineal gland, Descartes thus absorbed physiognomy into the tradition of anatomical and physiological inquiry. While Descartes' physiological theories were influenced by contemporary ideas of circulation and also humoral medicine, it was his emphasis on the relationship between body and mind and body and soul that was central to physiognomists. Descartes highlighted the importance of movement and voluntary facial expressions, acknowledged the possibility of deception in physiognomical observation and, most importantly, recognised the body not as an unalterable object that can be read as a written text, but as an impermanent and changeable unit that has to be observed in its variability, like the spoken, rather than the written, word.

The founder and director of the *Académie royale de peinture et de sculpture* in Paris, Charles Le Brun (1619–90), expanded upon Descartes' concept of the legibility of passions, focusing on the visual representation of facial expressions. In emancipating it from divination, Descartes and Le Brun root physiognomy in the observation of the mechanical body as it changes over time, rather than in its immobile and immutable essence, and shift its epistemology onto causality rather than the analogy of the physiognomical syllogism. Thus, bodies are no longer meaningful in that they resemble something (e.g., an animal), but because their traits and movements are caused by their physiology (e.g., the humours) (Courtine and Haroche 2007).

Johan Kaspar Lavater (1741–1801) gained prominence for his contributions to physiognomy, particularly through his work *Physiognomische*

Fragmente, zur Beförderung der Menschenkenntniss und Menschenliebe, published from 1775 to 1778 (and translated into English in several different abridged versions, the most successful of which were Hunter's and Holcroft's). He revolutionised the field by proposing that physiognomy could discern specific character traits in individuals rather than merely categorising them into general types. Lavater argued that a person's character could be revealed by analysing their facial features, especially the lines and contours of the face. He thus considered silhouettes as particularly important to study physiognomy (Lavater 1794, 219–21). Physiognomy, Lavater (1794, 24) posits, is 'the science or knowledge of the correspondence between the external and internal man, the visible superficies and the invisible contents'. Physiognomy is the science of making the invisible, inner, reality, visible, of making it surface, a (pseudo)science that will soon have a central role in making madness visible in the context of the nascent psychiatry. According to Lavater, physiognomy is concerned with the permanent traits of the face at rest:

> The head, especially the face, and the formation of the firm parts [...] The eye, the look, the cheeks, the mouth, the forehead, whether considered in a state of entire rest, or during their innumerable varieties of motion,—in fine, whatever is understood by physiognomy—are the most expressive, the most convincing picture of interior sensation, desires, passions, will, and of all those properties which so much exalt moral above animal life. (Lavater 1794, 22)

A different (pseudo)science, which he calls 'pathognomy', is 'the knowledge of the signs of the passion', which reveals 'character impassioned [as] manifested by the moveable parts in motion' (Lavater 1794, 24–25). Most importantly, Lavater inaugurates, indirectly, the era of craniometry and thus phrenology, on which I will return shortly:

> I consider the system of the bones as the great outline of man, and the scull as the principal part of that system. I pay more attention to the form and arching of the scull, as far as I am acquainted with it, than all my predecessors; and I have considered this most firm, least changeable, and far best defined part of the human body, as the foundation of the science of physiognomy. (Lavater 1794, 62)

Lavater's editions in English had variable fortunes and, most importantly, were both (Holcroft's and Hunter's) abridged editions, based on a French translation of Lavater's work, but both translators took substantial liberties (Erle 2010, 134–37). Neither includes reference to the XVI *Fragmente* of Lavater's original (in his second volume) for example, entitled 'Schwariche, Thörichte Menschen' ('Weak and Foolish Men) (Lavater 1775, 181–90). According to Lavater, foolishness, stupidity, idiocy and madness emerge in the field of the visible as 'deformity, animal dullness, twitching convulsions, crooked smile, inconsistency, indeterminacy, stiffness, looseness' (Lavater 1775, 181), all characteristics that, as we have previously seen, ascribe to the insane an air of vagueness, indistinction and closeness to the animal. In commenting on an illustration of four heads of fools, Lavater quotes a 'perceptive friend' of his, who states that 'around the temple is the seat of [...] folly, where the spirits without smoke pathetically work' (Lavater 1775, 183), showing once again the persistence of the trope of madness as a gaseous entity, with or without smoke. Later illustrations represent other mental disorders, including 'quiet, closed-off, inaccessible, incurable melancholy. This is especially evident in the folds above the cheekbones, the uneven eyebrows, the astonished gaze, the small nostrils, and the closed dry mouth' (Lavater 1775, 185). The *Fragment* concludes with Daniel Chodowiecki's famous plate that 'catalogues' illnesses and deformities (Fig. 32). It displays 18 people, among whom there is a hunchback, a giant, a dwarf and a figure who looks like a classic *insipiens*: he wields a staff of madness and is dressed in torn clothes. Lavater concludes with a rather inclusive plea:

> Almighty God! How diverse are your people, and their forms so manifold. You have created them all wisely and wonderfully, and each is a spectacle of your grace and kindness! Even the worst, most spoiled, most miserable—is an embodiment of your grace and kindness! [...] They all live—and delight in life—and defend themselves against those who would rob them. [...] Therefore—healthy, upright, intelligent, noble human, look upon your weaker fellow beings, but do not scorn them! You are human, and they are no less, and in the eyes of higher beings, you are what they are to you—The Lord enlightens all eyes. They breathe our air, and warm themselves in the rays of our sun. (Lavater 1775, 189–91)

Lavater is not exclusively concerned with mental disorders, but when he does apply his physiognomic considerations to madness, we face the same issues we encounter in other tropes of its visualisation: namely, different mental disorders are often lumped together in the discussions, and put alongside foolishness, stupidity and other characteristics and disabilities, and the visible signs of such features are

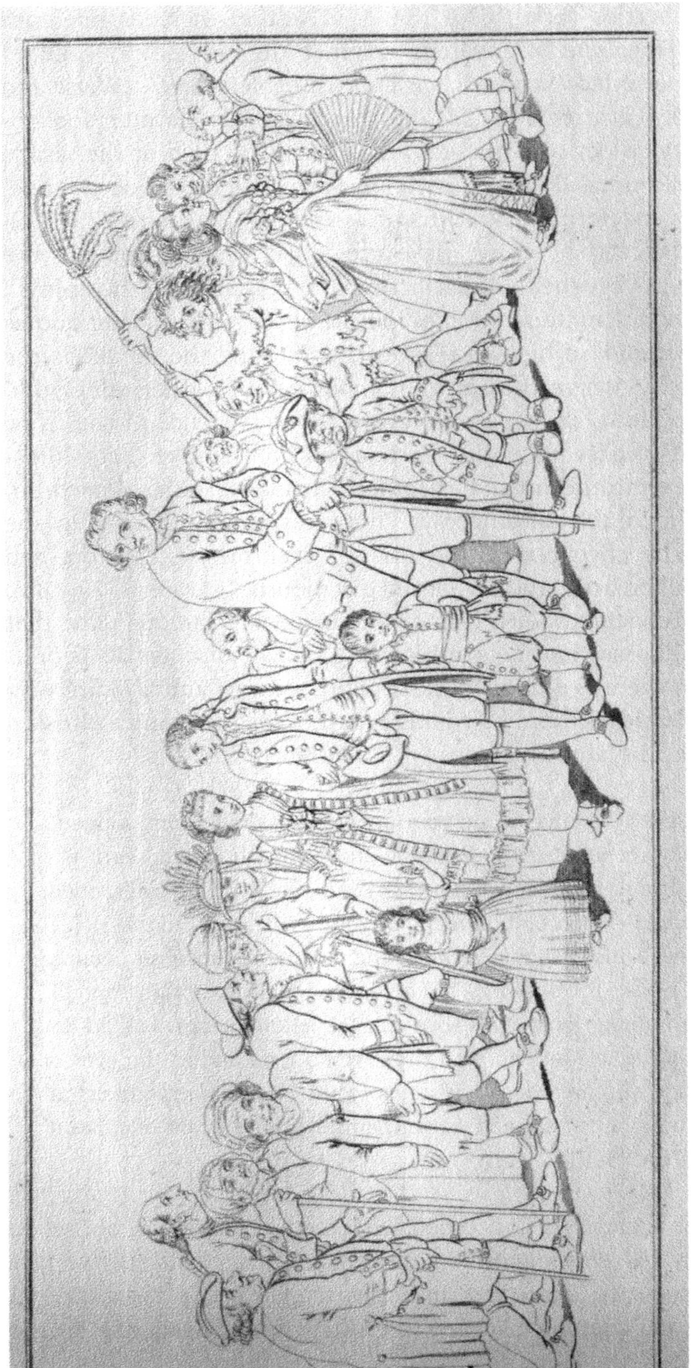

Figure 32: Daniel Chodowiecki's illustration to Lavater's XVI Fragment (1776), page 43. Courtesy of Victoria University (Toronto).

equally brought together without discrimination. Chodowiecki's plate and Lavater's conclusion of *Fragment* XVI sum this up very well: 'how diverse are [the] people!', and only the keen and trained eye of the physiognomist can appropriately distinguish the visible characteristics of such diversity. The almost esoteric aspect of physiognomy, with its contradictory and confusing descriptions of widely different characteristics and disorders, is second nature to this pseudoscience. It will continue to characterise physiognomy throughout its history also, and perhaps especially, when its study begins to concentrate exclusively on the shape of the cranium, with Gall's phrenology.

Some years later, in 1785, Johann Engel published *Ideen zu einer Mimik*, which, as Gilman (2014, 67) notes, shifts the attention from physiognomic study to the whole body, and to posture. With the seventh figure shown in his book, Engel illustrates a 'slothful, inactive soul'—a man, standing slouched, mouth semi-open, looking down with a bulging belly. 'Only the extremely dumb and lazy', he comments (Engel 1785, 114), would display such a posture. While I would not go as far as Gilman in considering this a physiognomic description of madness (or idiocy, in this case), it does indeed, in its image and words, overlap the definitions of dumbness/stupidity with laziness and idleness by means of postural considerations, a characteristic overlap that recurs throughout history and to which I will return later in this chapter.

Physiognomy, Phrenology and Medicine

At the turn of the nineteenth century, the study of physiognomy, which analysed facial and bodily traits, expressions and postures to infer character and psychological states, inspired what we could consider a new, more focused specialism, known as phrenology. While physiognomy relied on the outward appearance of the body and face to draw conclusions about a person's nature, phrenology exclusively examined the shape of the head. It posited that the shape of the skull was a reflection of the underlying shape of the brain, specific regions of which corresponded to distinct personality and behavioural traits. Phrenologists believed that by examining the bumps and depressions on the skull, they could map out an individual's mental faculties and tendencies with scientific precision, thereby transforming the study of human character from an art, based on observation, to a science grounded in anatomical analysis. Despite being almost immediately discredited, phrenology left a long-lasting influence on craniometric (and anthropometric) analyses that would be central in the medical (psychiatric) visualisation of madness over the course of the nineteenth century.

Phrenology was created by Franz Joseph Gall (1758–1828) and his assistant and close collaborator Johann Spurzheim (1776–1832). Gall had been fascinated by the appearance of the head since his youth, and some of his very early observations as a child might even have been the seeds for his future work. He observed, for example, that his classmates who excelled at memorising lengthy passages often had prominent eyes and large foreheads, and from this observation deduced that the region behind the eyes must contain an organ responsible for verbal memory. He further speculated that if one's cognitive ability could be linked to a specific external feature, other abilities, in turn, might also be indicated by outward physical traits (Finger and Eling 2019, 12).

According to Gall, the brain was composed of a series of distinct regions or organs, each responsible for different mental functions. Along with his collaborator and colleague Spurzheim, he dissected more than 120 brains, thus providing empirical support for the pair's theories on the brain's anatomical and functional segmentation. They argued that the size of each brain region was directly proportional to the strength of its corresponding mental function, much like muscles grow with use and shrink with disuse. They mapped various psychological traits and sensory abilities, like sight and hearing, onto specific brain areas and they observed that, since the brain develops in early life, the skull bones adapt to its shape, allowing one to infer a person's character and mental abilities from the shape of their head (Finger and Eling 2019, 36). They called the theory behind these observations 'organology' and the method of observation 'cranioscopy'. These two names would later give way to the better known 'phrenology' (Fig. 33).

In their *Anatomie et physiologie du système nerveux en général, et du cerveau en particulier* (Gall and Spurzheim 1810), Gall and Spurzheim discussed madness and mental illness on several occasions.[1] They had no doubt that mental illnesses were disorders of the organs of the brain, and that the brain's size and shape were thus affected. For instance, they discussed some dissections by Willis, Bonn and Pinel of brains and skulls of 'born imbeciles', and noted that they all had

1 For instance: vol. 2: 190–212, 254–55, 261–67, 270–96, 334–43, 353–55, 417–52; vol. 3: 122–33, 157–59, 174–75, 187–90, 217–44, 269–75, 301–7, 329, 334–37; vol. 4: 49–51, 83–86, 102–3, 152, 187–88, 221, 258–63.

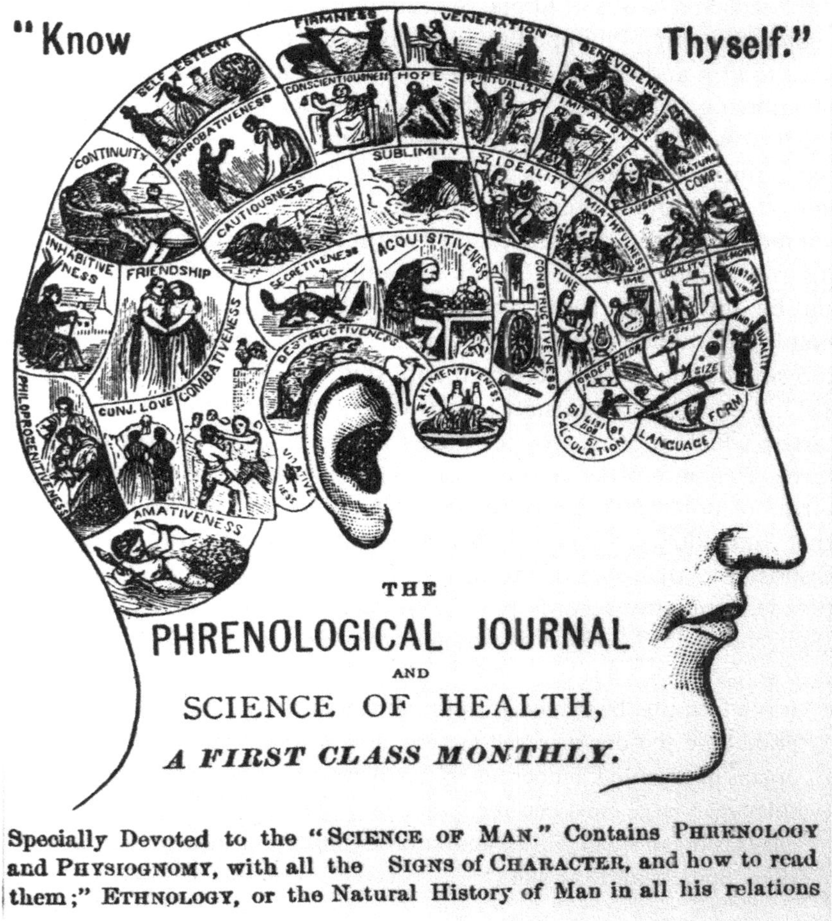

Figure 33: Phrenology: Chart. Source: Wellcome Collection.

less than a quarter of the grey matter than 'normal' brains. They also noted, however, that in cases of mental illness, the shape of the skull was not necessarily only affected by the abnormal changes in the organs of the brain, and thus a diagnosis based on phrenology could be confused with other factors, such as ethnicity.

In 1817, independently of his teacher Gall, Spurzheim (1817) published the treatise *Observations on the Deranged Manifestations of the Mind, or Insanity*. It was a study on the possible ailments of the brain, ranging from migraines to insanity, and their treatment, and included considerations on what a mental hospital should look like. The treatise includes four copper plates, of which two are studies of the heads and skulls of idiots. Spurzheim notes, however, that several people, including Philippe Pinel (to whom I will return shortly), attributed to him and Gall the idea that one could 'maintain the possibility of knowing by the external shape of the head whether any one is predisposed to insanity or not' (Spurzheim 1817, 140). 'That this is our opinion is merely imaginary' (Spurzheim 1817, 140), he rebuts, but like with other organs, he continues, 'we find that certain brains are more disposed to disease, and certain configurations more liable to insanity' (Spurzheim 1817, 140). The only conclusion Spurzheim feels can be drawn with certainty, in relation to how any form of insanity manifests in outer traits, in particular the shape of the head, is that 'a too small brain is unfit for the manifestation of the mind' (Spurzheim 1817, 142). This conclusion is particularly relevant to 'idiotism from birth', which the two copper plates at the end of the treatise illustrate. The only other observation that Spurzheim feels is needed in terms of potentially applying phrenology to the study of insanity, is that 'individuals of a certain character predominant from infancy are disposed to that sort of insanity [...]. The natural conduct of insane people frequently accords with their natural temper and disposition' (Spurzheim 1817, 143). For instance,

> It is a fact, that by far the greatest number of those who are insane by pride have the organ of self-esteem large in proportion to the other organs of the mind. It does not follow, however, that every one who has this organ large must become insane by pride, nor that every one who has this organ small will be absolutely exempt from such an hallucination. (Spurzheim 1817, 144)

Somewhat diplomatically, Spurzheim concludes: 'in insanity, the configuration of heads is neither to be overlooked, nor to be overrated' (Spurzheim 1817, 146).

Phrenology experienced alternating periods of acceptance and rejection, but importantly, it contributed to solidifying variants of the pseudoscience that visualised inner characteristics and mental disorders through outer, permanent traits. I will return shortly to the extent of its legacy in psychiatry and indeed we should note that some of its findings that were quickly dismissed at the time would later be confirmed, such as cerebral localisation and the function of the cerebral cortex, initially validated by Broca's studies in 1861. Gall and Spurzheim's method of brain dissection—preserving it in alcohol, slicing it from the base up and following its fibrous parts—also proved significant, contrasting with Vesalius's technique of slicing unpreserved brain horizontally from the top. Simpson (2005, 480) rightly considers these to be fundamental contributions to neuroscience, and one of the paradoxes in the history of phrenology, namely that their pseudoscience was more successful than their actual discoveries. Alongside this, phrenology also had a profound impact on the arts and literature, with authors using phrenological and physiognomic ideas to describe the characters in their novels or in the depiction of subjects in their paintings (see, e.g., Boshears and Whitaker 2013; Gilman 2014, 120–31; Rivers 1994; Tytler 2014; Van Wyhe 2004).

Phrenology, the study of the shape of the cranium, is certainly not the only form of physiognomy that takes root in Europe over the course of the nineteenth century. If the cranium provides the permanent shape for the equally permanent characteristics of the human being, it is in the face, and its varied expressions, that the physiognomist can grasp the fleeting details of feelings, emotions, affections and thus also forms of madness, whether they were considered temporary or permanent. Studies on facial expressions often overlapped with the fine arts, in texts that could be considered the heirs of emblem books. Such texts described facial expressions to aid the representation of emotions and conditions, such as madness and mental disorders, in painting. One such work is Charles Bell's *Essays of the Anatomy and Philosophy of Expression* (first edition 1806). With this work, Bell openly hoped to give

> a new impulse [...] to the cultivation of the fine arts, by explaining their relation to the natural history of man and animals; and by showing how a knowledge of outward form, and the accuracy of drawing which is a consequence of it, are related to the interior structure and functions. (Bell 1847, 2)

In the essay of the volume dedicated to 'Pain', Bell recommends that the insane should only be represented if strictly needed, for moral purposes. If it cannot be avoided, they should be represented as 'strong and muscles rigid and distinct, the skin bound, the features sharp, the eye sunk' or 'as of a pale sickly yellow, with wiry hair' (Bell 1847, 179). To distinguish the insane from the passionate, Bell recommends the avoidance of any representation of 'mental energy' and movements of 'all those muscles which indicate sentiment', as the aim is 'to convey this peculiar look of ferocity amidst [the] utter wreck of the intellect' (Bell 1847, 180). The painter should 'have recourse to the lower animals, and study their looks of timidity, of watchfulness, of excitement, and of ferocity' (Bell 1847, 181). Even though he is referring to the expressions of the face and posture, Bell is here clearly drawing on traditional physiognomics and animal resemblances. The overlap between the fine arts and medicine does not mean physiognomy was considered less of a science though. As Schopenhauer (2015) put it in his discussion on physiognomy, 'each human face is a hieroglyph which truly can be deciphered, indeed whose alphabet we bear within us ready-made'.

Medical treatises on insanity started to incorporate illustrations informed by such phrenological, and in particular physiognomic, studies only later in the nineteenth century, and more frequently in its second half. Philippe Pinel (1745–1826), who achieved an almost mythical status as the founder of modern psychiatry by 'freeing' the insane from the chain of the Salpêtrière hospital, could also be regarded as one of the pioneers of the medical illustration of madness. In the *Traité medico-philosophique sur l'aliénation mentale ou la manie* (published in 1801), Pinel includes two illustrations, in which he compares the skulls and the appearance of a 'normal' subject, of an idiot and of a maniac. He provides a detailed description of the idiot's appearance, emphasising the disproportionate size of the face compared to their small cranium, their lack of animation, and 'lines' that indicate, he says, 'the most absolute stupidity' (Pinel 1806, 126). He also notes the great disparity between the height of the head and the body, the depressed crown and temples, the heavy looks, a wide-open mouth and a limited capacity for knowledge and speech. He remarks that the patient's physical and cognitive abilities are severely impaired, noting that they have difficulty feeding themselves and responding to basic needs, have a feeble, tottering step, and have no interest in motion or reproduction. He contrasts this with the maniac, whose skull is better proportioned and more in line with classical standards of beauty, implying that their condition is temporary and not permanent. Pinel uses these physiognomic descriptions as a potential basis for diagnosis, suggesting that such detailed observations can be applied to other similar cases, even though he does not explicitly establish a physiognomic diagnostic method (Pinel 1806, 127–33).

Another prominent psychiatrist of this era was Jacques-Louis Moreau de la Sarthe (1771–1826), known for his contribution 'Mental Medicine' in the *Methodological Encyclopaedia* (1816). In 1807, he completed an eight-volume translation of Lavater's work, adding three appendices, the first of which on the 'physiognomy of madness' and the other two on the physiognomy of disease more generally. The first appendix on the physiognomy of madness includes two illustrations: one is Hogarth's Bedlam (see Fig. 53) and the other reprints

Pinel's heads of an idiot and a maniac, alongside the head of Victor, the feral child of Aveyron, from Jean Marc Gaspard Itard's 1801 study. Moreau de la Sarthe discusses how the physiognomy of the insane and idiots form a distinct classification within the morbid physiognomies, as highlighted by Lavater. He suggests that the shape of the head and character are related to insanity and idiocy, based on the degree of the former's physical alteration. The first skull described is from a maniac who was ultimately cured, showing that there was no direct link between skull shape and intellectual ability; indeed the second skull, despite its roundness, belonged to a young man with good judgement. Born idiots, he posits, often have smaller, asymmetrical skulls, a trait noted among the cretins from the Pays de Vaud, and an example of an idiotic child with significant skull deformities is also given. Moreau de la Sarthe then provides a detailed analysis of an idiot from the Bicêtre asylum, whose disproportionate face and cranium indicate a severe intellectual deficiency. This individual, the son of a farmer, had limited verbal expressions as well as no memory or emotional connections. Pinel identified physical defects in their skull, such as asymmetry and thick cranial structures, both of which were linked to idiocy. Moreau de la Sarthe then describes a child with such traits, noting that the physiognomy of the insane varies with the type and severity of the insanity, reflecting either an exaltation of ideas or a profound melancholy. Finally, the portrait of the feral child of Aveyron, treated by Itard, is described as displaying expressions of savagery, unease and mental deficiency, marked by facial features and scars from a life in the wild. Moreau de la Sarthe's work does not add much to Pinel's ideas, but his thoughts display an interesting mix of craniometric considerations and more physiognomical considerations on facial expressions (Lavater and Moreau de la Sarthe 1809, 223–33).

Jean-Etienne-Dominique Esquirol, a pupil of Philippe Pinel, published a series of essays on psychopathology in the *Dictionary of Medical Sciences* (1812–22). These are supplemented by numerous illustrations depicting mental disorders, such as demonomania and mania, that highlight both 'restless' expressions and specific facial angles. Other images, like those for melancholy and raging mania, depict stereotypical traits such as hidden hands and dishevelled hair. These illustrations are based on specific cases rather than being generic depictions of insanity, and were collated into the first ever visual guide to madness, which complemented Esquirol's 1838 work *Des maladies mentales considérées sous les rapports médical, hygiénique et médico-légal* (Esquirol 1838). This volume featured 27 illustrations that provided a representative cross-section of the patients at the Salpêtrière asylum.

These illustrations reflected Esquirol's detailed case studies, focusing on several different visual considerations, including fleeting ones such as expression, posture and demeanour, and permanent ones such as head shape.

Contrary to his predecessors and mentors Pinel and Esquirol, Étienne-Jean Georget (1795–1828), in his 1820 treatise *De la folie, ou aliénation mentale*, considers physiognomy as a set of characteristics, in particular expressions, whose nature is too fleeting to become a diagnostic tool of reference when it is not paired with constant and detailed observation.

> It is difficult to describe the appearance of the mentally ill; one must observe it to retain the image. People are unrecognisable; their facial features have changed direction, and their overall appearance is completely deformed. The faces are almost as different as the individuals themselves; they vary according to the passions and various ideas that occupy or agitate them, the character of the delirium, the stage of the illness, etc. In general, the faces of idiots are silly and insignificant; those of maniacs, as agitated as their minds, are sometimes tense and convulsed; in the stupid, the features are dull and have no expression; the faces of melancholics, contracted, bear the imprint of pain or extreme preoccupation; the monomaniac king has a proud and high air; the devout one, humble, prays while fixing the sky or the ground; the fearful one flees while looking to the side, etc. I limit myself to this simple statement, as only seeing it can give an idea of the rest. (Georget 1820, 133)

Georget also remarked that 'one could write entire volumes on the expression, the intellectual appearance of the insane; but it would be without any useful purpose for treatment. The various alterations that can occur in the exercise and manifestation of intellectual faculties are extremely numerous' (Georget 1820, 87). He seemed to be more convinced of the use of physiognomic observations in the 1823 edition of the same treatise, however, where he states that

> The appearance is often very expressive and quite well indicates the nature of the mental disorder. Joy, contentment, fear, sadness, despair, anger, agitation, fury—all these passions have their signs on the face of the insane just as they do in reasonable individuals; they are only much more pronounced in the former because the passions that characterize the delirium, acting continuously and with intensity, must leave deeper traces. (Georget 1823, 19)

Georget is clearly not dismissing the study of physiognomics of the insane, but he does stress how difficult it is, given that it is grounded on a vast amount of fleeting movements and expressions.

Famously, Georget commissioned ten portraits of the insane from his friend the painter Théodore Géricault (1791–1824). It is still a matter of debate whether these were commissioned to illustrate the fleeting physiognomy of madness according to Georget or as a remedial activity for Géricault himself during his breakdown of 1819 (Snell 2018, 115). They might even have been made to illustrate a new, never-published edition of Georget's *De la folie* (Snell 2018). Dating them is also complicated, but they were likely painted around 1820 (Kromm 2002, 237). What is important is that these portraits differ greatly from previous physiognomic drawings as they feature three-quarter, half-length views of faces lit against dark, simple backgrounds that rarely hint at specific settings. The subjects wear their own clothes, varying from the neat to the dishevelled, and the faces are illuminated and painted with thick strokes around the eyes, giving a softer effect compared to traditional drawings. The expressions show a degree of tension and unease, the heads and torsos are subtly misaligned, and the eyes avoid a direct gaze with the viewer. There is also a sense of introspection and discomfort that is emphasised with furrowed brows and downturned mouths. While the men appear more formally dressed, suggesting a private care setting, the elderly women's red eyes and sagging features indicate prolonged distress. Their unkempt hair and exposed necks mark them out as Salpêtrière inmates, contrasting with the more dignified presentation of the men. Overall, this series of paintings (of the ten commissioned only five survive) neither shows the viewer individual portraits that necessarily characterise a particular disorder nor shows univocal signs of insanity, possibly reflecting Georget's ambivalence towards physiognomics.

Esquirol, and with him the 'Salpêtrière school' of physiognomics, appeared in Britain with Alexander Morison (1779–1866), director of the County of Surrey asylum. According to Morison (1826, 125) there is no doubt that 'the appearance of the face [...] is intimately connected with, and dependent upon, the state of the mind' due to the 'repetition of the same ideas and emotions, and the consequent repetition of the same movements of the muscles of the eyes, and of the face', which 'give a peculiar expression'. Other, more permanent, external features, such as the shape of the skull as suggested by Gall's phrenology, continues Morison, might have a connection to mental disorders, but this remains to be ascertained. Before going into

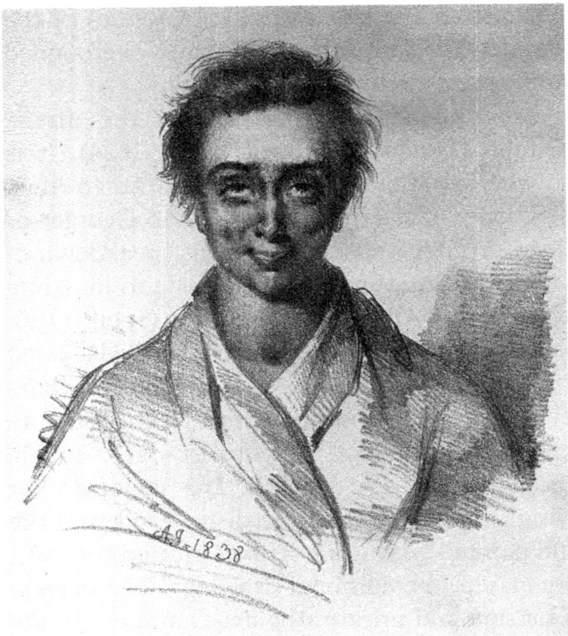

Figure 34: The physiognomy of mental diseases / [Sir Alexander Morison]. Source: Wellcome Collection.

an in-depth description of the 13 illustrations included in the second edition of his *Outlines of Lectures on Mental Diseases,* Morison thanks his friend and colleague Esquirol for allowing him to consult his extensive collection of busts and drawings. Morison's plates in this second edition are very similar to Esquirol's, with deep tones to emphasise the shadows, and contours that best detail the expression of the patients. In the third edition of the *Outlines* and in Morison's 1840 treatise *The Physiognomy of Mental Diseases,* however, lithographs rather than etchings appear, and, while the difference is noticeable and more 'impressionistic', as Gilman (2014, 92) aptly notes, in their substance the portraits continue to display, with emphatic chiaroscuro tones, the changing of expressions (Fig. 34). Morison is particularly interested in portraying how expressions change from the florid period of mental disorder to remission, pre-empting the comparative albums of mental asylums such as San Clemente in Venice, which I analyse in the next chapter. Also, in this later treatise the underlying stance on physiognomics remains the same as that from the *Outlines*:

> There is no class of diseases in which the study of Physiognomy is so necessary as that of Mental diseases. It not only enables us to distinguish the characteristic features of different varieties, but it gives us

> warning of the approach of the disease in those in whom there is a predisposition to it, as well as confirms our opinion of convalescence in those in whom it is subsiding. (Morison 1840, 1)

I might not fully subscribe to Cagnetta's view that such an approach to visualisation 'becomes, in the absence of a "real anatomy", in which illness originates, the "mythical" anatomy of psychiatry' (Cagnetta 1981, 33). There is, however, a fundament of truth to this assertion, insofar as psychiatrists indeed find in physiognomy and phrenology a (pseudo)scientific way to make madness visible and to enable it to surface. Phrenology, as we will see, despite being a pseudoscience, played an unexpected yet crucial role in the development of modern neuroscience. By its proposing of the theory that the brain is divided into distinct 'organs', each one responsible for different mental functions, phrenology inadvertently paved the way for the scientifically valid theory of brain localisation. This concept, according to which, roughly, specific mental functions happen in particular brain regions, has revolutionised our understanding of the brain and mental disorder. Brain imaging technologies, such as fMRI (functional magnetic resonance imaging) and PET (positron emission tomography) scans, have emerged from this discovery, enabling a new way of visualising mental functions, and thus mental disorder. I will return to this in the following chapters.

Posture

Permanent traits of the skull or fleeting facial expressions are not the only features that visually conveyed inner traits and madness. At the entrance of the infamous Bedlam hospital in London, which we have already seen inside thanks to Lens and Strut's abovementioned print (Fig. 25), the statues by Caius Gabriel Cibber (1680) stand as powerful visual summaries of the two key postures of madness (Fig. 35). These sculptures, representing 'Raving Madness' and 'Melancholy', visualise the dichotomy that has shaped our understanding of mental illness for centuries. The figures not only represent the polar extremes of mania and melancholia, but also embody the contrasting physical postures that have become central to the visual and cultural representation of mental disorders. These postures, which reflect the external manifestations of internal states, are integral to the physiognomy of madness and have become deeply embedded in the visual arts as much as in psychiatry (Harrington 2019, 218–19).

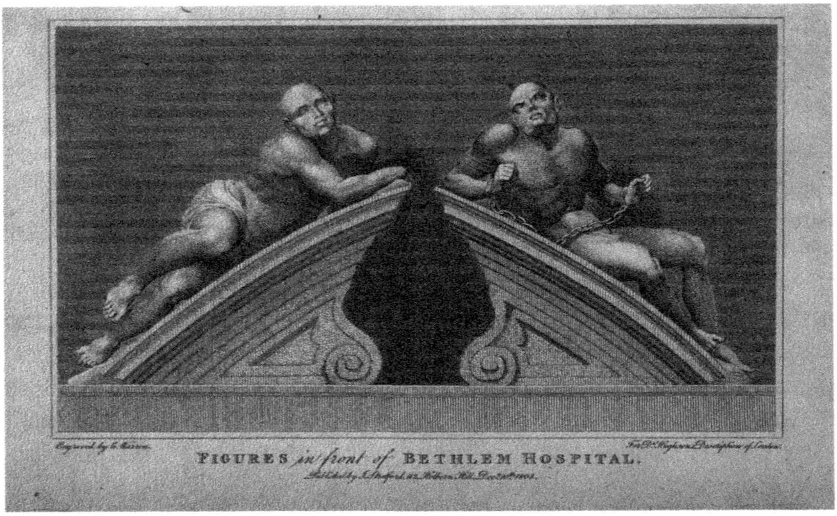

Figure 35: Statues of "raving" and "melancholy" madness, each reclining on one half of a broken segmental pediment, formerly crowning the gates at Bethlem [Bedlam] Hospital. Engraving by C. Warren, 1808, after C. Cibber, 1680. Source: Wellcome Collection.

Cibber's *Raving Madness*, in turn, conveys violent energy; its limbs are contorted and strained, pushing against the chains that bind it. The body is twisted, the muscles taut and the head thrown back, as if caught in a scream of uncontrolled rage or despair. This extended posture, with limbs thrown outward in a desperate attempt to escape or resist, is characteristic of the visualisation of mania. The figure embodies a chaotic, outward-reaching energy that seems to be tearing the body apart from within. This is a posture of violent externalisation, where the body is depicted as if being forced to act out the disorder of the mind. Gilman (2014, 20) mentions Pieter Xavery's 1673 *Two Madmen* terracotta, which is another similar example of a raving maniac, the uncontrolled movements of mania emphasised by the chain at his feet (Fig. 36). Equally, the examples discussed above of the raging maniacs in Lens and Strut's print of Bedlam for Swift's book (Fig. 25) and in Goya's depictions of the asylum (Fig. 26) depict the same outward frenzied postures.

The opposite is true in Cibber's *Melancholy*, which depicts a figure that is collapsed inward, closed off from the external world. The melancholic sits with his head bowed, shoulders slumped and his hands hidden from view, as if weighed down by an invisible burden.

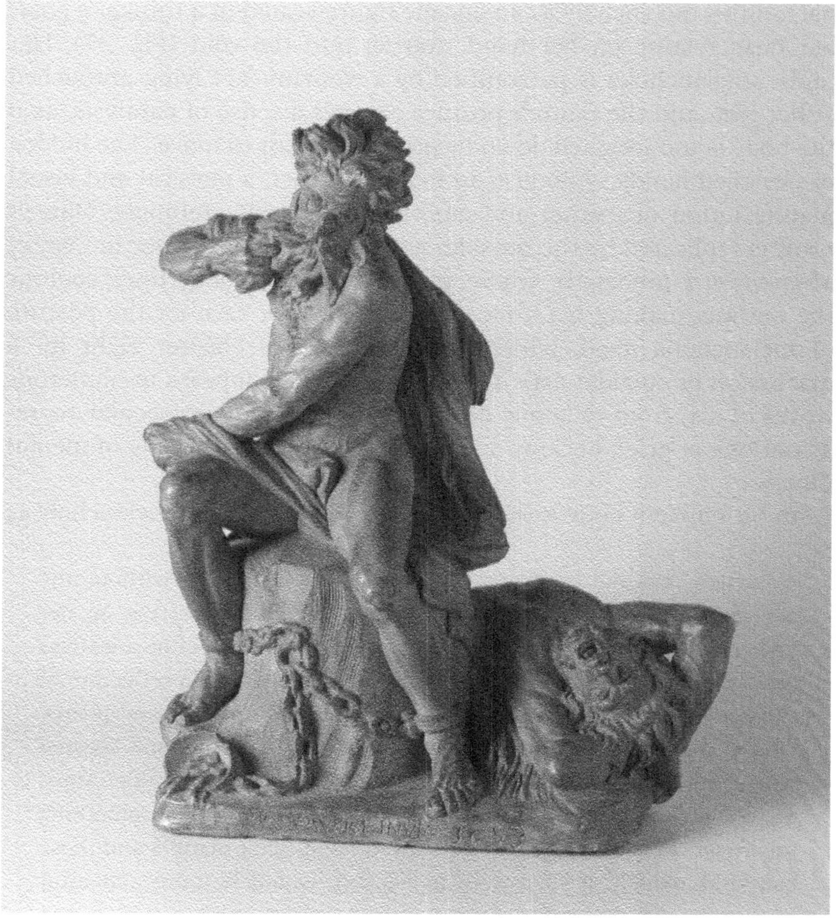

Figure 36: Pieter Xavery, Two Madmen, 1673, terracotta.
Courtesy of Rijksmuseum, Amsterdam.

This posture of contraction, of limbs drawn inward and the body folded in upon itself, reflects the withdrawal and passivity associated with depression. The melancholic's posture is one of stasis, where the energy that drives the maniac outward seems instead to be turned inward, trapping the sufferer within their own mind. The hidden hands symbolise inactivity and ineffectuality, as if the melancholic is incapable of taking any meaningful action. This posture, like that of the maniac, externalises the internal state of the sufferer, making visible the invisible suffering of the mind. The most striking illustration of depression is Albrecht Dürer's 1514 print *Melancholia I*, which personifies melancholy as an angelic figure seated in a thinker's pose, her head resting on her hand, staring into the void (Fig. 37). Her tools—melancholia is personified by a woman—are lying untouched at her feet, and the figure's posture conveys a sense of paralysis, as if the body is too weighed down by grief or despair to move. The hidden or clenched hands symbolise an inability to act, a physical and visual manifestation of mental and emotional paralysis. Tellingly, Dürer's print is replicated by the outsider artist Oswald Tschirtner in *Copy of Melancholia I* (undated), where simple and continuous lines contour the outline, making her almost unrecognisable, save for the posture of melancholia itself, which is preserved (see chapter eight for a discussion of outsider art). This posture, which appears in numerous works of art, from religious depictions of mourning to secular representations of grief, became a key image in the iconography of mental illness.

In his emblem book *Iconologia*, Cesare Ripa describes melancholy as

> A woman, sad and sorrowful, dressed in shabby clothes without any adornment, [who] will sit upon a stone, her elbows resting on her knees, and both hands under her chin. Nearby, there will be a leafless tree among the stones. Melancholy has in man (who is a reflection of the entire world) the same effects as winter has on trees and plants, which, shaken by various winds, tormented by the cold, and covered with snow, appear dry, barren, naked, and of the lowest value. Thus, no one avoids the conversation of melancholy men as something unpleasant. Their thoughts always dwell on difficult matters and those bad risks, which, if they were to happen, would be pure and utter misfortune. They imagine these dangers as present and real, as shown by the signs of sadness and pain. She is poorly dressed, without ornament. (Ripa 1593, 384)

The traditional iconography of melancholy often overlaps with that of acedia or idleness; the melancholic figure is frequently depicted as idle and listless. In *Iconologia*, Ripa describes acedia as 'an old, ugly woman, poorly dressed, [who] sits with her cheek resting on her left hand [...], her elbow placed upon her knee, and her head bowed' (Ripa 1593, 6), attributes that also align with his depiction of melancholy.

The posture is often replicated in the history of art, and is more emblematic and recognisable than that of mania. For instance, in the 1615 painting entitled *Melancholia*, Domenico Fetti represents her as a woman in a pensive position contemplating a skull. Like in Dürer's print, in Fetti's painting melancholia is also paired with an

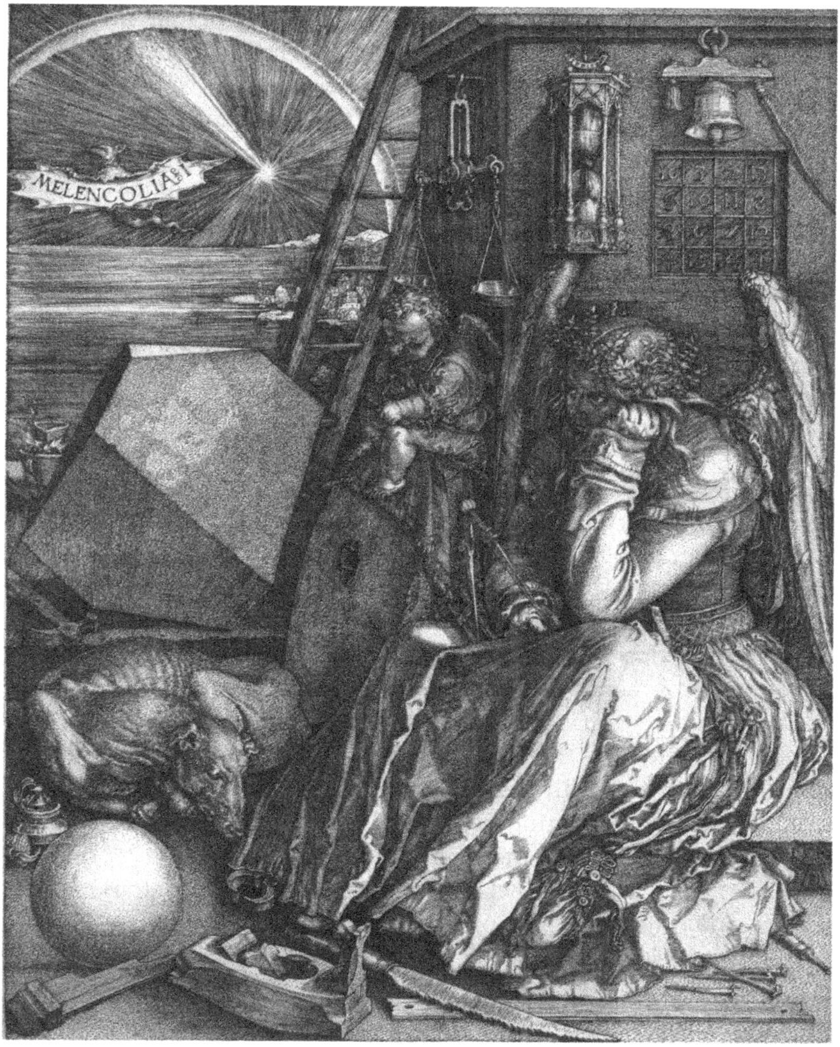

Figure 37: Albrecht Dürer, Melancholia I, engraving 1514. Courtesy of MET Museum (New York).

idle and indolent dog. Edvard Munch, in his variations on melancholy (1891–96), invariably depicts a person, this time a man, sitting, idle, contemplating the horizon, head resting on the hand, in the pensive position. Though rarer, we even come across this posture in medieval illumination: the abovementioned diagram for cauterisations in Rogerius's manuscript of the thirteenth century, in fact, depicts (bottom left) the melancholic with their head resting on their palm (Fig. 2). I will return to the posture of the melancholic in chapter seven, to see it also at work in photography and photoreportage.

In addition to the two opposite extremes in the representations of mania and melancholia, another posture that became central to the visual vocabulary of madness is the *arc de cercle,* or opisthotonus. Opisthotonus is an extreme spasm, defined as 'dramatic abnormal posture due to spastic contraction of the extensor muscles of the neck, trunk, and lower extremities that produces a severe backward arching from neck to heel' (Shahade and De Jesus 2024). Typically, the trunk is elevated off the ground and the sufferer stands on their heels and head, body arched. Several medical conditions can cause it, but it is considered typical of tetanus. In iconography, the opisthotonus is often used to visualise those possessed by demons. We can find it in a range of images of possession and exorcism as far apart as Girolamo di Benvenuto's sixteenth-century painting of St. Caterina exorcising a woman (Fig. 16) and the famous 'spider walk' scene of the 1973 film *The Exorcist* by William Friedkin. Again, the page of Rogerius's medical manuscript, in its top right, shows an epileptic, also in the position of the *arc de cercle* (Fig. 2). Pieter Xavery's abovementioned terracotta features a maniac in the foreground but also a madmen contorted in the *arc de cercle* position in the background (Fig. 36). Most importantly, the *arc de cercle* became the iconic posture of the hysteric attack with Charcot's *Iconographie,* which features Augustine in several positions typical of tetanus (e.g., the tetanic hands), including the opisthotonus (Fig. 22).

These postures—whether the violent extension of the maniac, the inward collapse of the melancholic or the dramatic arch of the hysteric/possessed—serve once again as a means to visualise mental disorders and allow them to surface and become recognisable as 'other' in contrast to 'normal' postures. They also embody broader cultural anxieties about the body, control and the boundaries of sanity. The body, in these representations, becomes a site of both diagnosis and meaning, where the physical form mirrors the psychological state, and where the body performs under the influence of forces well beyond conscious control. These are anxieties that we have already seen at play in the dances of madness.

Conclusions

The exploration of physiognomy in this chapter has traced the ways in which madness has been visually encoded onto the body, reflecting centuries of pseudoscientific belief that physical appearance, particularly facial features, expressions and posture, can reveal inner psychological states. Physiognomy served as a tool for categorising and differentiating individuals who were deemed to suffer from mental illnesses, thus visually distinguishing the 'insane' from the 'sane'. One of the key contributions of physiognomy, as we have explored in this chapter, is its role in reinforcing the boundary between mental illness and normalcy by rendering madness visible and legible through the body. The deterministic view that one's external appearance can reveal the truth of one's mental state allowed physiognomy and its derivatives, such as phrenology, to flourish as a means of identifying and categorising people with mental disorders.

Physiognomy extended beyond the face to also codify the posture of the body, in the arts as much as in medicine. The stark contrast between the rigid, contorted posture of the maniac and the slumped, withdrawn stance of the melancholic, as exemplified in Cibber's statues, offers what we could deem a visual shorthand for understanding a very deep-seated dichotomic thinking of mental disorders, that is between mania and melancholia.

As we have seen, the legacy of physiognomy extends beyond the pseudoscientific methods of the past. The desire to render madness visible, to make it legible through the body, continues to shape modern psychiatric thought and visual culture. The physiognomic tradition, though now discredited, has left an indelible mark on how we understand and represent mental illness. By emphasising the body as the site where madness becomes visible, physiognomy has perpetuated the view that mental illness is something that can be observed, categorised and controlled. In the next part, I will discuss how these considerations apply to medicine, with a particular focus on the adoption of specialised medical tools to visualise mental disorder.

PART THREE

Medical Othering / Medical Imaging

CHAPTER FIVE

Madness through the Lens: Psychiatric Photography

I WILL NOW SHIFT THE FOCUS to the evolution of the tools employed to capture medically meaningful images of the bodies of the insane: first photography and then brain and neuroimaging. In this chapter in particular, I move on to discussing how the introduction of photography marked a continuation, and even a reinvigoration, of the study of physiognomics. Photography, however, also introduces new tropes into the visualisation of mental disorders that go beyond physiognomics and individual portraits. I thus also study the photographic archive and its impact on the visualisation of mental disorders. The aim of this and the next chapter is to discuss how specialised tools contribute in unique ways to the visual othering of the individual who is suffering from a mental disorder. If in previous chapters I have asked how madness emerges in the field of the visible by etching itself on the very body of the insane, in these two chapters I ask how specialised tools make madness visible.

In the mid-nineteenth century, the advent of photography profoundly shook visual culture and visual representation, significantly influencing the sciences and medicine. It goes without saying that photography also revolutionised visual representation in psychiatry, changing the way mental illness was documented and perceived. It did not necessarily enhance diagnosis or understanding, but it did alter the methods and tools used in psychiatric practice. After discussing Hugh Diamond's pioneering use of photography in lunatic asylums, this chapter focuses on an understudied corpus of images. We will examine the psychiatric photography in post-unification Italian asylums (1860–1900), specifically the two largest surviving archives from Venice and Reggio Emilia. Although geographically limited, this corpus showcases well the primary uses of photography in psychiatry, highlighting how the medium was used to depict mental disorders through the portraiture of the insane. This more localised and focused approach also allows us to explore the material significance of photographs, illustrating how they enabled the establishment and flourishing of a network of knowledge.

In the golden era of positivism—when only 'verifiable scientific knowledge about natural phenomena' was the 'authentic source of truths about the world' (Sturken and Cartwright 2017, 25)—photography seemed to be the perfect instrument for scientific investigation, in that it is a 'method of producing representations through a mechanical recording device rather than relying solely on the scientist's subjective eye and hand (using pencil to sketch a view on paper, for example)' (Sturken and Cartwright 2017, 25). As Marien (2021, 143) notes, 'photography participated in the production of evidence in many fields. Geology, biology, botany, medicine, astronomy, and chemistry used photography to collect and exhibit evidence'.

From its inception, photography had a privileged epistemic status (Cohen and Meskin 2004) and was regarded as a transparent medium (Mizrahi 2021). This contributed to generating a deep-seated faith in photography as an objective and fully realistic medium, often overlooking its subjective and artistic aspects. As Sturken and Cartwright (2017, 349) have it, 'despite its status as a black-boxed technology (one that hides away its mechanisms and design choices in a single, closed unit), the camera requires its user to make subjective and culturally informed decisions'. In spite, or perhaps precisely because, of this faith in it, photography had a crucial impact on the sciences and medicine. It revolutionised the visualisation of natural phenomena, allowing scientists and medical professionals to document the details of the natural world and human anatomy with what they believed was unprecedented accuracy. Photography also became an indispensable tool for teaching and explaining procedures, offering clear, illustrative guides that could be shared widely. It also played a critical role in documenting microscopic structures for instance, unveiling a hidden world that was previously inaccessible. The use of photography in psychiatry is rooted both in the long-standing relationship between madness and visual representation that we have been looking at, and in this early, enthusiastic and uncritical adoption of photography as a tool for scientific investigation.

Thus, the advent of photography marked a significant moment in the visualisation of mental disorders. Photography's power to freeze fleeting expressions and gestures, and, as was believed, to capture portraits without any subjective bias, provided a powerful new tool for psychiatrists. It also offered a new instrument to support the study of physiognomics, since it allowed for a seemingly objective examination of the physical manifestations of mental states. This development bridged the gap between early pseudoscientific practices and the emerging medical approaches to psychiatry, even though the presumed objectivity of photography was often more a matter of belief than a reality. The portrait photography of psychiatric patients was enthusiastically adopted for its purported demonstrative capabilities (e.g., to show the healing properties of the asylum through before/after treatment comparisons); for illustrative purposes (e.g., to depict the typical appearance of certain mental disorders); for its therapeutic value (e.g., to show patients their progress); and for its objectivity (e.g., to identify patients in case of escape or relapse). However, the fervour for psychiatric photography was both intense and short-lived. By the early twentieth century, the inclusion of photographs in medical records and psychiatric treatises became standard practice, but as this became more common, psychiatrists seemed less interested in exploring the actual relationship between mental disorders and the portraits of the affected. While portrait photography became widespread in psychiatric contexts, its specific significance for psychiatry diminished; photographs identified patients but were soon recognised as insufficient for conveying the nature of their mental disorders. It became apparent that photography alone could not make mental disorders visible and psychiatrists had to seek other sources, which medicine provided (these will be explored in the following chapter). As in different contexts, such as criminology, ethnology and anthropology, 'the camera was [...] a scientific tool for constituting groups of people as Other' (Sturken and Cartwright 2017, 355), bringing its alleged objectivity and novelty to an overlap with other forms of visual representation that strove to other the insane.

Psychiatric Photography

The British physician and amateur photographer Hugh Welch Diamond (1809–86) was a pioneer in many ways. He was one of the founders of the British Photographic Society, one of the first to experiment with the wet-plate collodion process (which allowed better sensitivity and faster exposure times than previous processes) and one of the first, if not the first, to develop a 'systematic theory and practice of clinical photography' (Gilman 2015, 5). Diamond succeeded Morison at the

Surrey County Lunatic Asylum in Springfield, where he worked as superintendent of the female wards from 1844 to 1858. After perfecting the wet collodion technique, he used it to photograph the inmates of the lunatic asylum, where he established a permanent photographic laboratory in 1851, the very first photographic laboratory installed in a medical facility, let alone in an asylum (Fig. 38). On 22 November 1856 he delivered a paper to the Royal Society entitled 'On the Application of Photography to the Physiognomy and Mental Phenomena of Insanity', giving birth to the diagnostic use of photography in psychiatry. In his paper, subscribing to the physiognomic theories that dominated the field at the time, Diamond argued that photography aids the study of insanity because it permanently records the appearance of the mentally ill. It also serves two other purposes: it assists treatment, in that it gives patients an accurate depiction of what insanity is doing to them; and it also assists identification, in case the need of readmission should arise. The photograph, says Diamond (in Gilman 2015, 19), 'speaks for itself with the most marked pression and indicates the exact point which has been reached in the scale of unhappiness between the first sensation and its utmost height'. 'The photographer', continues Diamond (in Gilman 2015, 20), 'secures with unerring accuracy the external phenomena of each passion, as the really certain indication of internal derangement, and exhibits to the eye the well known sympathy which exists between the diseased brain and the organs and features of the body'. This 'known sympathy', which Diamond takes for granted, finds a 'perfect and faithful record' in photography, free as it is of the 'painful caricaturing which so disfigures almost all the published portraits of the Insane as to render them nearly valueless either for purposes of art or of science' (Gilman 2015, 24).

According to Diamond, photography is the perfect realistic record of the external features of the human being, which he believed to sympathetically reflect the diseased brain. He also assumed that mental disorders ultimately stem from brain diseases. Therefore, to the discerning eye, photography is considered a perfect and faithful record of mental disorder and the diseased brain. However, each of these statements demands critical scrutiny—that is, the objectivity of photography, the tenuous link between facial features and brain characteristics, and the assumption that mental disorders always and only originate from brain diseases. The strong bond between visual representation and mental disorders is the leitmotif and object of study of this monograph and, as we have seen, it can be traced back even to the prehistory of humans. We cannot therefore consider Diamond's statement a founding one. It is, however, one of the most explicit and

Figure 38: H.W. Diamond. Portrait of a mad woman. Albumen print after collodion glass negative. 1852-1854. Courtesy of MET Museum (New York).

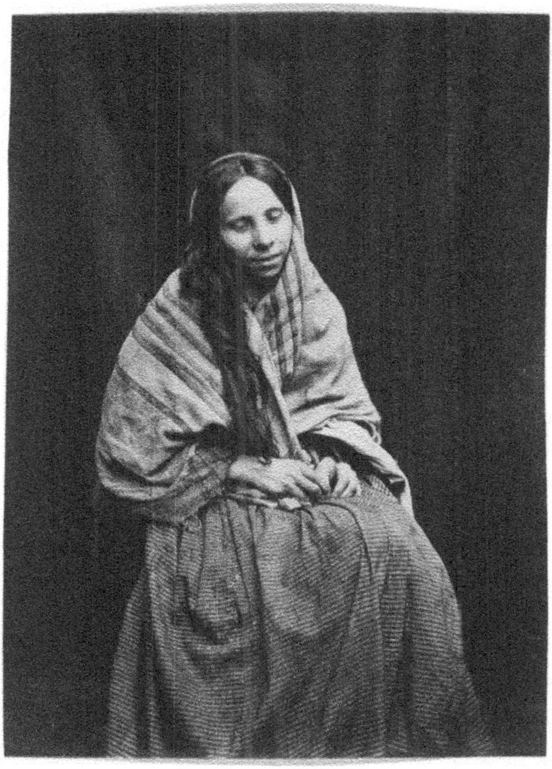

interesting, one that, unwittingly perhaps, resonates still in most contemporary studies of brain imaging: it sanctions, by means of some acritical turns in the argument, the very possibility of seeing the diseased brain, and thus the production of a permanent record as to what madness looks like.

Two of the three uses of photography in psychiatry (for diagnosis and for identification), according to Diamond, map onto the two main early uses of photography in medicine and the social sciences, according to Sekula (1986, 17): namely the nominalist and the realistic approaches. These are exemplified by Francis Galton's composite portraiture and Alfred Bertillon's 'bertillonage'. Between 1880 and 1890, Bertillon created a system for criminal identification known as *bertillonage*, the predecessor of the mug shot. Arrested persons were photographed from different angles and identifying details, such as tattoos and scars, were documented. These photographs were then accompanied by records describing the personality traits of the individual. Sekula notes that Bertillon, through these precise measurements and classifications, reinvented physiognomy in non-metaphysical, ethnographic terms, since these photographs captured only the individual's external appearance, which was used to identify them. In contrast, Galton believed that the body as a whole revealed an individual's true nature, and so he developed a composite portrait technique as part of a eugenic project to classify (and grade) humans. This method involved photographing multiple subjects, underexposed, on a single plate. The overall composite photo had the correct exposure and was a combination of everyone's traits. Sekula describes Bertillon's work as relying on the indexical nature of photography, emphasising its ability to record a physical trace of a concrete object. Galton's work, however, aimed to elevate his composite photographs to a symbolic level, by expressing general laws through these specific cases. Galton saw composite portraits as symbols referring to a universal category, while Bertillon's system simply linked each photograph directly to its subject, without implying any hidden truth. According to Sekula, Galton and Bertillon represent the contrasting, yet complementary, ways photography was used in the social sciences and medicine in the late nineteenth century. Bertillon's archives functioned as indexes, where photographs and personal records verified an individual's identity. For Bertillon, the role of photography was to confirm a one-to-one correspondence: one criminal, one photograph. His approach prioritised the contingent nature of the photographic image over the theoretical ambitions of physiognomy. Bertillon aimed to create a science of the individual, establishing specific rules governing appearance and behaviour, where photography identified, explained and understood individuals.

Therefore, according to Diamond, photography worked within a nominalist framework; it aided diagnosis by illustrating in the particular what the universal looks like. Yet, photography worked as a 'realist' tool as well; it represented a single individual who could be recognised, indexically, by their resemblance to their own image; no universalism was involved. To this extent, Diamond's work, albeit pioneering as far as photography and psychiatry are concerned, is part of a larger picture: a new technology (photography) interfacing with new or developing practices and sciences.

The third use of photography is possibly the most innovative. Diamond praised photography as an aid to therapy, to show patients how insanity 'crooked' them and/or how much they improved thanks to their regimens in the asylum (Pearl 2009). According to Di Marco (2015, 13), 'for Diamond, photography was not just an index of a body: it recorded an identity and a history, and thus it was conceivable to use it as a therapeutic tool'. This was possible because Diamond looked beyond the physiognomy of the face, to include hair and clothes, an overview of which could give to the patient a clearer sense of deviation from the norm, and thus of their insanity, urging them into a healing process (Pearl 2009, 292–93). This is the first recorded use of photography within the context of therapy and, even though this idea emerges in parallel to, but independent of, the 'discovery' of 'outsider art' (which I will discuss in chapter eight), it is part of a cultural climate in which madness is made visible not only for the benefit of 'sane' society, as a tool of othering, but also as a conduit for the expression of the self.

The year before delivering his paper, Diamond had already exhibited three of his pictures in the Paris *Exposition Universelle* of 1855. The journalist Ernest Lacan lamented that so few of Diamond's pictures were shown: 'This magnificent collection already contained numerous specimens, so we were surprised to see only three displayed at the world's fair' (Lacan 1856, 74). Lacan (1856, 74) held Diamond in high esteem, considering him 'one of the most skilled amateur photographers' and praising how he 'had the courage to reproduce the features of the unfortunate individuals entrusted to his care'. Lacan hoped his example would be followed, and indeed his hopes were soon realised.

The first textbook to feature photographs (reproduced as lithographs) was Dietrich Georg Kieser's *Elemente der Psychiatrik* (Kieser 1855), which reproduced photographs taken in Jena by C. Schenk and J. Schnauss in the previous years. These images accompanied detailed case studies and images of brain specimens, and Kieser believed that the photographic portraits complemented the written case studies, providing a visual representation of what was described in words. As such, he did not delve into physiognomic considerations, assuming the images spoke for themselves.

In 1858, ten of Diamond's pictures were published for the first time as lithographs after photographs by William Baggs, and were printed by Hullmann & Wallon for the first volume of the *Medical Times and Gazette* of 1858. These illustrated a series of 'communications' by the psychiatrist John Conolly (1794–1866), a promoter of the non-restraint approach in psychiatry, and then resident of the Middlesex County Asylum in Hanwell. The first of these communications, entitled 'The Physiognomy of Insanity', gives the name to the series. With 'the new and important art of photography', says Conolly (1858, 3), 'in the course of a few seconds, the form and fabric of material things are copied and fixed with a fidelity scarcely attainable by graphic skill or by the painter's art'. No one, he continues, has mastered this art in an asylum as well as Diamond:

> This proficiency has also enabled Dr. Diamond to enrich his portfolios with curious portraits of the insane, which are not only truthful as portraits, but revive in those whose various forms of mental peculiarity had made their characteristic stamp; thus furnishing representations highly interesting, generally singular and striking, sometimes amusing, sometimes, it must be confessed, awful, but always suggestive of useful thought. When we contemplate such portraitures of the human face, strained or disfigured by the mysterious workings of a disordered brain [...] we are reminded of the havoc ever making—by evil thoughts, evil habits, or evil passions—or by want and distracting care. (Conolly 1858, 3)

In this very eloquent paragraph, Conolly is subscribing to the standard nineteenth-century approach to physiognomy, whereby it is taken as a fact that the 'workings of a disordered brain' have a noticeable effect on the human face. He is also, however, raising an issue which will not be one for much longer: that is, there was no easy and economical way to include photographs in printed books at this time, until photolithography. Including inserts on albumen print was comparatively very expensive, so the elected method was therefore normally to engrave a lithograph *after* a photograph, thus manually contouring it ahead of mass printing. The perceived realism of the photograph was preserved only in the caption (lithograph/print *after* daguerreotype/talbotype/photograph, etc.). In Conolly's words, 'there is so singular a fidelity in a well-executed photograph that the impression of very recent muscular agitation in the face seems to be caught by the process, which the engraver's art can scarcely preserve' (Conolly 1858, 3). In a paper on the medical uses of photography, published in the journal of the photographic society founded and presided by Diamond, Wright praises Conolly's essays and compares Diamond's photos with their lithographic reproduction. He comments: the lithograph 'is entirely destitute of all those minute points of expression which alone could give any value to such an illustration' (Wright 1867, 204). The differences between the lithographic reproductions and their photographic sources are certainly noticeable, and this is to be expected in comparing the same subject reproduced by two different media. To the contemporary eye, however, physiognomy having been discredited, the differences are purely aesthetic and have no semantic value; they do not alter the meaning of the picture. It is not as if the photograph of an individual affected by senile dementia would illustrate senile dementia better or more univocally than the lithograph taken from it.

The late 1850s were just the beginning of the widespread use of photography in mental hospitals, and Diamond's photos, thanks to his involvement with the photographic society and his paper, were just the most famous. In Bedlam, Henri Hering photographed the insane and so did Brushfield, director of the Chester County Lunatic Asylum. Brushfield wrote a short letter in 1856 to the *Journal of the Photographic Society,* which was published in volume three of 1857 under the title 'Application of Photography to Lunacy'. In this letter he noted that, even without having read Diamond's paper, the importance of photography to psychiatry was patent to him.

> Patients are very much gratified to seeing their own portraits [...] in our worst female ward I have had a positive (on glass) framed and hung up for nearly eighteen months, and it has never yet been touched by any of the patients [...] Last week a patient, who was formerly one of our most violent cases, begged for a portrait of herself, that she might send to her son [...] to show how much better she was [...] In the case of criminal lunatics it is frequently of great importance that a portrait should be obtained [...] if they do escape from the asylum [...] they may frequently be traced by sending their photographs to the police authorities [...] the photographs would thus cause them to be identified. (Brushfield 1857, 289)

Like Diamond, Brushfield found photography useful for identification but also for therapeutic purposes.

Photography was rapidly adopted in asylums, sometimes independently of Diamond's work. In 1851, the journal *La Lumière: Revue de la photographie* announced the

> successful application of photography to medicine. It was Dr. Baillarger who had the idea of using it to transmit faithful images of some unfortunate individuals with cretinism, whom he was able to study during his travels. We examined these portraits and found them remarkable from the point of view of daguerreotype, but of such deformity in relation to human nature that we almost wished for the reestablishment of the law of the Spartans or that of the Twelve Tables: *Insigni deformitate puerum, cito necato.* (Govi 1851, 5)

Govi's chilling final words find an unfortunate echo in the numerous applications of photography to psychiatry and neuropathology that would follow in the decades to come, giving rise to eugenics and the Nazism that flowed from it. The French doctor Govi mentions, Jules Gabriel Françoise Baillarger (1809–90), was to become famous for his studies on pellagra and cretinism, and his pictures were included in the atlas of Benoit August Morel's infamous *Traité des Dégénérescences* as a visual confirmation of his theory of degeneration. According to this, mental (and moral) disorders are hereditary traits that tend to worsen through the generations—in other words, degeneration can be thought of as the negative counterpart to evolution.

Photography was widely adopted in French asylums. The 1867 *Société medico-psychologique* conference was themed 'De l'application de la photographie à l'étude des maladies mentales' and was the first of its kind. It gathered together all the major psychiatrists who employed photography in their studies, such as Baillarger and Morel, and also Brière de Boismond, Moreau de la Tour and Valèry Combes. In 1869, the *Revue photographique des Hôpitaus de Paris* was released for the first time and would run until 1876, presenting semiotic photographs for the diagnosis of illnesses. It included numerous neuropathological examples, taken in the photographic laboratory of the Hôpital Saint-Louis. In 1876, for example, Henri Dagonet, pupil of Morel, published 33 physiognomic photographs, gluing them one by one into his volume *Traité élementaire et pratique des maladies mentales* in order to avoid their reproduction through lithographs and the consequent loss of detail mentioned above. One of the most important French photographic books on mental disorder is Charcot's abovementioned *Iconography*, in which the performative aspect of the images takes centre stage along with the visual.

Photographic Archives

Psychiatric treatises only represent the surface of psychiatric photography and the visual representation of mental disorders through photography. To a certain extent they are the most interesting as they were supposed to be shown and seen, and thus they presuppose a level of circulation. The archives of lunatic asylums, however, contain a wealth of portraits of patients that are often overlooked. The examples I have chosen for this section are archives from asylums in Italy from the second half of the nineteenth century. I have done so for a number of reasons. First of all, they have not been widely studied, especially in an international, cross-cultural and trans-historical context. Secondly, some of them are very well preserved and catalogued. This stems from a 2014 nationwide project called *Carte da legare*,[1] which was meant to 'safeguard the archival heritage of the former psychiatric hospitals after their permanent closure and to enhance their cultural content from a medical-psychiatric and social perspective' (SIUSA 2014). Thirdly, they are very representative of the kind of photographic materials that can be found in well-preserved psychiatric hospital archives.

According to the traditional history of Italian psychiatric photography, the first person to use a camera in an asylum was Augusto Tamburini, director of the *frenocomio* San Lazzaro in Reggio Emilia around the 1870s (Schinaia 2005, 33). It is likely this mistaken view originated from the seminal exhibition *Nascita della fotografia psichiatrica*, in whose catalogue the curator, Cagnetta, affirms that 'the first use of psychiatric photography in Italy is attributed to Augusto Tamburini (1848–1919), who introduced it in 1878 at the San Lazzaro Asylum in Reggio Emilia shortly after being appointed director (1877–1907)' (Cagnetta 1981, 42). From San Lazzaro, it was said, photography would be widely adopted in asylums throughout the peninsula. The first actual use of photography in an asylum in Italy, however, did not happen in Reggio Emilia. As Fornaciari (2005, 107) aptly noted, 'in Italian psychiatric institutions, the first experiences occurred during the last quarter of the nineteenth century, almost simultaneously in Aversa and Venice'.

Despite the traditional historiography, an 1878 publication had already declared that it was not Tamburini in Reggio Emilia who introduced psychiatric photography in Italy. This publication, which appeared in the periodical of San Lazzaro asylum, the *Gazzetta del Frenocomio di Reggio*, was the first and only scholarly publication in Italian entirely dedicated to the use of photography in asylums. The article, entitled 'La fotografia nel nostro manicomio', penned by Arrigo Tamassia, Cesare Lombroso's successor as chair of forensic medicine in Pavia, praises the use of photography in psychiatry in the manner Diamond had laid out, whose work Tamassia had very likely read. In the editorial note to the article the editor affirms that 'we publish […] this article […] on the *photography of the insane*, that we introduced in our asylum, imitating what our bemoaned colleague Salerio, in the male asylum in Venice, and dearest friend Dr Virgilio

1 The name of the project, *Carte da legare*, is a pun. *Matti da legare* (literally: 'the insane to be tied up') is an expression that could be translated as 'batshit crazy'; *carte* means papers, documents; and *legare* on its own can mean both to tie up/secure with a rope, but also to bind (itself a double meaning with rope and paper). The pun thus evokes the madness that was meant to be tied up, as documented in the papers that are now being bound and catalogued.

in the asylum of Aversa started a long time ago' (Tamassia 2011, 101). Unfortunately, during the survey by the *Carte da legare* project, no photographic archive was found in Aversa, whereas the Venice one, which also predates Tamburini's photographic work, was, and still is, very well preserved.

Venice: Comparative Album, Admission Registers and Medical Records

San Servolo is a small island in Venice's Lagoon. Initially it was a military hospital managed by the Fatebenefratelli friars from 1715, and then transitioned to housing the mentally ill in 1797 following Napoleon's arrival. By 1804, it became the *Manicomio Centrale*, serving several provinces (Galzigna 2007). During the *Regno Lombardo-Veneto*, Father Prosdocimo Salerio (1815–77) became director, introducing Pinel and Esquirol's moral therapy and improving facilities, including a library with works on photography. Although Salerio's photographic activities are not directly documented, references in later works confirm his efforts in photographing patients (Battanoli 1881). The earliest images in the San Servolo archives date back to 1874, the final year of Father Prosdocimo Salerio's life and career. These images, found in various albums, include patients admitted and discharged in 1874, and while photos do appear in the medical records from the 1874 folder onwards, they do not appear for every patient. Some records, ordered either by the discharge or death date of the patient, refer to admissions from several years prior, thus complicating the dating process, but it is believed that Salerio initiated the use of photography at San Servolo in the final decade of his career. The evidence points to its first use between 1870 and 1874, most likely around 1873 or 1874, and photography became more common in medical records and albums from then on.

While Father Prosdocimo Salerio initiated the use of photography at San Servolo, more substantial records survive for San Clemente, where the female section of the Veneto asylum was established in 1873. Directed by Cesare Vigna (Giuseppe Verdi's doctor), San Clemente holds the richest collection of early psychiatric photography albums in Italy. Vigna—unlike Salerio, who bought photography books to train his assistants—hired professional photographer Oreste Bertani in 1882 to document patients. Bertani, known for his work on *La basilica di San Marco in Venezia*, was paid 350 lire for his services,[2] highlighting the significant role of photography in the asylum's operations.

2 Conto consuntivo del Giornale di Uscita Reg. 5/472 e Registro di Cassa 1881–1883 n. 3/58, Archivio Fondazione San Servolo IRSESC.

The holdings of photographic interest in the archive of San Servolo and San Clemente (created in 1873 together with the inauguration of San Clemente itself (Cagnetta 1981, 43–44)) consist of two albums of portraits of male patients (San Servolo), five albums of portraits of female patients (San Clemente), numerous medical records with photos glued into them and a number of albums of exterior and interior views of both asylums.

The first album from San Servolo, titled *Album comparativo,* contains 519 photos of 264 patients, showing photos of each patient upon admission and discharge (Fig. 39). The photos are paired: admission on the left, discharge on the right, arranged in two columns of four rows per page, with each page displaying eight patients (16 photos). The columns are labelled 'ammalati' (sick) and 'guariti' (healed). The pairs are in numbered grids, captioned by diagnosis, and each photo is marked with the admission (En.) or discharge (U.) date in month/year format; the photos are standard 5x8 cm albumen prints. Diagnoses are omitted after the first row of page 30, and pages 31 to 33 lack grid numbering. This is perhaps the most interesting album preserved in the Venice archives: it is the only 'comparative album' in Italy and across the globe it is a rarity. There is no reference to this album in the *Relazioni statistiche* or elsewhere in contemporary literature, probably meaning that it was not considered a particularly exceptional or peculiar effort. Cesare Lombroso knew about the album or, at least, was well aware of the efforts of the San Servolo asylum to use photos to compare the visual appearance of patients upon admission with their appearance upon discharge. He writes: 'S. Servolo had a wonderful idea, which was to photograph the patients upon entry and after they had recovered. Now the difference in many cases is so great that without absolute certainty of good faith, one would struggle to believe it was the same person' (Lombroso 1890, 61).

This comparative album seems to be crafted to give a reassuring image of the asylum. The album's title itself suggests a narrative of transformation, as it shows how patients entered the asylum in one state and left it improved or healed. This apologetic intention can be seen in the photographs taken between 1873 and 1887. Starting in 1874, this practice involved placing a photograph of each patient upon their admission into their medical records, and occasionally including these photos in the triennial statistical reports compiled by the asylum's directors. This initiative coincided with the final years of Prosdocimo Salerio's tenure, which ended in 1877. Even though in most comparisons a contemporary viewer would not struggle to see the same person in the two photos, as Lombroso affirmed, the album

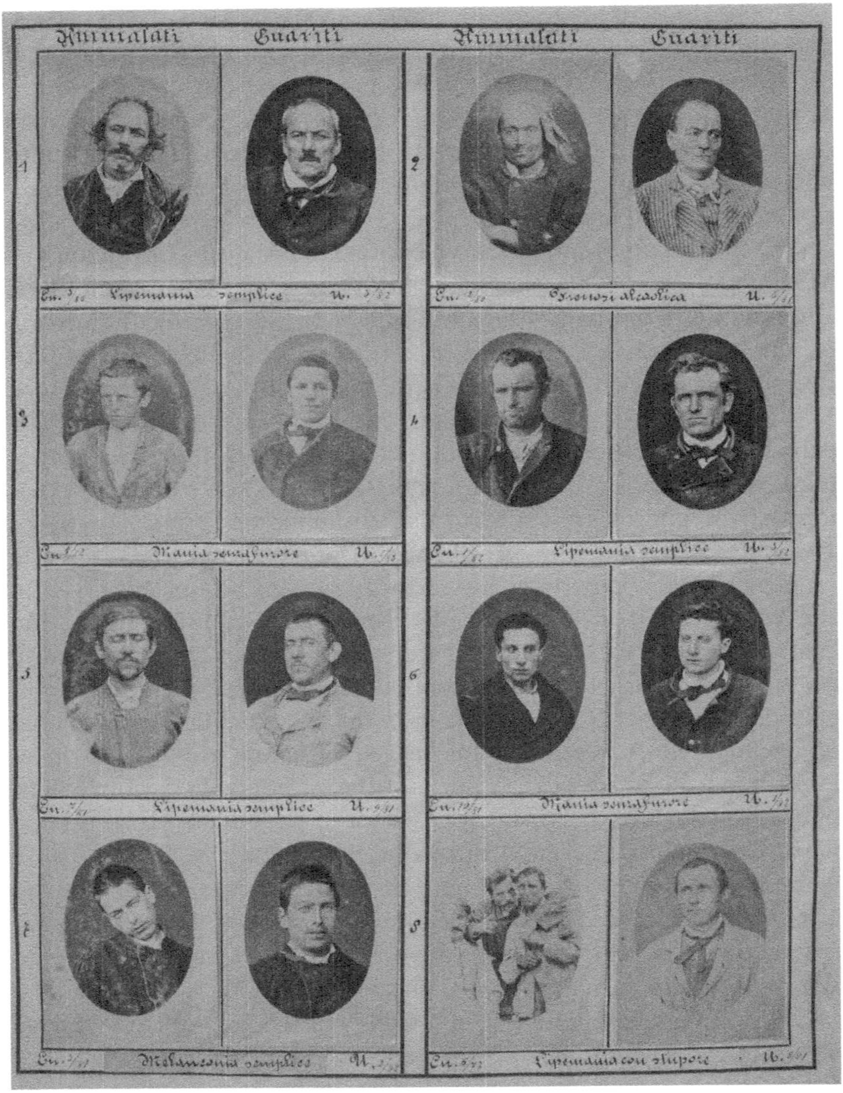

Figure 39: First page of the Album Comparativo of San Servolo. Courtesy of Archivio storico di San Servolo – San Servolo srl – Città metropolitana di Venezia.

serves as a testament to the medical community's desire to legitimise and humanise the asylum's work, providing a visual and statistical narrative that underscores the institution's role in the perceived improvement of mental health care during that era.

The second album, *Album delle presenze figurate*, is not comparative and is accompanied by a text-only 'Indice delle presenze figurate'. It includes 619 male portraits taken upon admission. The photos are sewn into the pages that contain five rows and columns, totalling 25 images per page, and the pages and images are numbered, corresponding with the 'Indice'. Most portraits are captioned with the patient's name and admission date, these spanning from 1874 to 1902. Unlike the first album, which compares patient appearances before and after treatment, this album likely served as an admission register to aid in recognition and identification.

The first album from San Clemente, titled simply *Fotografie*, has 80 pages with 1,578 portraits of female patients. The photos are 5x9 cm *carte de visite* albumen prints, arranged in four rows and five columns, for a total of 20 portraits per page. Each page and photo is numbered, the pictures are captioned with the patient's name, and 'M. Bertani Oreste. Fotografo' is signed at the bottom of each page. This album likely served as a photographic addition to an admission register, similar to the second album of San Servolo. The pictures date to 1881 and 1882, as Bertani was initially paid in August 1882, with the first pictures appearing on records from 1881–82, and the second album is dated to 1883 (Fig. 40).

The second album from San Clemente, titled *Ritratti fotografici delle dementi nel manicomio di S. Clemente negli anni 1883–1887*, has 80 pages with 1,578 photos; the photos are *carte de visite* format, 5x9 cm albumen prints. Some pages have blank spaces and some photos are missing. This is the most difficult album to interpret as most portraits are numbered without names or diagnoses. Occasionally, notes such as 'Morta' (Dead) or 'Uscita' (Discharged) are added. Dates are added sparingly and the numbering of the pictures is not always sequential. Only a few portraits have a precise discharge date for the patient annotated in their captions. On the second page, number 28 is likely missing, leaving at least two spaces blank between numbers 27 and 29. Following number 31, there is a second picture of patient number 29 with the note 'Uscita', likely indicating discharge. After this, there is a different picture of number 11 with no note in the caption. The portraits then continue without blanks, but the next portrait is numbered 34, skipping 32 and 33. There is no portrait or blank space between numbers 35 and 37, and this is followed by a

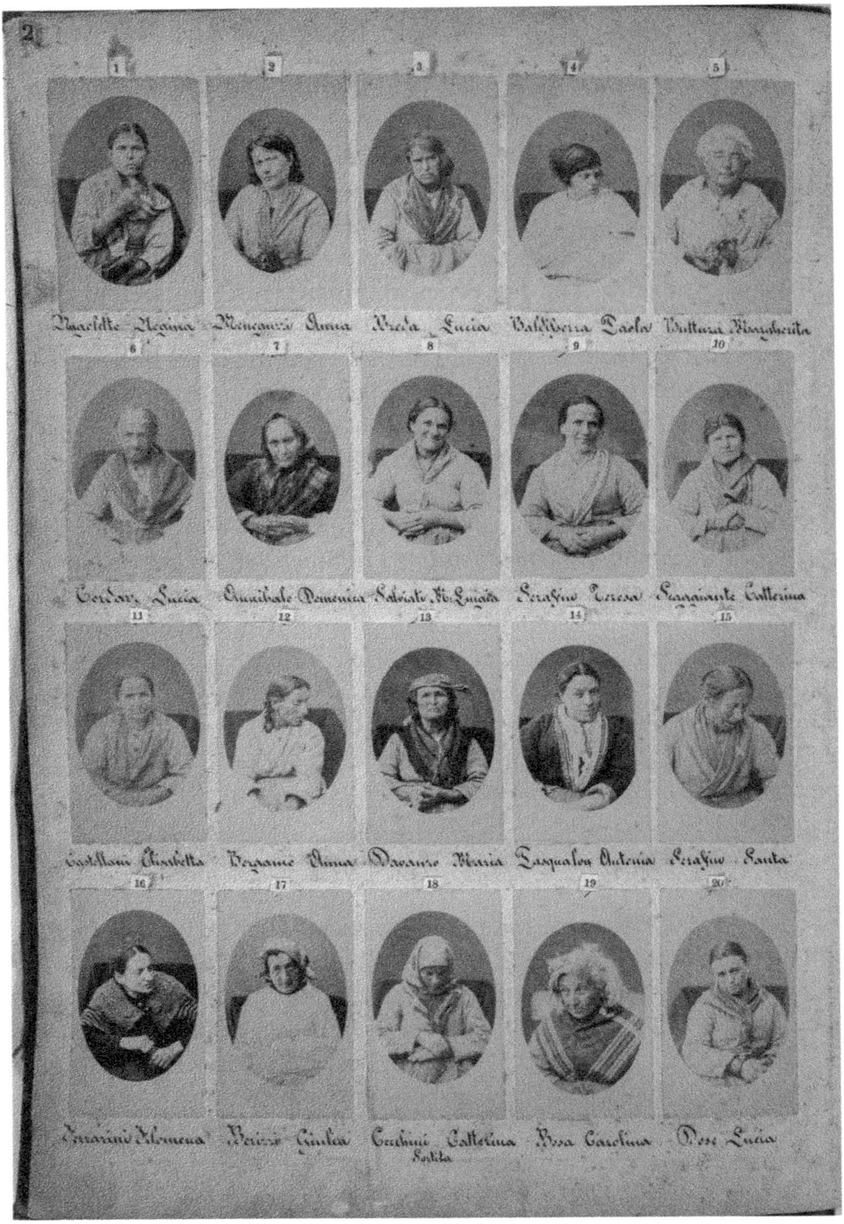

Figure 40: First page of the first album of San Clemente. Courtesy of Archivio storico di San Servolo – San Servolo srl – Città metropolitana di Venezia.

discharge picture of number 15 with the note 'Uscita'. After a blank space, the numbering continues with 38 and 39. Without blanks, the sequence includes the portrait of number 44, noted as 'morta', and then a discharge picture of 24, noted as 'sortita'. On page 3, the first picture is number 32, followed by 40, 46, 47, with then continuous numbering. Page 4 continues this sequence, interrupted only by some discharge pictures of previous patients and a hole where a portrait was crudely removed with a sharp blade. This pattern of continuous numbering interrupted by discharge pictures persists throughout the album. Occasionally, there are full-print images of patients in their environment, sometimes with their trade instruments (e.g., p. 12, third picture in the first row, uncaptioned; p. 14, row 3, picture 3), half-length portraits not in an oval (e.g., p. 15, row 1, picture 2) or full-length ones (e.g., p. 21, row 2, picture 1). Some full-length portraits hint at the diagnosis, such as the praying attitude of the patient on page 26, row 2, picture 1. From page 16, the album is organised as a comparative one, with each admission picture paired with a discharge one on the right. However, several photos were probably never taken, resulting in numerous gaps. Additionally, many photos are the same as those in the first album. The album could seemingly be regarded as a transitional album from individual portraits to a comparative style, pairing admission and discharge photos. Many gaps indicate missing discharge pictures. The album is not signed by Bertani, although he was likely the photographer. This album appears more experimental, with staff assembling it from 1883 onward, unlike the earlier, more systematically arranged album.

The third album from San Clemente has the same binding as the first. A badly scratched label bears the title *Ritratti fotografici delle dementi per gli anni 1888–1890* and it is divided into annual sections. Each page has four rows of three pictures, most of which are incomplete. Each picture is captioned with the patient's name. In the pages for 1888 (1–16), the first column of each page always has pictures captioned with '1 F', meaning first photo, sometimes followed by a second picture of the same patient, captioned '2 F', or a blank space, or a different patient's picture. Starting from page 17, the first of 1889, the original idea of the album's format becomes clear. Each two-page spread contains four rows of pictures arranged in six columns, totalling 12 pairs of admission/discharge pictures per spread. Not all patients have both pictures and there are numerous blank spaces. From page 45, the captions '1 F' and '2 F' disappear, leaving only the names, with occasional out-of-place pictures (e.g., at page 51, where Fioravanti's portrait replaces the expected discharge picture of Mietto

Teresa). The style of the pictures is comparable to those in previous albums, suggesting they were still taken exclusively by Bertani.

The fourth album from San Clemente has the same binding as the second and features portraits in the *carte de visite* format. It contains 887 photographs arranged in 74 pages, with three rows of five pictures each per page. Photos are glued directly to the page without a frame. Many pictures are missing and the album is generally less organised than the previous ones. Only a few portraits are captioned, in pencil, likely with the patient's surname. While some pictures might be admission/discharge pairs, the lack of captions makes this difficult to confirm. Some patients appear to have two consecutive portraits, but these do not seem to be comparative pairs as both depict a florid period of their 'insanity'. Closer inspection revealed that this album consisted solely of duplicates from previous albums, and likely served as a repository for duplicates or outtakes, as suggested by the missing, unglued pictures.

The fifth and final preserved album from San Clemente is notably different. Bertani received his final photographer fee on 10 January 1891, the same year the asylum's director, Vigna, resigned. The photos in this album were clearly taken by a different, less-experienced photographer, resulting in several overexposed, out-of-focus pictures with inconsistent framing and poorly curated poses. The photos are also printed on lower-quality paper, harshly cut and glued without frames in four rows of four pictures per page. Pencil guidelines for aligning the pictures and space for captions and comments are present, but no photos have captions. The album contains a total of 295 portraits, with some photos missing.

The other medical records held in the archive of San Servolo and San Clemente provide an interesting picture of the relationship, or lack thereof, between the photo of the patient and their medical information.

San Servolo's medical records evolved significantly over the years. In 1842, the *Tabella da appendersi al letto del maniaco* was introduced and was renamed to *Tabella del maniaco* in 1843. By 1857, a more detailed template was introduced, incorporating extensive patient information such as name, birth details, occupation and marital status, and also included sections for a historical summary of the illness and details of treatment progression, alongside a space for the diagnosis. The influence of Esquirol's nosology was evident in the nomenclature used, and an area at the bottom right of the page was reserved for discharge or death dates. The inclusion of patient photographs began with records from 1874, with Odorico Bortolo's case, admitted for 'mania orgogliosa per amor deluso' in 1870. Oval albumen prints, approximately 7x5 cm in size, were affixed to the records, possibly upon admission but more likely upon discharge for easier patient identification. Following Salerio's tenure, under Giacinto Videmari's direction, San Servolo's medical records adopted a more structured approach and began to note physical constitution, nutritional state and a detailed phrenopathic diagnosis that started to include considerations related to heredity and organic conditions. Subsequent years saw further refinements in the templates, coexisting with earlier versions, and a gradual increase in the inclusion of patient portraits, both upon admission and discharge. Only in 1916 was a standardised template with a designated space for patient photographs adopted.

In San Clemente, the medical records were rather different. The asylum opened in 1873, with Vigna, a pupil of Salerio, as its first director. While Salerio had already started using photography in San Servolo, Vigna did not adopt the practice until nine years into his tenure. The earliest preserved photographs in San Clemente date to 1881 or 1882, confirmed by the first payment to the professional photographer Bertani on 9 August 1882 and the appearance of portraits in the 1881–82 medical records. The first medical record with a photograph is that of Meduna Antonia, admitted on 20 September 1881 with a diagnosis of 'demenza consecutiva'; she was discharged on 20 June 1882 (Fig. 41). Her portrait also appears in San Clemente's first album, at page 3, portrait 3, with the note 'sortita' (exited). Sadly there is no direct reference made between the medical record and the album's numbering, making cross-referencing challenging. Most charts in the folder relate to patients admitted in 1881 or 1882 and discharged in 1882, but some exceptions complicate the dating and scope of the photographs. For example, Businelli Teresa's record features a portrait in Bertani's style, although she was admitted on 20 March 1876 and discharged on 19 February 1885. Her portrait appears in San Clemente's first album, at page 12, photo 5, and suggests that Bertani's task was to photograph all patients, whether upon admission, discharge or mid-stay, although this was likely not done systematically. From 1883, Bertani seems to have focused on taking admission and discharge photos for the comparative albums. Unlike San Servolo, from 1882 onwards, most San Clemente medical records featured patient portraits, and by 1905, a record template with a dedicated space for the photograph was adopted.

Perhaps the most striking feature of the medical records from both San Servolo and San Clemente is how little they correspond

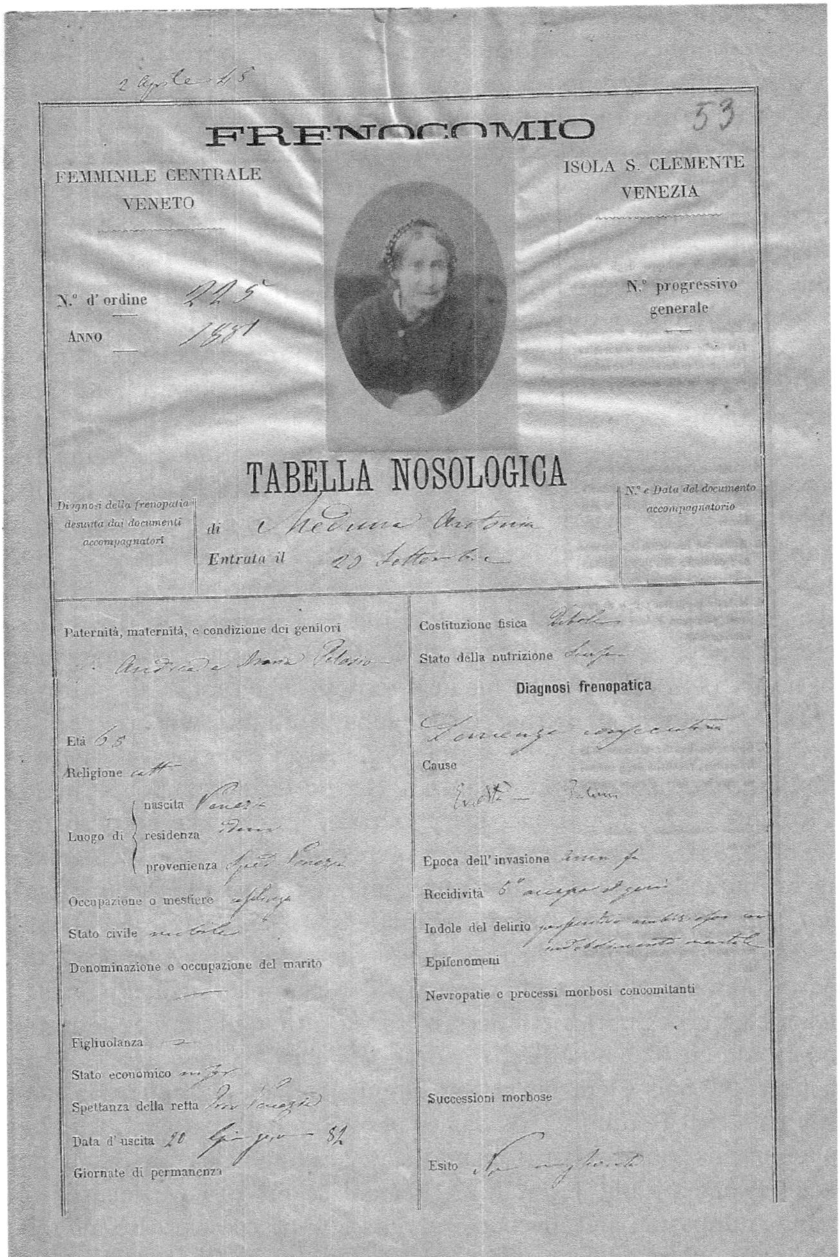

FRENOCOMIO

FEMMINILE CENTRALE VENETO

ISOLA S. CLEMENTE VENEZIA

N.° d' ordine

ANNO

N.° progressivo generale

TABELLA NOSOLOGICA

Diagnosi della frenopatia desunta dai documenti accompagnatori

di

Entrata il

N.° e Data del documento accompagnatorio

Paternità, maternità, e condizione dei genitori

Età

Religione

Luogo di: nascita, residenza, provenienza

Occupazione o mestiere

Stato civile

Denominazione o occupazione del marito

Figliuolanza

Stato economico

Spettanza della retta

Data d' uscita

Giornate di permanenza

Costituzione fisica

Stato della nutrizione

Diagnosi frenopatica

Cause

Epoca dell' invasione

Recidività

Indole del delirio

Epifenomeni

Nevropatie e processi morbosi concomitanti

Successioni morbose

Esito

Figure 41: Sample medical record from San Clemente. Courtesy of Archivio storico di San Servolo – San Servolo srl – Città metropolitana di Venezia.

to the photographic albums. Apart from the patient's name, it is almost impossible to quickly cross-reference the two sets of visual data. This remains true even for those records from the last decade of the nineteenth century, when the use of photography in psychiatric medical records in Venice was well established. Therefore, regardless of whether the albums were intended as simple visual supplements to an admission/discharge register, as an admission/discharge register themselves, as an archive of duplicates in case a picture was lost or simply as a tool for facilitating identification, the organisational system in place made it very difficult to actually use them effectively. This indicates that photographic albums in Venetian asylums existed somewhat independently from the medical records and should be considered cultural artefacts in their own right. While most, if not all, pictures in the comparative albums also appeared in the medical records, within the albums they assumed an independent significance, not necessarily linked to the patient's identity or the institution's need to identify them. In the comparative album, each photograph of each patient loses the individuality and singularity required for identification purposes; instead, it becomes part of a sequence of data, where the patient's identity is obscured. The only features that matter in the picture are the visual manifestations of the illness and the healing power of the institution. The illness is visually interpreted as chaos, unkemptness and disarray, while the institution's power is understood as the ability to restore order and reason to the irrational chaos of madness.

Reggio Emilia: The Diagnostic Album and Physiognomics

Among the first asylums to employ photography, second only to Venice and Aversa, was Reggio Emilia's San Lazzaro asylum. The buildings of the San Lazzaro mental asylum in Reggio Emilia, like many similar structures across Europe, originally served as a leper colony. San Lazzaro transitioned into a mental asylum in the seventeenth century, and in the 1820s, director Antonio Galloni renovated the facility. Inspired by advancements in French alienism, he abandoned physical coercion in favour of moral therapy and ergotherapy. However, Galloni's golden age was short-lived and conditions worsened until Carlo Livi took over in 1873. Under Livi, San Lazzaro gained a vast library, a craniological museum, a histological lab, a lab for experimental psychology, a new pharmacy with a lab for chemical analysis and an electrotherapeutic cabinet. The asylum became a major centre for psychiatric research in Italy, collaborating closely with the University of Modena and launching the journal *Rivista sperimentale di freniatria* in 1875,[3] which is still in publication.

San Lazzaro's development as both a hospital and a research hub peaked under Livi's successor, Augusto Tamburini, who directed the asylum from 1877 to 1907 while serving as a professor of psychiatry in Modena. Tamburini expanded the use of ergotherapy, introduced therapeutic singing and drawing lessons, and implemented one of Italy's first outpatient care systems, the *Società di assistenza per malati dimessi o convalescenti* (Society for the Assistance of Discharged or Convalescent Patients), along with a foster care system. He also established a professional school for psychiatric nurses and custodians at San Lazzaro.

Tamburini's most significant innovation for us was his creation of a photographic studio in 1878, initially managed by Emilio Poli, who joined San Lazzaro in 1872 as a copyist, then became a cloakroom attendant in 1876 and from 1877 onward was a self-taught photographer. Poli's equipment was rudimentary, producing albumen prints in *carte de visite* (CdV) format, as was customary at the time. After Poli's death in 1899, Giovanni Morini, a former patient, took over the role of photographer.

In reference to Poli's work as a photographer in San Lazzaro, Tamassia authored the only paper specifically addressing the use of photography in psychiatry in Italian, which I mentioned above. This article appeared in San Lazzaro's journal, *Gazzetta del Frenocomio di Reggio*. After noting that Tamburini was following in Saverio and Virgilio's footsteps, Tamassia praises photography for permanently capturing the physiognomies of patients in various phases of their illnesses, thereby supporting the study of the semiotics of mental illnesses. Tamassia begins with a description of San Lazzaro's idyllic premises and lists the innovations introduced over the years, including the telegraph and later the telephone. Among these innovations, Tamassia was most interested in photography, which, at San Lazzaro, he remarks, is devoid of the exotic and mysterious art of portraiture and *tableaux vivants*. There are no 'perfumed antechambers [...] decorated with liveries and precious tapestries' or the 'dark, mysterious cell' in which to contemplate 'shy beauties', as Tamassia (2011, 11) puts it. In Reggio Emilia, asylum photography is done in daylight, without a studio, and the darkroom is amateurishly assembled by the

3 *Frenatria* was used to refer to psychiatry to avoid any reference to the 'psyche', which sounded too spiritual. The root *phrenos*—broadly speaking 'the nerves' in ancient Greek—suggested a more organic and scientific approach (Donnelly 2003, 30).

'good' Mr Poli, as Tamassia calls him. Poli's 'clients' are the patients, who demand no idealisation of their physiognomies and repay the services of the 'good Poli' either with a 'cheerful cry of genuine joy' or with a curse (Tamassia 2011, 11). What is significant about their attitudes in front of the camera is that, according to Tamassia, the patients behave more genuinely and present themselves as they truly are, rather than posing in the 'buffoonish or tragic positions in which most photographs of the sane are draped': 'madmen simply do not know these diplomatic lies' (Tamassia 2011, 12). Because of the patients' ingenuousness and naivety, the camera can capture the essence of insanity, which cannot be faked or posed. If madness is thus self-evident and transparent, then photography is the perfect medium to reveal this self-evidence. It is because of this transparent, genuine and open behaviour of madmen in front of the camera that their pictures become such an important scientific instrument: 'from this natural and spontaneous pose of the madman emerges the great value of the images obtained, for from these we can often trace the hidden and tyrannical idea that crushes a poor mind' (Tamassia 2011, 12). The symptom is thus fixed onto paper and the illness becomes evident in the picture: from the praying position adopted by those affected by religious monomania, to the tense face and semi-open, immobile eyes of those tormented by hallucinations, to the exposed breast of the girl suffering from erotic monomania, the candid smile of the euphoric maniac or the vapid one of the fatuous, and so on. Each diagnosis is assigned specific visual characteristics that can be captured by the camera.

If, for the sane, photographs serve as memories, for the insane 'who vegetate', what utility can they possibly have? First of all, remarks Tamassia, the insane are not always alone and their families cherish the tranquil pose they naturally assume in front of the camera. For the family of the insane, perusing a picture of their beloved is a consolation, even more so if it is the picture taken upon discharge, the last one in the comparative pair: 'the last photograph arrives: it is that of the healed man!' (Tamassia 2011, 14), although, strangely enough, no comparative album or pair of pictures is preserved in the archives of San Lazzaro. Photography is also useful for the patients, mostly as a 'reward' and as an instrument of 'moral therapy': 'one of the many moral means by which the alienist tries to guide those poor minds, or to restrain deliriums' (Tamassia 2011, 14). Where photography truly excels, however, is when used as a scientific tool. Tamassia recalls Darwin's and Duchenne's studies on human expression, which revealed the 'sublime law of the transformation of living types' (Tamassia 2011, 14). Where can evolution best reveal itself if not in a collection of pictures of the mentally ill? Tamassia argues: 'here the expression is completely spontaneous, unaffected by anything conventional or imposed [...] thus we are faced with a true physiological experiment offered by nature' (Tamassia 2011, 14). Therefore, photography has several uses in psychiatry and science in general, according to Tamassia. First, it forms the basis for physiognomic investigations, capturing spontaneous expressions and offering a permanent record for study. This reveals, by unspecified means, 'the traces of very remote atavisms' (Tamassia 2011, 15) written on the face and the evolutionary paths from animals to humans. Second, it grounds the alienist's diagnosis in visible evidence and serves as an important teaching aid. Third, it aids in identification, allowing the asylum director to instantly recognise 'his patients' and create an 'iconographic census'. Tamassia's article, albeit in more emphatic, even poetic terms, displays similarities with Diamond's: photography aids diagnosis through physiognomy, helps the patients and enables identification.

Photography might have arrived in San Lazzaro after the pioneering work of San Servolo; however, its archives, in terms of its photographic material and variety, compare favourably with those from San Servolo and San Clemente. They amount to 27 albums of different sizes and contents, totalling more than 1,500 photos, which include portraits of patients, group photos, pictures taken at conferences and architectural images of the premises, and range in date from the late 1870s to the late 1930s. The most relevant for us here are the first five albums (A1 to A5) and the albums that collate the photos for display (C1 to C4).

Albums A1 to A3 can only now be consulted in digital format as the originals are in such poor condition. Album A1 is a small photographic album containing 48 CdV albumen prints of female patients' portraits, one per page, and most pictures are cut into an oval shape and mounted on cardboard. With a few exceptions, such as with Zanelli Esterina, admitted on 22 October 1877 (page 6), the photos are uncaptioned. This, along with the fact that the albumen prints vary in their states of preservation, displaying different levels of fungal colonisation, makes precise dating challenging. It is likely that the photos were taken at different times and possibly with different emulsions, but we do know that all were taken by Poli and were among his earliest works. Notably, some of the cardboard mounts for the photos are bright white, indicating a restoration attempt in recent years. The portraits are mostly medium-level close-ups, with some close-ups of the face, while the women portrayed exhibit a variety of expressions but are all posed. Technically, one picture is out of focus and two are motion-blurred due to camera movement.

Album A2 is a larger collection, containing a total of 100 photographs in various formats, cut into irregular rectangular shapes and pasted onto the pages in different arrangements (Fig. 42). The first eight pages are captioned by hand, while the following pages are not, but according to them all the photos were taken between October and November 1892 and are attributed to Poli. Although the photos are catalogued as 'aristotypes', the loss of detail over time, the tone of the images and the amateur level of the printing suggest they are more likely albumen prints. The photographs are diverse in nature; several were taken outside and depict female patients either alone or in groups, in natural poses and settings. The first page features a 'Group of Idiots' with shaved heads, seated in front of a door-window in the courtyard, and the subsequent pages display individual portraits of female patients posing naturally against a wall, outside in daylight. Several pictures are out of focus, motion-blurred by camera or subject movement, and/or overexposed. The captions include the patient's name, diagnosis and sometimes admission date. What stands out most about these pictures is how the poses clearly relate to the diagnoses. In the centre of page 2, Leonide Vandelli, diagnosed with 'acute recurrent mania', is portrayed standing and moving her arms, similar to Maria Sgarbi on the following page. On page 3, top right, Maria Boiardi, diagnosed with lypemania, appears to be weeping in an out-of-focus mid-close-up. On page 4, Regina Bratti is kneeling with hands joined in prayer, and is described as being diagnosed with 'religious paranoia'. On the following page, Ersilia Babbini, elegantly dressed, is featured in a counter-*plongée* portrait with her chin up, not looking at the camera, and is diagnosed with the 'delusions of grandeur' phase of 'progressive paralysis'. From a photographic technique perspective, it is interesting to note that several darker pictures on the following pages are captioned 'by magnesium light', indicating the use of the first form of flash photography.

Two main considerations can be drawn from this album. The first is that the inconsistency in technique, pose and subject may suggest that these were test photos. Given that Poli had been working as a photographer for at least ten years by 1892, it is plausible that these were experiments with new equipment or a trial to systematise the visual admission registers, as the album's organisation is rather incoherent. The second consideration concerns the correspondence between gestures/poses and diagnoses. This visual language and the use of photography to 'document' the

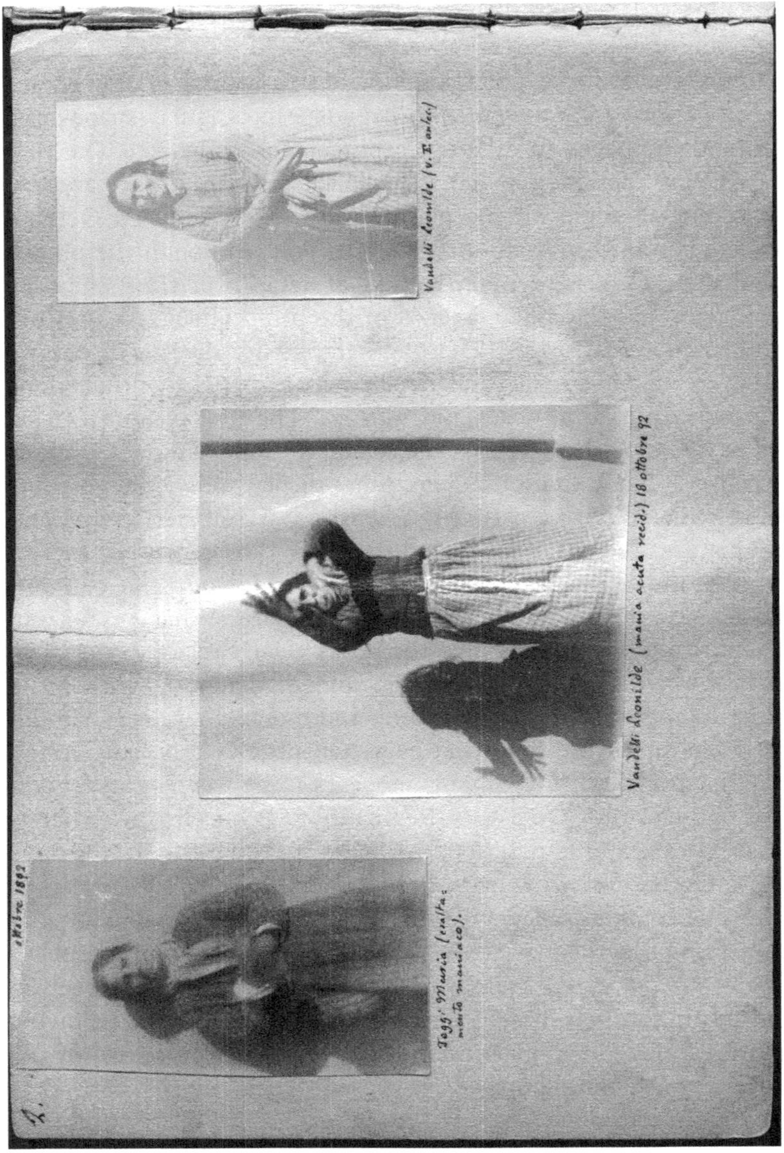

Figure 42: First page of San Lazzaro's Album A2. Courtesy of Archivio dell'ex ospedale psichiatrico San Lazzaro di Reggio Emilia – Ausl RE.

demeanour of the insane is reminiscent of Charcot's iconographic work at Salpêtrière 30 years earlier. The roots of this visual language date back well before psychiatry and photography. They are rooted in occupational photography first of all: portraits of workers from various social strata, commissioned by the workers themselves, featuring specific props to instantly indicate their line of work. Numerous such pictures are found in Bertani's portraits of San Clemente. Here, gestures and demeanour become the 'props' of specific diagnoses, forming a visual system of symbolic reference that connects psychiatry to photography, following the tradition of classic physiognomy. At the same time though, occupational photography itself drew from established conventions in painting, where the use of carefully placed props was meant to reveal otherwise hidden traits and characteristics of the subject.

Album A3 is in a very poor state of preservation. Each page was originally designed to contain four photos in pre-cut cardboard ovals, but several are torn and many photos have been lost. The first picture in the album, taken by the Plaff brothers from La Spezia, portrays a construction site, likely at San Lazzaro, but all the other pictures are most likely taken by Poli and are oval-shaped albumen prints of both male and female patients. Some of these photos are captioned directly on the image with the patient's name and admission date, and some also include the diagnosis. These captions are revealed only on the torn pages, as otherwise they would be covered by the cardboard mounts of the album. Notably, this album contains fewer out-of-focus or motion-blurred pictures compared to the previous ones.

Of greater interest for our purposes are the archival units referred to as albums C1 to C4, which include photos of patients mounted on cardboard, complete with captions. These photos were intended for display, either at conferences or during lectures. Indeed, some might have been noteworthy cases to showcase at international exhibitions or to present at conferences, or exemplary cases to illustrate diagnostic theories. Album C1 features two photos: a frontal, slightly-to-the-right profile and the back of the head of a male patient, both in the usual CdV format, mounted on oval cardboard. The title is 'Imbecillità epilettica' and the caption reads: '[Name Redacted] di anni 15. Frattura al cranio a due mesi di età. Scopertura del cervello nella regione parieto-occipitale destra, per un'estensione di cm 18,5x6,5. Emiepilessia, emiatrofia, emiparesi sinistra'. Album C2 features six portraits of patients (five men and one woman) which are albumen prints, arranged in three rows of two pictures each. The top row is captioned 'Paralitici', the middle row 'Pellagrosi' and

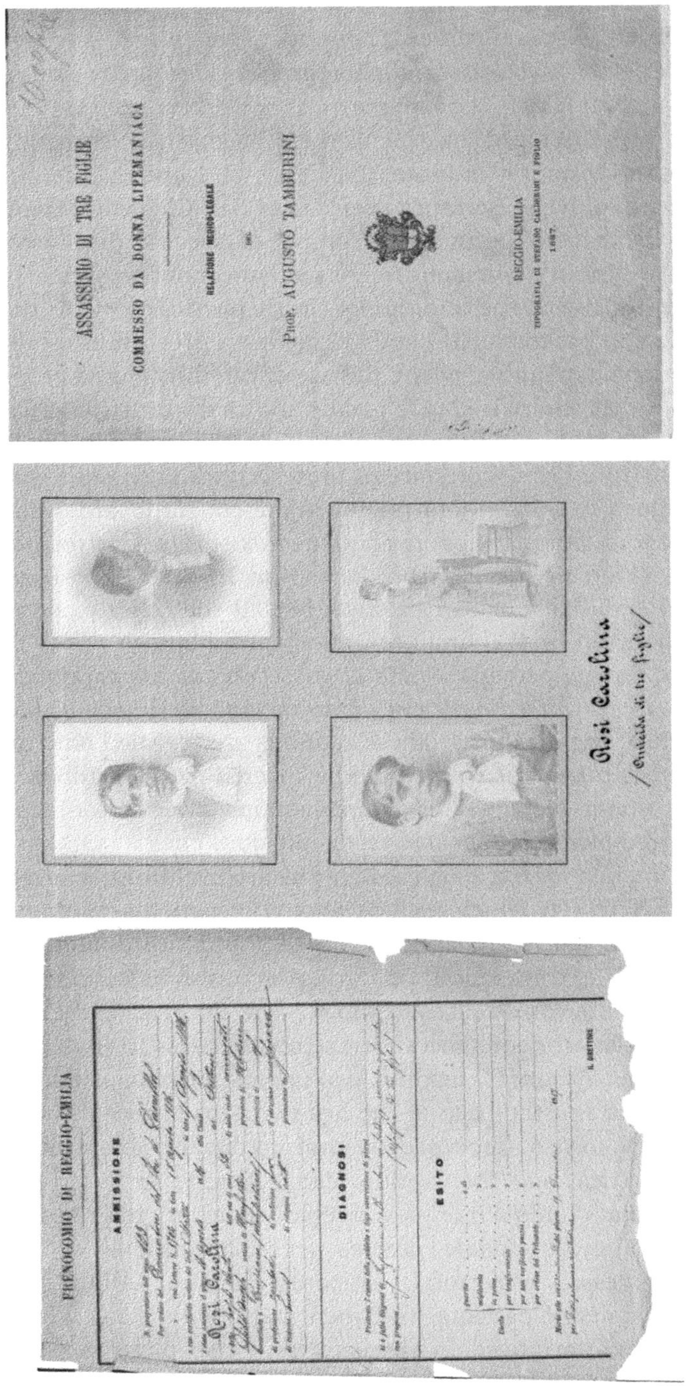

Figure 43: Rosi Carolina from left: medical record, framed photos, forensic expertise. Courtesy of Archivio dell'ex ospedale psichiatrico San Lazzaro di Reggio Emilia – Ausl RE.

the bottom row 'pazzi morali'. Album C3 is another single sheet of cardboard, entitled 'Pazzia Periodica', and features five oval portraits of women, arranged in a manner slightly reminiscent of 'trophies'. A smaller caption at the bottom right reads: 'fotografia del frenocomio'. Album C4 consists of two sheets of cardboard, one with nine portraits and the other with eight, all of male patients in CdV format and oval shape. Some portraits are frontal, while others are profile shots and there are no captions.

Another similar set of display pictures is held in the archive. It is a framed sheet of cardboard in which four CdV portraits of the same patient are mounted: a full frontal in oval, a profile in oval, a mid-close-up demi-profile filling the entire picture and a full-body profile of the patient leaning on a chair. The subject is Carolina Rosi, who, as the caption reads, was 'omicida di tre figlie' (Fig. 43). Augusto Tamburini himself wrote the forensic expert witness report (relazione medico-legale), which was published in issue twelve of the *Rivista sperimentale di freniatria* and as a standalone text in 1887. According to her medical record, Carolina was admitted in 1886 by request of the public prosecutor, with a diagnosis of hallucinatory lypemania with homicidal tendencies. She died in the asylum at the end of 1887 from tuberculosis. Carolina Rosi's medical record includes another portrait of her, a mid-close-up against a wall, in a larger format, framed in cardboard (not glued). Carolina Rosi's is an exception though, since the majority of medical records in San Lazzaro did not feature a picture, unlike those of San Servolo and San Clemente. Only from 1904–1905 onwards do some medical records include a glued portrait of the patient (for instance, Fortunato Bernardoni, admitted in 1905 for senile melancholic dementia, and Vittorio Ferrari, admitted in 1904 for paralytic dementia). On the medical record template, there is no dedicated space for the photo, however, which is glued to the right of the second section, titled 'Diagnosis'.

The ovals attached to medical records are the same as those that appear in albums A4 and A5, which are admission registers and diagnostic albums of male patients, admitted in 1903–1904 and 1905–1906 respectively. These are large albums, containing 144 and 409 photos respectively, arranged in three rows of five pictures per page. The photos are catalogued as aristotypes and each photo is captioned with the name, admission date and diagnosis of the patient. The author of the photos is Giovanni Morini, a former inmate who succeeded Poli as the photographer of the asylum in San Lazzaro. Album A5 shows clearly that on some pages some of the pictures have been glued on top of other, similarly sized pictures.

Portraits, Photography and the Archive

Even within the rather niche field of psychiatric photography, canonical historiography often dictates the interpretations. Italian studies of both Italian and international psychiatric photography have largely adhered to a Foucauldian narrative to explain the surge in the use of photography in psychiatry, a trend that emerges also in studies beyond Italy (Godbey 2000). This adherence to Foucault is likely influenced by the strong reformist, radical and 'anti-psychiatric' movement that emerged in Italy from the 1960s onwards, which brought the country into the international spotlight. This movement profoundly affected the visualisation of mental disorders and had a significant impact on visual culture in general, so I will return to it in chapter seven in more detail. In concluding this section on photography, I will just focus on this canonical interpretation. Doing so allows us to understand how a historical corpus of images has been integrated into more recent discussions, particularly within the context of the radical shifts in psychiatric practice and visual representation that have shaped contemporary perspectives.

In the nineteenth century, psychiatry was trying to establish itself as a scientific and medical discipline, which necessitated an organic basis for diagnosis, study and intervention to justify its place in medicine. The brain and nervous system were the chosen areas of focus for this. However, they were not tangible enough, and insufficient progress was made to convincingly connect them to the aetiology of mental disorders (more on this in the next chapter). Critics agree that photography was the observational tool psychiatrists adopted to probe the body and identify signs of mental disorders. Bollati, for instance, asserts that 'in order to make a diagnosis of social danger scientific, it was necessary to anchor [photography] to measurable gestures, and only the body is measurable' (Bollati 1979, 7). Terzian (1981, 24) argues that 'at the moment the camera shutter clicked, the entire individual and collective history of the photographed subject was automatically erased [...] the resulting image, whatever it was [...] returned mechanical phenomena caused by the anatomical or functional damage of the hypothesised disease'. 'All this', he continues, 'through two continuous processes: distancing from oneself and scientific manipulation of the image' (Terzian 1981, 22).

Dalla Palma adds, 'the photographic eye, in the act of seeing and fixing the madman, circumscribes a world of possibilities, but also annihilates certain conditions of communication, turning the subject back into an abstraction, the patient into a disease, within a practice of classification and comprehension that is not always fully aware of its procedures and aporias'. Dalla Palma (1981, 10) thus notes that photography is used to abstract the subject and focus only on the diseases, while Fornaciari (2005, 107) argues that photography short-circuited 'empirical observation and nosological entity'. Bolis comments that photography allowed psychiatrists to create catalogues of mental disorders and showcase madness as manageable by the institution (Bolis 2009). Muzzarelli (2009, 21) adds to this that photography was used to distance the subjects suffering from mental disorders.

This thesis likely originated from the seminal exhibition held during the Venice Biennale in 1981, *Nascita della fotografia psichiatrica,* curated by visual anthropologist Franco Cagnetta. In the catalogue, he writes,

> when psychiatry was born with the pretension of being a medical and naturalistic science, which sought in the body the origin of the disorders it dealt with, it had to seek an anatomical basis that originated them: an organ. When it was realised that it was not possible to demonstrate with certainty what the organic site and anatomical basis of the 'disorders' were, psychiatry began to take an interest in 'physiognomy', which suggested a diagnosis through the 'organ' of the face. From the beginning of the nineteenth century, it began to study drawn portraits of madmen, that is, an image of the madman. (Cagnetta 1981, 33)

This thesis became so widespread that it can be considered the canonical interpretation of psychiatric photography. The most prominent proponent is Schinaia, who asserts that

> the reproduced image, replacing the bodily substrate, gives the illusion of a 'natural substrate'. This illusion was decisively favoured by the emergence of photography as a medium, considered in the mid-nineteenth century as an objective and certain reproduction of nature. In the absence of a 'real' anatomy in which the disease originates, the photographic image of the madman became the mythical anatomy of psychiatry. (Schinaia 2004, 460)

This thesis is deeply rooted in a Foucauldian conception of psychiatry as a form of disciplinary power, and suggests that psychiatry turned to physiognomics because it could not find other organic substrata. However, this interpretation overlooks the research on the biological origins and treatments for mental disorders which had been taking place before and after the rise and fall of psychiatric photography. In Italy, such photography primarily took place in asylums and most scholarly publications on psychiatry avoided discussing it or physiognomics, focusing instead on other aspects of mental disorders. According to the canonical history, this 'iconographic fervour', as Tagliabue (1993, 30) calls it, fades 'in step with the decline of the theories that supported its utility', such as an exclusively organicist approach to psychiatry and physiognomic studies. According to this standard interpretation, what primarily remains is judicial photography used to identify mental patients. The focus also shifted to architectural shots of asylum facilities, highlighting their organised and well-equipped nature, occasionally also featuring blurred images of patients and staff. Such portrayals remained largely unchanged until the 1960s when photography began to expose the harsh realities of asylums, capturing images of restraint beds, straitjackets, peepholes, dilapidated rooms and the degrading daily lives of patients (Tagliabue 1993, 30–31).

Since the advent of psychiatric photography, portraits of the mentally ill have been collected in asylum archives for alleged scientific purposes, namely: to facilitate prolonged study of diagnoses, to compare the progression of illnesses across successive images and to compare portraits of various patients. This diagnostic aspect is a continuation of the physiognomic and phrenologic tradition; instead of drawings of reference, now we have photographs. To this extent it is interesting to note that in the context of psychiatry, Galton's composite photography was hardly used. Photography was not a universalising tool, but a way to illustrate and exemplify the general theory of physiognomics.

The asylum photographic archive adds a new dimension to photography and the visualisation of mental disorders. It possesses a control mechanism that, although claimed to be strictly 'medical', is inherently administrative as well. It is not incidental that the use of identification photography to monitor individuals and social groups originated in asylums before being officially adopted by the police and courts, after Bertillon (1890) postulated its importance. Diamond had already praised photography as an instrument to identify patients in case of relapses and readmissions, for instance. He did not seem, however, to advocate for a systematisation of this, and thus his pictures did not seem to exercise this function. The creation of administrative records in state and public asylums, such as the Italian ones we explored above, introduced a political purpose for institutional use and misuse, and by the 1880s, psychiatric photography began to be commonplace in asylums almost worldwide. The purpose of these portraits shifted predominantly towards identification and classification, to recognise those previously institutionalised and to track them in case of escape. Psychiatric photography evolved from a diagnostic tool that continued the tradition of physiognomy, to a judicial instrument aimed at the individuation and identification of those who deviated from the established norm. As Tagg (1988, 17) noted, the camera became entangled with institutional practices and their disciplinary purposes. Identification photos removed individuality and agency from the insane and the criminal to the point that they can be considered forms of cultural subordination.

As D'Autilia (2012, 114) notes,

> it will take a hundred years for what is now treated as a 'photographic object' to return to being a 'subject'. The psychiatric case is indicative of the cultural and social constraints that determine what is photographable: faces do not change, their reading does, then they invited us to read madness, later social exclusion.

Schinaia concurs, stating that in the 1960s with documentary photography 'the original relationship facies/madness is replaced by the all-encompassing symmetry *facies*/social exclusion' (Schinaia 2004, 471). Although this reading is not entirely incorrect, it is a vast oversimplification that relies on a Foucauldian reading of Italian psychiatric history in connection with the notion that Italy lags behind other countries. While certainly peculiar—as I will continue to show in chapter seven in reference to anti-psychiatry and the visualisation of mental disorders—the use of psychiatric photography was also rather reflective of the international context. Additionally, even though a Foucauldian reading is certainly appropriate, further arguments can contribute to the shaping of a more nuanced view of the use of photography in the visualisation of mental disorders, as I have shown in this chapter.

Conclusions

The use of photography in psychiatric institutions is an important milestone in the visual representation of mental disorders, in making madness visible and thus in the visual othering of the insane. The appearance of photography in the mid-nineteenth century reinvigorated the discipline of physiognomics, providing a seemingly objective tool to capture the physical manifestations of mental states.

Photography allowed for the creation of detailed and reproducible images, which were perceived as more reliable than artistic illustrations. This technological advancement brought about new tropes in the visualisation of mental disorders, extending beyond individual portraits to include the systematic documentation of patients within the context of their psychiatric institutions. Photographic images were used to promote the beneficial effects of the asylum, and the order that therapeutic practices could bring both to society and to individuals. We also witness the first therapeutic (or at least pseudo-therapeutic) use of images, namely from such photography.

My analysis of these archives brings us to two main concluding considerations. First, there is a certain level of inconsistency in the photographic techniques, subject matter and criteria for assembling the albums that suggests that these images and archival practices were often experimental. Second, the link between gestures, poses and diagnoses reflects a continuation of the physiognomic tradition, where the visual language of psychiatry borrowed from occupational photography and painting conventions to create a symbolic reference system. This system, as seen in the posed and captioned images, aimed to make the invisible realities of mental disorders visible and comprehensible.

The adoption of photography in asylums, as traditional historiography has it, was likely influenced by a desire to legitimise psychiatry as a medical discipline. Moved by the intention of finding a visual and physical appearance to mental disorder to make psychiatry a serious medical discipline, photographers played an integral part in the visual othering of the insane. As Sturken and Cartwright (2017, 355) note, ‘the camera was [...] a scientific tool for constituting groups of people as Other, different from the socially accepted norm’.

As we noted at the beginning of this chapter, as the interest in the use of photography in psychiatry waned, and became pervasive but devoid of deeper meaning and potential interpretation, psychiatry as a medical discipline sought other means of picturing mental disorders, and scientific and technological progress provided them. This is the topic of the next chapter.

CHAPTER SIX

Madness through the Looking Glass: Visualising Mental Disorders Inside the Body

IN THE PREVIOUS CHAPTER, I analysed the medical attempt to connect the outer appearance of individuals to their inner lives—including mental disorders—by means of photography. This, I argued, continued the tradition of physiognomics. In this chapter, I study a seemingly opposite medical tendency: attempting to make madness visible by looking inside the body. Obviously, these are not opposites; on the contrary, there are numerous continuities and overlaps. Firstly, we could argue that by looking inside the body instead of looking at apparent features we are just shifting the surface to a different layer. This layer is much more concealed than outer features and requires more specialised tools to be observed, but it remains, nevertheless, a surface of visibility onto which the otherwise invisible mental disorder is made visible. Secondly, there is a historical matter that cannot be denied. Despite being discredited, phrenology, as I have mentioned in the previous chapter, established the study of brain localisations, paving the way to the epistemological premises of brain imaging: that cognitive functions, and even personality traits, can be mapped onto different areas of the brain, whose activity can be seen and visualised. Finally, photography itself paved the way to a series of imaging techniques—starting with X-ray—that enabled humans to make visible the insides of the body in a mechanical and non-representational way.

Following Sturken and Cartwright's example, in this chapter I hold good that 'scientific, technical, and informational images and looking practices are no less historically and culturally situated than are other images and media' (Sturken and Cartwright 2017, 340). Studying scientific visualisations of mental disorders as situated within their cultural context is one aspect of this chapter; the other is to study them to comprehend

> how contemporary ideas about 'truth' in scientific practices are often the product of particular visual discourses and practices. Social and cultural meanings are assigned to that which is visible and measurable, and those meanings change over time; we nonetheless rely on these meanings to make claims about universal facts and bodily truths. (Sturken and Cartwright 2017, 355)

From Phrenology to Brain Imaging

As discussed in chapter four, Gall's phrenology was one of the earliest attempts to link brain function to behaviour. Gall also believed that the brain was composed of multiple distinct organs, each responsible for different aspects of personality and behaviour. Despite its popularity, phrenology lacked any scientific validity and was discredited rather quickly. By examining the bumps on a person's skull, it became clear that phrenologists could not determine character traits or mental abilities. However, the notion that the brain was made of discreet organs, each presiding over different functions, paved the way to brain localisations, and with it, to the quest for representing or, better still, *observing* and photographing the brain and its centres in action and in vivo. Famously, in 1848, John Martyn Harlow documented what is considered neuroscience's 'patient 0' (Macmillan 2001, 2004; Macmillan and Lena 2010). It was the incident in which Phineas Gage's frontal lobe was penetrated by an iron rod during an accident while blasting rocks for a railway line. This incident became pivotal in developing brain localisations for two reasons. The first is that despite a large part of the brain being destroyed, the patient survived and retained most cognitive, sensory and motor functions. The second is that his personality changed radically, suggesting, at the very least, that the brain is indeed compartmentalised. In 1861, Paul Broca encountered a patient at Bicêtre Hospital who had experienced a 21-year gradual loss of speech and movement, but without losing comprehension or cognitive abilities. Upon conducting an autopsy on the deceased patient, he discovered a lesion in the frontal lobe of the left hemisphere of their brain. In 1865, he published his findings from 12 patient autopsies, encouraging further research to try and correlate various brain regions with sensory and motor functions. A similar discovery had been made by Marc Dax a generation before. Broca's hypothesis was later supported by Gustav Fritsch and Eduard Hitzig in 1870, who discovered that electrical stimulation of the motor cortex induced specific involuntary muscle contractions in dogs. Broca's theory was also subscribed to by John Hughlings Jackson, also in the 1870s, who observed the sequence of seizures in epileptic patients and deduced the organisation of the motor cortex. Carl Wernicke expanded on the theory, highlighting the specialisation of brain areas for language comprehension and production. The brain's architecture was initially made visible through staining techniques, and Otto Deiters was the first to describe nerve cells in their current form in 1865. In the 1870s, Italian physician and scientist Camillo Golgi invented a revolutionary technique known as the 'black reaction' or Golgi staining. This method involved hardening brain tissue in potassium dichromate and then impregnating it with silver nitrate. Golgi's technique allowed for the visualisation of individual neurons in their entirety, and he used this technique to support the reticular theory, according to which the nervous system was a continuous network of fibres. Spanish neuroscientist Santiago Ramón y Cajal refined Golgi's staining technique and used it to provide evidence for the neuron doctrine. This doctrine proposed that neurons are discrete, individual cells that communicate with each other through synapses.

The localisation of brain functions and the study of neurons was initially a postmortem study. Angelo Mosso (1846–1910) in Turin created a specialised scale to weigh the head and assess blood flow to different parts of the brain, enabling the study of brain activity in vivo and establishing one of the principles of brain imagining: brain activity corresponds to increased blood flow (which would later be refined to brain activity corresponding to the increased presence of oxygenated blood in the area). Mosso's interest in brain function localisation started with temperature measurements of the scalp and the brain (Mosso 1894), a practice that was rather common at the time (Zago et al. 2009; Lanska 2019). He then used a specialised plethysmograph to record brain pulsations (normally observed in the fontanelles of newborns) and measure changes in cerebral blood flow. This method, applied on the scalp and even to patients with skull openings, allowed Mosso to study cerebral blood flow variations during cognitive and emotional activities in vivo (Sandrone et al. 2012; Mosso 1880).

Mosso then moved on to study blood flow to the brain by weighing the head. Mosso's 'human circulation balance' consisted of a table on which the patient would lay. This was very delicately balanced and

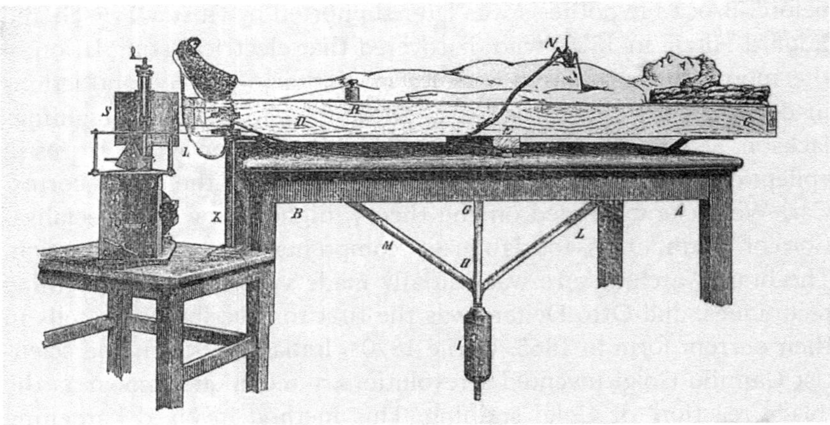

Figure 44: Illustration of Angelo Mosso's Human Circulation Balance Machine to weigh blood flow to different areas of the brain. Courtesy of Marco Rodolfo Galloni.

would tilt with changes to blood flow (Fig. 44). At the same time, Mosso recorded changes in breathing and pulsations to the hands and feet. He found that cerebral blood flow increased with the complexity of the task at hand. For instance, a simple auditory stimulus caused the balance to shift towards the head. However, more complex tasks, such as reading a difficult text, or more emotionally charged ones, such as listening to a letter written by one's spouse, led to a quicker tilt towards the head compared to reading simpler materials like newspapers or novels (Sandrone et al. 2014; Mosso 1880, 1882). Mosso's study of brain circulation in vivo was not only 'innovative with regard to the tool used and the number of variables taken into account' but also 'in the design of neuroimaging experiments' (Sandrone and Lorusso 2022, 172). This renders his work still 'extremely relevant in contemporary neuroimaging' (Sandrone and Lorusso 2022, 172) even though 'we cannot directly prove that the balance could factually quantify task-related alterations of cerebral blood flow [...] a definitive piece of evidence linking increases in blood flow to a detectable increase in brain weight is lacking' and 'the precise anatomo-functional details of the neurovascular coupling are still elusive' (Sandrone and Lorusso 2022, 173; see also: Krieger et al. 2012; Logothetis 2008; Drew 2019; Iadecola 2017; Bright et al. 2020).

What Rose calls the imperceptible shift 'from one epistemology and ontology to another' (N. Rose 2016, 147), the shift from the structure of the brain to its function, did not happen (as he argues) with the later invention of positron emission tomography (PET) but was already present in the first studies of the brain in vivo, which were already concerned with the measurement and *visualisation* of brain functions in their presumed *loci*. Mosso's human circulation balance is a successful attempt at *measuring* brain activity. There were, however, still several pieces of the jigsaw missing to produce an *image* of the living brain that discerns its (presumed) active centres: a proper 'engine of visualization' as Maynard (2018) calls them.

Another piece of the jigsaw is X-ray. The invention of X-ray technology is attributed to Wilhelm Conrad Röntgen (1845–1923), who, in 1895, while experimenting with cathode rays and gas discharge tubes, discovered X-rays. A fluorescent screen in his lab began to glow when exposed to an unknown type of radiation emanating from a Crookes tube (a partially evacuated gas tube with a cathode and an anode that produces cathode rays when electrified). He found out that these rays traverse the body at different rates depending on the density of the matter they encounter, and thus can image the inside of the body. Röntgen's work earned him the first Nobel Prize in Physics in 1901 (Glasser 1993; Kevles 1997, 9–32). X-ray, however, is able to capture only solid matter, such as bones, and the brain is entirely composed of soft tissue, is radio-opaque and is surrounded by bones (the skull), making it invisible to X-ray (with the exception of calcified tumours, and larger brain calcifications which I have discussed in chapter two). In 1918, the American neurosurgeon Walter Dandy developed air ventriculography precisely to make the brain (more) visible to X-ray. Dandy (1918) injected air into the ventricles of the brain, thus creating a contrast that allowed for a visualisation of the brain's ventricular system under X-rays. This method allowed for the study of tumours and hydrocephalus. Air ventriculography was followed by cerebral angiography, a technique for visualising the blood vessels in the brain. Introduced in 1927 by the Portuguese Egas Moniz (who became famous for the invention of the lobotomy and psychosurgery), cerebral angiography consisted of injecting a contrast medium into the carotid artery to produce X-ray images of the cerebral vasculature. It allowed for the diagnosis of vascular diseases, aneurysms and arteriovenous malformations (Artico et al. 2017).

Electroencephalography, invented by Hans Berger in 1929, allowed for a non-invasive measurement of electrical activity, but it did not directly impact brain *imaging*. The next milestones were made between the 1970s and the 1990s with computed tomography (CT), magnetic resonance imaging (MRI) and positron emission tomography (PET). Meanwhile, Wilder Penfield in Montreal developed a procedure to map brain functions in vivo, in real time and on the organ itself. This method involved performing a craniotomy on awake patients, followed by electrical stimulation of the cerebral cortex to identify functional areas. Patients' responses to stimulation helped Penfield pinpoint the epileptic focus for surgical removal. His work indeed provided some crucial insights into brain function, revealing for instance the somatotopic organisation of motor and sensory regions and the role of the hippocampus in memory (Penfield and Boldrey 1937; Penfield 1958).

Computed tomography (CT) was pioneered in the early 1970s by Godfrey Hounsfield and Allan Cormack, for which they shared the Nobel Prize in 1979. CT consists of firing narrow X-rays into each section of the brain and reconstructing the overall image with a computer. This is particularly useful for brain imaging as it goes past the skull and differentiates between different tissue densities in the brain. CT scans allow for the diagnosing of tumours, haemorrhages and traumatic injuries (Hounsfield 1973). The inventors of magnetic resonance imaging (MRI), Paula Lauterbur and Peter Mansfield, were also awarded the Nobel Prize, albeit only in 2003, almost 30 years after their invention. MRI does not fire radiation, but rather uses strong magnetic fields and radio waves to create sections, which detail different tissue densities (Lauterbur 1973). One of the key advantages of MRI over CT is that it does not use ionising radiation and the results feature superior contrast resolution, particularly in soft tissues, making it better suited for brain imaging.

So far we have been talking about imaging the brain in vivo: distinguishing between pools of blood (haemorrhages), swollen blood vessels (aneurysms) and masses (such as tumours). We are not talking about imaging the activity of the brain, what happens to it when it is working in one way or the other. Brain function in vivo and in (almost) real time can be imaged by functional MRI (fMRI), which allows for the measuring of changes in blood flow in the brain. This is made possible by Ogawa's realisation that, since active brain cells increase their absorption of oxygen from blood, where blood becomes deoxygenated there is activity taking place. The difference between oxygenated and deoxygenated blood, Ogawa argued, could be imaged, since blood without an oxygen molecule is paramagnetic, in other words it changes the magnetism around it when placed in a magnetic field and thus affects the magnetic resonance of water protons in the vicinity. This is what he called BOLD (blood-oxygen-level-dependant) contrast imaging (Ogawa et al. 1990). I will return to the limits of this in psychiatry in the next section.

Positron emission tomography (PET) scans image metabolic processes of the body and allow for molecular-level study. Michel Ter-Pogossian, Michael E. Phelps and their colleagues at Washington University in St. Louis (Phelps et al. 1975) developed PET in the 1970s. PET scans work by injecting a patient with a radioactive tracer (e.g., a glucose analogue such as fluorodeoxyglucose) which, as it decays, emits positrons that collide with electrons in the body. This produces gamma rays that are detected by the PET scanner. The resulting data is processed to generate images that reflect the tracer distribution, highlighting areas of high metabolic activity. By being able to measure metabolic functions, PET allows for the imaging of brain activity (Raichle 1998).

Similarly to PET, single-photon emission computed tomography (SPECT) scans are variants of nuclear imaging that allow for the measurement of blood flow and functional processes in the body, particularly the brain. Like PET, SPECT also works by injecting a gamma-emitting radioisotope into the bloodstream, and this tracer is typically bound to a molecule that targets specific tissues or organs (Kuhl and Edwards 1963). As the tracer decays, it emits gamma rays, which are detected by a gamma camera rotating around the patient. The data collected is reconstructed into 3D images of the tracer distribution within the body (brain) by a computer. Like PET, SPECT can be used to map brain activity (Wernick and Aarsvold 2004, 39–40).

Diffusion tensor imaging (DTI) was developed in the 1990s as a specialised form of MRI that enables the visualisation and measurement of the diffusion of water molecules in biological tissues, primarily in the brain. DTI exploits the fact that water diffusion is anisotropic, meaning it varies depending on the direction, particularly in highly structured tissues like white-matter tracts in the brain (Basser, Mattiello and Le Bihan 1994). In DTI, MRI scanners are used to track the movement of water molecules along nerve fibres; by measuring the rate and direction of water diffusion, DTI can generate detailed images of white-matter tracts, revealing their integrity and orientation (Mori and Zhang 2006). The quantitative data obtained from DTI, such as fractional anisotropy and mean diffusivity, are used to assess the microstructural properties of white matter (Beaulieu 2002b).

The latest non-invasive brain imaging technique is near-infrared spectroscopy (NIRS). Much like fMRI it measures cerebral haemodynamics by detecting changes in oxygenated and deoxygenated haemoglobin concentrations. NIRS operates by emitting near-infrared light (700–900 nm) into the scalp and detecting the light that is either absorbed or scattered by brain tissue. The differential absorption of light by oxygenated and deoxygenated haemoglobin allows NIRS to infer brain activity based on blood oxygenation levels (like fMRI, it's based on BOLD). This method provides real-time monitoring of brain function (Obrig and Villringer 2003).

These are the most important instruments used to picture the inner workings of the body, and in particular brain and neural activity. Needless to say, these have been, and continue to be, invaluable tools for medical research, but also for correctly diagnosing patients and checking the effectiveness of therapies. All of these instruments have proven, and are proving, pivotal for understanding brain and neural activity. What we need to bear in mind though is that while X-ray (and to a different extent CT and MRI scans as well) produces images more or less directly, like a photograph, all other methods, including fMRI, produce *data* that is subsequently made visible in the form of colourised 3D images. This is key to understanding where cultural processes can interfere with (and be influenced by) scientific imaging. In the next section, I will discuss their application in the context of psychiatry, that is to say, their use as tools to visualise mental disorders.

Picturing Mental Disorders

The application of such brain imaging techniques in psychiatry is both promising and contentious. On the one hand, these techniques provide valuable insights into brain function and thus into some of the underlying mechanisms of psychiatric disorders. On the other hand, there are significant concerns about the over-generalisation of results, the socio-cultural impact of brain imaging and the epistemological premises of the use of brain imaging in psychiatry.

Is there, as Rose and Abi-Rached (2013, 74) maintain, an 'epidemic of visualisation' in reference to brain and neuroimaging techniques? Rose and Abi-Rached cite Logothetis's study, in which he claims that a Web of Science query for '"fMRI," or "functional MRI" or "functional magnetic resonance imaging"' returned over 19,000 peer-reviewed articles (Logothetis 2008). When Rose and Abi-Rached repeated the exercise in 2010 it returned 53,662 results of which almost 7,000 were published in 2009 alone (Rose and Abi-Rached 2013, 74). I repeated the search in the summer of 2024 (the exact query was, searching in 'all fields': 'fmri OR "functional MRI" OR "functional magnetic resonance"'). This indeed returned almost 100,000 articles, with some discrepancies however compared to Rose and Abi-Rached's report (e.g., 3,476 results in 2009 instead of the reported almost 7,000, and no result prior to 1997), although these discrepancies are not particularly relevant to the present study. While indeed there has been an impressive growth in studies in this area, we actually see a steady 5,000–6,000 articles published every year after 2013 with the above keywords. Adding 'AND brain' to the query does not narrow down the result (approx. 97,000 vs approx. 99,000) and returns a similar yearly trend of publications. This is, at best, anecdotal evidence, and while I am not comfortable calling it an 'epidemic', it does support the notion that the interest in imaging the brain via fMRI (and we haven't even considered other methods such as DTI, NIRS and PET) grew up to 2013, and for the following 11 years remained steady at an average of 5,500 publications per year.

What impact do these imaging techniques have on our understanding of mental disorders and, in particular, in what ways do they give us the impression (and often the illusion) of being able, finally, to make madness visible? Are the vast (and clinically invaluable) datasets that are gathered via imaging techniques translatable into easily viewable and thus 'readable' images of mental disorders? What engenders the 'uneas[e]' of translating 'quantitative data into pictorial form' that Rose and Abi-Rached (2013, 74) individuate?

My objective is not to validate or invalidate the feasibility of visualising brain activity, especially in the context of mental disorders, nor to question whether brain and neuroimaging can, could or should contribute to clinical psychiatry. Rather, it is to comprehend the process of visualisation as a political and aesthetic phenomenon. This process attracts critique, engenders contentious debates and is both influenced by, and contributory to, cultural dynamics. The representation of the brain, particularly when depicting mental disorders, inherently carries political implications and becomes a politicised image.

In the next section I will discuss the uses (and/or lack thereof) of brain and neuroimaging in psychiatric practice and research, as well as the potential limitations, room for interpretation and criticisms that it has attracted. In the following section I will discuss the use of brain and neuroimaging of mental disorders in popular media.

Psychiatry and Functional Brain Imaging

The brain and neuroimaging techniques described above have been pivotal in our understanding of how the brain is structured and how it works/functions. In this section, I will focus on functional brain imaging and its use in psychiatry: as a diagnostic tool, as a tool to aid treatment and finally as a research tool to study the etiopathogenesis of mental disorders.

Thomas Insel, director of the US National Institute of Mental Health (NIMH) until 2015 and one of the most prominent proponents of brain imaging as the foremost source of knowledge in psychiatry, maintained that

> Patterns of regional brain activity associated with normal and pathological mental experience can be visualized [...] and ultimately, biomarkers for mental disorders may not be proteins or neurotransmitters but may emerge from neuroimaging (functional magnetic resonance imaging (fMRI), single photon emission computed tomography (SPECT), etc.). Logically, if these are disorders of brain systems, then the visualization of abnormal patterns of brain activity should detect the pathology of these illnesses. (Insel and Quirion 2005, 4)

Functional brain imaging has also shown promise—according to many, more than just 'promise'—in improving diagnostic accuracy in psychiatry. For example, SPECT and PET can distinguish between traumatic brain injury (TBI) and post-traumatic stress disorder (PTSD), conditions that often overlap in their clinical presentations. Henderson and colleagues (2020, 12) highlight that functional brain imaging can differentiate these conditions. As they argue (Henderson et al. 2020, 3), the inadequacies of the DSM (the *Diagnostic and Statistical Manual*, the diagnostic manual of reference crafted by the American Psychiatric Association and widely employed internationally) in its categorical diagnostic strategies have been highlighted by the relative failures of multiple large treatment trials, including the STAR*D, STEP-BD and the CATIE (Warden et al. 2007; DePaulo 2006; Rush et al. 2006; Lieberman et al. 2005). The *Diagnostic and Statistical Manual*, widely used in psychiatry, is in fact entirely based on observable symptoms rather than biomarkers (that brain images are alleged to be), favouring reliability over validity, as Insel (2013) pointed out. Brain imaging promises to bring validity to DSM diagnoses.

DTI seems to be promising for psychiatric diagnosis (Podwalski et al. 2021), in particular to assess white-matter pathology as a presumed common feature of several mental disorders (Sagarwala and Nasrallah 2020). Several studies show promise in relation to schizophrenia: brain imaging parameters predict the risk in developing the illness with a good probability of 0.75 and above (Koutsouleris et al. 2012); it helps to distinguish between affective and nonaffective psychoses (Koutsouleris et al. 2015), and DTI can also identify groups with a good or fair outcome (Koutsouleris et al. 2015).

Mayberg (2014, 31–32) uses brain imaging to distinguish between subtypes of depression. As Insel (2022, 137) remarks,

> While scans in children have not yet revealed a diagnostic biomarker, studies in adults with depression appear more promising. Research using imaging of brain connectivity at rest suggests that the DSM category of major depressive disorder is at least four distinct disorders with different brain signatures, or biotypes. In biotype I there is reduced connectivity between the frontal cortex and the amygdala, areas associated with fear and the assessment of emotion. Biotype II shows reduced connectivity in the anterior cingulate and orbitofrontal areas, part of that default mode network, supporting motivation and decision-making. Biotype III shows altered connectivity in thalamic and frontostriatal networks, circuits that support reward processing and action initiation. And biotype IV shows a combination of features of I and III. These subtypes cannot be identified by clinical features or severity alone, but they are associated with different symptom profiles. While people with different biotypes differ in measures of anxiety and anhedonia (lack of pleasure), these studies of brain connectivity give more precision than the clinical symptoms.

Falkai, Schmitt and Andreasen (2018, 180–81) are more cautious in reviewing the outcomes of using neuroimaging in diagnosing bipolar disorder, depression and schizophrenia, and while they question whether the results can be interpreted as 'a possible substrate for organic psychosis' (Falkai, Schmitt and Andreasen 2018, 183), they also believe that 'it is premature to claim that brain imaging methods are not useful' (Falkai, Schmitt and Andreasen 2018, 185).

Imaging techniques do indeed seem to be very useful to *improve* diagnosis, rather than to diagnose mental disorders outright. As Henderson and colleagues (2020, 4) remind us, 'the absence of evidence is not the evidence of absence'; we cannot discard the probability that one day it might be possible to diagnose mental disorders precisely and swiftly via brain imaging. However, as Insel (2022, 127) himself recently remarked, 'while biological psychiatrists have spent five decades searching for a laboratory test to rule in a psychiatric illness, as opposed to ruling out a medical cause, there is still no clinically useful diagnostic test'.

One of the most significant results of brain imaging in psychiatry is its potential to guide treatment. Neuroimaging can predict which patients are likely to respond to specific medications or interventions. For instance, patients with depression who show increased perfusion in the ventral frontal cortex and anterior cingulate gyrus are more likely to respond to selective serotonin reuptake inhibitors (SSRIs) (Henderson et al. 2020, 12). This approach would be a contrast with the traditional trial-and-error method of prescribing medications, which can be time-consuming and frustrating for patients. According to Mayberg (2014, 31–32), brain imaging can be effectively used to confirm treatment outcomes by picturing how brain activity changes thanks to adherence to a psychopharmacological regime or after a psychotherapeutic cycle.

According to Insel (2022, 137), initial studies correlate the biotypes that neuroimaging identifies in depression to treatment response: 'Roughly 80 percent of people in biotype I responded to transcranial magnetic stimulation. For the other three biotypes, the response rate was below 50 percent. In a similar study of brain connectivity and PTSD, the fMRI predicted accurately that certain patients would not respond to psychotherapy'.

Brain imaging used in the context of psychiatric diagnosis can serve a purpose similar to the way portrait photography was seen by Diamond: patients can *see* their disorder and thus be more compliant with treatment. Likewise, having a visible, biological substrate for their disorder, patients might feel less the stigma still widely associated with mental illness. As Henderson and colleagues (2020, 13) point out,

> In our collective clinical experience, patients tend to be less interested in the 'diagnosis,' compared to physicians. Rather, patients tend to be most interested in learning what can be done for their condition, whatever it might be. SPECT and PET functional neuroimaging helps the patient by revealing the functional substrate of their psychiatric/psychological symptoms. There are two very fascinating outcomes we have observed. First, the patient, as well as their family, engages in less blaming and criticism since they now see the symptoms as the product of disrupted neurophysiology. Second, the patient often demonstrates improved compliance with treatment.

Brain imaging can also help identify the underlying biological causes of psychiatric symptoms that might otherwise have been missed. For instance, these techniques can reveal some of the neurophysiological cogs that relate to depression. According to Henderson and colleagues (2020, 2), functional neuroimaging has shown decreased activity in the frontal lobes and the anterior cingulate gyrus in patients with depression, which are critical regions involved in mood regulation. These findings underscore that depression results from multiple pathophysiological processes and the dysfunction of various pathways, suggesting that depression is the potential symptom of different disfunctions in brain activity. Henderson and colleagues (2020, 5–7) also review a vast and convincing corpus of literature that connects bipolar disorder, schizophrenia and depression to outcomes of viral and bacterial infection, toxicity, brain trauma, autoimmune diseases and other damage to the brain. Functional neuroimaging can detect these abnormalities, leading to appropriate treatments that address the root causes rather than just the symptoms. This approach can prevent misdiagnosis and mistreatment that often occur with non-visual psychiatric methods.

Ultimately, for brain imaging in psychiatry, it boils down to the holy grail of biomarkers and the correlated matter of the etiopathogenesis of mental disorders: are there biomarkers that identify a mental disorder? Is there a univocal causal relationship between abnormal brain activity and mental disorders? As Falkai, Schmitt and Andreasen (2018, 179–80) put it,

> The first successes in the attempts to identify structural imaging markers to support diagnostic, prognostic, and therapeutic processes are likely to be in Alzheimer disease because it is a classical neurodegenerative disorder with an established neuropathological basis. The search for such markers in so-called affective and non-affective psychoses, namely bipolar disorder, MDD, and schizophrenia, is likely to take longer because these disorders lack an established neuropathological basis.

Until recently the dominant etiopathogenetic model was that of a chemical imbalance. The typical example is serotonin, which was presumed to be lacking in cases of depression. These are thus treated with inhibitors of the reuptake of serotonin (SSRIs) that indeed increase the levels of bioavailable serotonin in the bloodstream (Harrington 2019). Imaging techniques have given way to a different etiopathogenetic model, that of 'mental illnesses as "connectional" or brain circuit disorders' (Insel 2022, 138). Even though the 'evidence for abnormal brain circuitry is not always consistent or specific' (Insel 2022, 138), a model based on brain activity expands the potential avenues of treatment, since brain imaging evidences that the 'plasticity or circuit change as the goal of treatment' can be achieved 'by medication, psychotherapy, experience, or a combination of these many factors' (Insel 2022, 138). This, perhaps not incidentally, responds to one of the main criticisms that has been laid on biological approaches to psychiatry, that is to say, that the workings of the mind cannot be reduced to a single biological process, be it neurotransmission or brain activity. According to Insel, the shift of focus from studying neurotransmitters to the study, via imaging techniques, of brain activity can help complexify the treatment of mental disorders and repudiate the mono-factorial view of their etiopathogenesis. The brain is plastic and responds to the environment; as such, its study is the opposite of a reductionist approach. On the contrary, this knowledge identifies in brain activity the seat where we can visualise and verify a properly multifactorial etiopathogenesis of disorders, and where we can equally tailor, visualise and ascertain a holistic treatment. The image of the brain is thus the image of the seat of the biopsychosocial approach, first theorised by Engel in 1977 and further developed in recent works, such as *Psychiatry Reborn* (Savalescu et al. 2020).

After 40 years of biological research in psychiatry, Thomas Insel's espousing of a biopsychosocial model in his 2022 book *Healing* feels almost like a u-turn. While he continues to advocate for imaging techniques to be used for psychiatric research, and continues to hope for the discovery of biomarkers for mental disorders, he is also aware that this cannot be the only response to mental disorder. This brings Insel's position much closer to Rose and Abi-Rached, perhaps the most famous critics of the biological approach in psychiatry and of Insel's own previous positions (Rose and Abi-Rached 2013, 15). Quite surprisingly perhaps, Insel's near-u-turn happened after visiting the epicentre of the Italian psychiatric reform movement, Trieste, which I will discuss in the next chapter, and which has also been central in Rose's numerous arguments against biological reductionism (N. Rose 2018, 146). While after Insel's near-u-turn, Rose and Abi-Rached's *Neuro* and Rose's individual works might seem somewhat outdated, they remain seminal to discuss the epistemological premises and socio-political implications of imaging techniques in psychiatry.

Localisation theory, for instance, remains under scrutiny and needs to be thought about more in terms of fluid connectivity rather than a strict mapping of mental disorders onto areas of the brain that do not seem to function like they do in the average population (Rose and Abi-Rached 2013, 75). Brain fMRIs are often treated as a precise map of how the brain works, much like phrenological schemes, overlooking the complexities and variabilities of brain function. The famous 'dead salmon' study by Bennett, Miller and Wolford (2009) showed brain activation in a deceased fish, highlighting the potential for false positives and the importance of rigorous statistical correction in interpreting imaging data. This study, albeit providing little more than anecdotal evidence, underscores the need for caution in translating quantitative data into pictorial form and drawing conclusions from these studies. Vul and colleagues (2009) also predicate caution, especially when drawing correlations between emotional states and relatively ample areas of the brain.

Several recent meta-analyses of neuroimaging techniques applied to psychiatric disorders again suggest caution is needed. Sprooten and colleagues (2017) analysed more than 500 fMRI studies and concluded that differences in brain activity could not specifically account for different diagnoses or symptoms. Wang and colleagues (2024, 157), in a meta-analysis of 31 studies on the combined use of machine learning and task-based neuroimaging data to diagnose schizophrenia, conclude that 'taken together, these results support the potential of using task-based fMRI data in combination with machine learning techniques to identify biomarkers related to symptom outcomes in SCZ, providing a promising avenue for improving diagnostic accuracy and treatment efficacy'.

Schumer and colleagues' meta-analysis of 205 studies on neuroimaging applied to bipolar disorder also revealed 'reproducible localization of prefrontal, parietal, and limbic differences distinguishing BD from control participants that are condition-dependent, despite heterogeneity, and point towards a framework for identifying reproducible differences in BD that may guide diagnosis and treatment' (Schumer et al. 2023). Even though promising, neuroimaging data reveals an ample heterogeneity and is still far from diagnostic accuracy. Zugman and colleagues' recent meta-analysis concerning anxiety disorders was also far from conclusive and revealed the heterogeneous nature of findings (Zugman et al. 2023). Whether it is for these reasons or due to an ideological resistance, as implied by Henderson and colleagues (2020, 4), the American Psychiatric Association maintains that neuroimaging has yet to demonstrate a role in psychiatry (First et al. 2018) and does not endorse its clinical use.

Logothetis's criticism on the limitations of fMRI and neuroimaging, especially when applied to mental disorders, still holds good, 16 years after being voiced (Logothetis 2008). No matter how precise neuroimaging becomes, i.e., how small the voxel (the smallest unit represented, that is to say the 3D version of the pixel) is,

> To understand the functioning of a distributed large-scale system, such as that underlying our memory or linguistic capacities, one must first know the architectural units that organize neural populations of similar properties, and the interconnections of such units. With 10^{10}

> neurons and 10^{14} connections in the cortex alone, attempting to study dynamic interactions between subsystems at the level of single neurons would probably make little sense, even if it were technically feasible. (Logothetis 2008, 871)

The caveats for the use of neuroimaging in psychiatry rest on its epistemological premises. One such premise is what makes an area of the brain active. We have seen above that fMRIs measure BOLD response; they measure, by virtue of their different magnetism, the flow between oxygenated and deoxygenated blood. As Roskies (2007, 864) remarks, however,

> the temporal relationship between the BOLD signal and neural activity is [...] complex. The BOLD response is significantly delayed (3–5 seconds) with respect to the neural activity that causes it, and the timescale of the response does not temporally mirror that of the neural activity. More often than not, the cognitive task of interest is complete long before there is an observable change in the MR signal.

BOLD signals are also indifferent to excitatory and inhibitory neural activity. In either case, in fact, neurons increase their metabolic demand and thus BOLD signals (Attwell and Iadecola 2002). In other words, we know where oxygenated blood becomes deoxygenated, but we cannot distinguish whether this means neurons in that area are becoming active or are being deactivated.

Roskies thus concludes that

> the visual properties of the image are not visual properties of the object being measured. Moreover, fMRI is not sensitive to brain activity, but to some of its causal effects. We infer the presence of brain activity from the change in the dephasing of the signal, and are warranted in doing so because of a general theory about the correlation between neural activity, metabolism, and blood flow. (Roskies 2007, 864)

Functional neuroimaging techniques return a wealth of data. This data needs to be processed and, to use the expression that is the central concern of this book, it needs itself to be made visible. The process of creating functional images of the brain that detail which areas are activated and when requires multiple stages with the potential of introducing biases and artefacts at any point. Dumit (2004, 59) identifies four key stages: experiment design, measuring brain activity, making data comparable and making the data presentable.

Each stage involves choices and assumptions that can affect the final images and their interpretation. Experiment design is a key area of contention in terms of biological reductionism. How can the complexities of real life be reproduced in the controlled environment needed for fMRIs? Patients need to stay still for half an hour or more inside the MRI tube, while being presented with stimuli that are meant to recreate real-life scenarios: social interactions, stressors, etc. Rose and Abi-Rached (2013, 79–80) bring the example of a study meant to measure the pain of social exclusion. To replicate social exclusion in a way that was compatible with having subjects inside MRI tubes, the experimenters used a virtual ball-tossing game, from which participants were excluded (Eisenberger, Lieberman and Williams 2003).

The complex process of the creation of images from the data collated during scans has been extensively scrutinised (Beaulieu 2002a; Roepstorff 2004, 2007). As Rose and Abi-Rached (2013, 78) put it,

> In the analysis and presentation of the scan data, computerized methods are used, involving choosing among a whole range of available algorithms to transform quantitative information into images of domains that can be explored spatially [...] The process involves transforming, smoothing, warping, and stretching the data on each individual to fit the standard anatomical space; this is necessary to make the images comparable and cumulable.

The final images of brain activity also tend to only feature the activity that is supposed to be relevant to the task at hand. Consequently, from the overall data collated, generic brain activity (e.g., being awake and vigilant) is subtracted, for instance by repeating the experiment on the same subject with a different task or using a control group. Such subtraction is an additional step that is added to the process of crafting the final image (Roskies 2007, 869).

A seeming continuity with phrenological maps of the head is undeniable: invisible functions of the mind are brought to visibility by 'projecting' them to a surface—that of the brain—which is then visualised. This continuity has been mentioned by several authors (Dumit 2004, 23; Hausken 2015, 69; Dobbs 2005), but I don't agree with Rose and Abi-Rached, though, when they affirm that the visual result is 'no different from that of the phrenologists of the nineteenth century' (Rose and Abi-Rached 2013, 79). While we need to acknowledge the artifice that is introduced in translating data into an image, biased as it might be considered, neuroimaging collects actual data, whereas phrenological maps were based on arbitrary observations.

Is This Madness Photographed?

The discussion in the previous section is as fundamental as much as it is inconclusive. The medical use of functional brain and neuroimaging should be considered the primary and most important use of such techniques. However, images have a life of their own and arguably circulate much more than the written text. Do brain and neuroimaging techniques allow medical doctors to make mental disorders visible (i.e., diagnosable)? No. Perhaps not yet, perhaps not ever. They can certainly be very useful in psychiatric diagnosis and therapy (e.g., to exclude organic damage to the brain and to predict therapy response in some cases), but we have so far not found biomarkers of mental disorders in such images.

The visualisation of brain activity, especially in reference to mental disorders, has profound socio-cultural implications beyond the medical. The images produced by brain imaging techniques can influence the public perception and understanding of mental health and, since these images often carry an illusion of transparency and truth, they might lead to a reductionist view of complex mental processes. Rose and Abi-Rached argue that the portrayal of psychiatric disorders as brain dysfunctions can stigmatise individuals and reduce the holistic understanding of mental health, which includes psychological, social and environmental factors. The increasing reliance on brain imaging in psychiatry can also affect how we perceive personhood and identity. Sturken and Cartwright (2017, 363) discuss how imaging technologies influence our understanding of what it means to be human. The reduction of complex mental experiences to brain activity can dehumanise individuals and overlook the rich, subjective aspects of mental health. This reductionist view can undermine the holistic approach to mental health care that considers the psychological, social and environmental factors influencing an individual's well-being. Insel argues for the exact opposite, as we have seen above: the brain can be the space in which biopsychosocial factors converge, where complexity, rather than simplification, is embodied and where non-biological treatments, such as psychotherapy, can find scientific proof. Either way, the image of the brain is not a neutral, scientific one (is there any such image?): it is an image built on aesthetic criteria, on and around which a social, cultural and political debate is structured. As Sturken and Cartwright (2017, 362–63) put it, 'while PET and MRI have been used to scan the body in whole and in part, brain images have produced strong cultural associations with personhood and have thus circulated through various social contexts such as advertisements and public service ads'.

Dumit (2004, 6) refers to the first appearance of brain scans in popular media, an article which appeared in *Vogue* in July 1983 titled 'High-Tech Breakthrough in Medicine: New Seeing-Eye Machines ... Look Inside Your Body, Can Save Your Life'. The piece included a graphic with three colourful, oval-like blobs labelled 'normal', 'schizo' and 'depressed' (these came from PET scans) (Fig. 45). Without needing to read the text, viewers could grasp that these images represented different brain scans, suggesting there are at least three distinct types of brains corresponding to three types of people. These images intuitively try to convince the viewer that brain imaging can differentiate between schizophrenic, depressed and normal brains. This visual logic leads to an implicit acceptance that different brain scans indicate fundamentally different kinds of people, and the labels reinforce societal assumptions about these differences, making them seem obvious and normal. Despite understanding that this is a categorical error—substituting a few scan differences for universal distinctions—the presentation persuades readers to believe in the essential difference between these three types of brains and people. The 'normal' brain in the article features a variety of areas, a balance between yellow and green with some red and blue areas. The depressed brain features no red areas and a vast portion of the brain in green or blue, whereas the 'schizo' brain displays a concentrated red area (around the occipital lobe). As

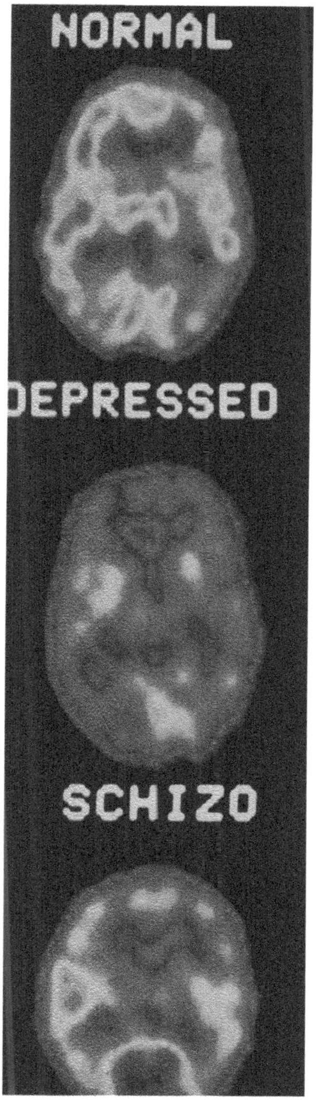

Figure 45: Excerpt from Vogue July 1983, p. 293. The image illustrates the PET scan differences between a 'normal', a 'depressed' and a 'schizo' brain. Courtesy of Condé Nast.

Dumit suggests, there is no need to read the article. Warm colours have always been used to indicate activity, chaos, passion (think of the sanguine temperament in humoral medicine for instance), whereas colder colours indicate inactivity, passivity, calm. The depressed brain is inactive, the schizo brain is overactive, the normal brain is normally active: it's almost tautological. There are numerous examples of uses of brain images in popular media towards the end of the twentieth century. For instance, a 1997 article in *The Times (Hammond, Indiana)* (Corcoran 1997) discussing the nature of mental illness in general features brain scans labelled as 'NORMAL BRAIN' and 'SCHIZOPHRENIC BRAINS' (capitals in the original). The 'schizophrenic brain' shows larger cavities than the normal ones, as per caption; however, the clinical significance of these differences is not explained in the article. As a result, the public is left to interpret the scans on their own, and given the common association of brain volume with intelligence, the depiction of these large voids in schizophrenic brains could easily lead to negative connotations. The images are not colourised, therefore the stark contrast between the bright areas of the 'normal brain' and the dark spaces in the 'schizophrenic brain' lends itself to a metaphorical interpretation of the schizophrenic mind. Well into the twenty-first century images of the brain are still used in news articles, such as Costandi's 2015 article for the *Guardian* reporting the findings of Bloomfield and colleague's study (Bloomfield et al. 2016), which conventionally uses warm colours to highlight glial activation in a brain PET scan.

The power of functional images of the brain and their potential to be used as images that make madness visible rests on what they conceal: the complex process discussed above to create the image on the basis of raw data. Yet, they also derive their power from their perceived proximity to photography, participating in photography's privileged epistemic status.

As Sturken and Cartwright (2017, 363) aptly remark, 'perhaps because of the positivist legacy of machine imaging, brain scans carry enormous power to suggest the "facts" of brain states and mental disorders'. In Roskies's words, it is the

> rough characterization of the commonsensical apprehension of neuroimaging data that explains the epistemic weight such data are accorded: Images are thought of as photographs of brain activity [...] While most neuroscientists familiar with neuroimaging techniques are not apt to mis-apprehend the evidential status of brain images in the ways I suggest, these images are disseminated far beyond the neuroimaging

> community, and it is here that such arguments become particularly relevant. (Roskies 2007, 861)

Given the privileged epistemic status accorded to photography, which I discussed in the previous chapter, its (misleading) association with neuroimaging short circuits the truth-value of functional brain images:

> When people look at an image of brain activation, they are inclined to think that they are 'seeing' brain activity: neuronal firing acts as sparks of light to 'light up' brain areas in which activity is present. This is an illusion, for there are no visible properties of brain activity to be instantiated in the image. The processes that comprise the generation of a brain image are distinctly different from those that feed us information about the visual world. Functional MRI is not transparent in the sense that photographs are, for the information we are interested in and that the technique is sensitive to is not visual information at all. What fMRI allows us to visualize directly are magnetic properties of the water in the brain. (Roskies 2007, 862)

This in turn generates what Racine, Bar-Ilan and Illes (2005, 160) called 'neuro-realism', the 'belief that fMRI enables us to capture a "visual proof" of brain activity, despite the enormous complexities of data acquisition and image processing'. Rose and Abi-Rached (2013, 78) conclude that 'the illusion of transparency is crucial to the effects of truth':

> Electroencephalographs, the CT scanners, the magnetic resonance imaging machines, and all the other technical devices of contemporary brain mapping are no more 'true to nature' than those produced by the other 'engines of visualization,' such as photographs, so tellingly analyzed by Patrick Maynard. But it is only through such artifacts that we have become able to see that which is not present to our un-augmented eyes. (Rose and Abi-Rached 2013, 55)

Numerous scholars (Carey 2006; Dobbs 2005; Racine, Bar-Ilan and Illes 2005; McCabe and Castel 2008) maintain that, regardless of the epistemological and aesthetic premises or fallacies of neuroimaging, including such images 'confers a great deal of scientific credibility to studies of cognition' (McCabe and Castel 2008, 344), whether they are meant for the scientific community or the lay public.

McCabe and Castel (2008) studied whether brain images enhance the perceived credibility of cognitive neuroscience articles. They hypothesised that such images would increase credibility by providing tangible representations of abstract cognitive processes. They conducted three experiments with participants reading fictitious articles accompanied by either a brain image, a bar graph, a topographical map or no image. McCabe and Castel conclude that brain images uniquely enhance the perceived credibility of cognitive neuroscience research. Michael and colleagues (2013) set forth to confirm McCabe and Castel's claim but ended up challenging their findings. They conducted ten similar experiments with nearly 2,000 participants. Their meta-analysis, which included McCabe and Castel's original data, found the effect of brain images on perceived credibility to be negligible (0.07 on a four-point scale). They suggested that the original study's effect was overestimated due to the novelty of neuroscience at the time, and as public scepticism grew, the persuasive power of brain images diminished. Additionally, they proposed that prior knowledge of neuroscience might moderate this effect. They thus concluded that the influence of brain images has been overstated and should be critically reevaluated: the addition of brain images 'exerts little to no influence on the extent to which people agree with the conclusions of a news article' (Michael et al. 2013, 721). Their findings suggest that while brain images may not significantly enhance perceived credibility, the careful presentation of scientific data still remains crucial, especially in contexts like the media and courtrooms. Regardless of whether brain images give more credibility or not to scientific articles and news items, and whether this is measurable or not, 'many cognitive neuroscientists have expressed frustration at what they see as the oversimplification of their data, and have suggested that efforts be made to influence media coverage of brain imaging research to include discussion of the limitations of fMRI, in order to reduce the misrepresentation of these data' (McCabe and Castel 2008, 351).

Through surveys conducted with both the general public and neuroimaging experts, a 2011 study (Wardlaw et al. 2011) found significant scepticism among the public regarding the use of neuroimaging for applications such as lie detection, consumer preference determination and use by employers or governments (among other concerns such as privacy and ethical implications). Experts, while also somewhat sceptical, were found to underestimate the frequency of neuroimaging being used as evidence in court cases, indicating a gap in awareness compared to the public. Both groups agreed on the importance of better informing the public to mitigate inappropriate uses of neuroimaging, though they differed on the need and method for regulation. Experts acknowledged the risks of inaccurate media portrayals of neuroimaging, but showed limited engagement with public communication, highlighting a need for improved frameworks for scientific outreach and media engagement.

Indeed, there is evidence of a growing caution in communicating the achievements of brain imaging in reference to mental disorders, perhaps also in consequence to Wardlaw and colleagues' recommendation that neuroscientists be held responsible for how their achievements are communicated in the press (Wardlaw et al. 2011). In 2016, *Psychology Today* reported that 'the science isn't there yet' to diagnose mental disorders with brain scans (Gillihan 2016), *MPR News* noted that brain scan studies might be too small to reveal anything relevant to psychiatry (Hamilton 2022) and *Science Daily* said that a new study (Segal et al. 2023) mapping brain regions has revealed the extraordinary diversity of brain activity in subjects affected by depression or schizophrenia, making diagnosis nearly impossible (Monash 2023). These articles feature either no image or stock/archival images of brain MRIs (*not* functional) being held and/or indicated by medical personnel. The images are presented just as 'eye candy' in the article and are not illustrative of its contents. This was also the case in a *Guardian* article of 2020, reporting on Onwordi and colleagues' study (Onwordi et al. 2020), entitled 'Schizophrenia study finds evidence of reduced links between brain cells' (Devlin 2020).

As discussed above, from the therapeutic use of photography to brain scans, there is a widespread understanding that visualising mental disorders by means of medical and expert imaging techniques increases compliance with, and trust towards, treatment, and decreases the stigma towards mental disorders, removing them from the limbo of invisible and untreatable diseases of the mind and giving them a bodily substrate. Schomerus and colleagues (2012) call into question this conception though. They systematically review and analyse the evolution of public attitudes towards mental illness over recent decades, with a particular focus on whether increased knowledge of the biological aspects of mental disorders has improved societal attitudes. Their study found that while there has been a significant increase in public understanding of mental health issues, particularly in terms of biological causes, this has not been translated into greater social acceptance of individuals with mental illness. The public is more accepting of professional help and treatment, but stigma and negative stereotypes persist or have even worsened. The study concludes that viewing mental disorders as brain diseases has not reduced their stigma, and recommends, much like both Rose and Insel, that a more balanced approach, incorporating both biological and psychosocial factors, is needed to improve social attitudes.

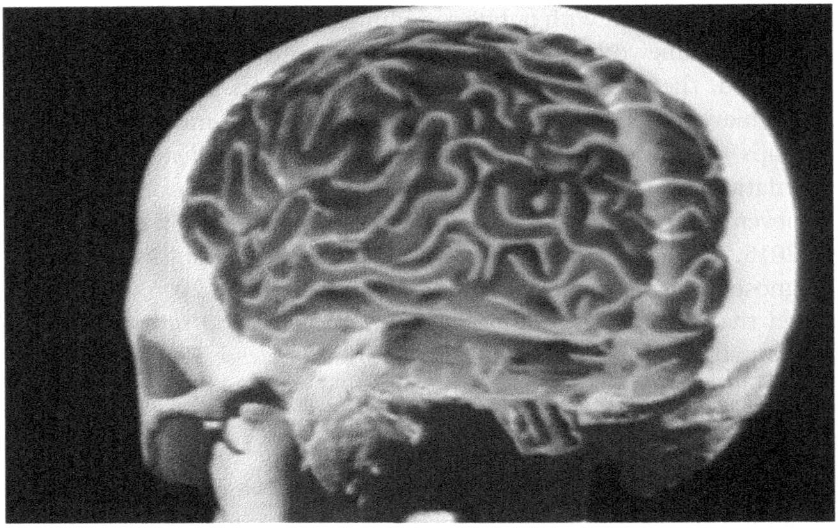

Figure 46: A frame from the trailer of Rampage (dir. William Friedkin, 1987). It depicts a crude reproduction of a brain scan.

The first film to feature a brain scan is Friedkin's crime thriller *Rampage* (1987), which follows a character named Alex who murders six people. The trailer intersperses images that should emulate brain scans (but are in fact rather different from real brain scans) between scenes of violence, while the voiceover comments: 'on the outside, he appears like the perfect boy next door. But on the inside, there is a murderer on a rampage'. Needless to say, the brain scan image (Fig. 46) appears on the 'but on the inside' part. In the same way phrenology unlocked hidden inner characteristics only to the eyes (and tools) of the experts, likewise brain imaging is here depicted as the tool that makes visible a hidden evil. The eyes deceive. It is very telling, albeit purely anecdotally, that *Rampage*'s director, Friedkin, had previously directed *The Exorcist* (1973), in which the possessed protagonist undergoes an MRI scan as part of her diagnostic journey. In *Rampage*, during Alex's trial, his defence lawyer requests PET scans to support an insanity plea; the scans, later analysed by a medical expert, apparently reveal Alex's schizophrenia. *Rampage* not only introduces to the big screen the forensic use of brain imaging, but it also uses it to legitimise the link between schizophrenia and violence. The courtroom scene suggests that Alex's violent acts are rooted in his schizophrenia, as evidenced by the abnormalities on his brain scan. This portrayal grants brain scans diagnostic authority (in the media), implying they can unequivocally prove the existence of mental illness. As argued by Dumit (2004, 151), the brain scan in *Rampage* becomes a pivotal piece of evidence, reinforcing the notion that an abnormal brain equals an abnormal person. The film thus conflates schizophrenia with violence and brain imaging with diagnostic certainty, leading to the misleading, but convincing, conclusion that violent tendencies in schizophrenic individuals are scientifically verifiable.

The sensationalistic popular depiction of brain imaging at the centre of legal matters is mirrored, if in more nuanced terms, in its actual use in forensic psychiatry. As Aggarwal (2009) notes, imaging techniques are increasingly employed in forensic settings, and these technologies are used to assess various mental states and even used as evidence in courtrooms. However, their application is fraught with challenges and, importantly, it cannot reliably measure complex sociolegal concepts, such as intentionality, which is crucial to ascertain criminal responsibility. Aggarwal regards the use of brain imaging in forensic settings as reductionist, posing significant ethical concerns, particularly regarding the concept of free will and individual agency. Like physiognomics and phrenology, the introduction of brain imaging in legal settings has granted the medical professional a further foothold in court, as it is only with medical authority that these images can be interpreted. Aggarwal concludes that the role of the forensic psychiatrist should not (or at least not only) be to interpret these images in court, but to advocate for a more nuanced and balanced use of brain imaging in forensic psychiatry.

The edited textbook *Neuroimaging in Forensic Psychiatry: From the Clinic to the Courtroom* (Simpson 2012) includes chapters on imaging and mental disorders as a predictor of violence and on the use of brain imaging in dangerousness assessment. These are just two of the examples used in what is clearly a work that supports the use of neuroimaging in legal contexts, but even this concludes with a cautionary chapter. Morse (2012, 341) highlights the need for 'scientific modesty' and 'genuine legal relevance' when such images are used in court, noting also that brain imaging is rarely used in criminal trials (Morse 2012, 342). Neuroimaging, he says, is often presented as evidence to support claims regarding a defendant's mental state (for example, scans showing abnormalities in the brain may be used to argue that a defendant lacked the capacity to control their actions due to a mental illness, thus supporting an insanity defence). This remains controversial since, as we amply discussed above, the relationship between brain abnormalities and behaviour is complex and not fully understood. One major issue with using brain imaging in the courtroom is that the interpretation of imaging data such as this does not necessarily explain the cause of any brain activity that deviates from the 'norm', or how such differences might influence behaviour. Brain imaging can also be misused or misinterpreted in courtrooms: Morse (2012, 341) refers to 'brain overclaim syndrome', whereby imaging evidence is overstated or misinterpreted, leading to exaggerated claims about its relevance in legal contexts. Morse warns that jurors and judges may be swayed by the seemingly objective and scientific nature of brain scans, without fully understanding their limitations. There is a risk that neuroimaging could be given undue weight in legal decisions, leading to outcomes that may not be supported by the broader scientific evidence (Morse 2012, 345). Morse (2012, 344) stresses that neuroimaging is still a relatively young science and many of the findings are correlational rather than causal, and that there are significant individual differences in brain structure and function, making it difficult to generalise findings from neuroimaging studies to specific legal cases. The reductionist potential for neuro-determinism—the idea that all behaviour can be reduced to brain function—returns in Morse's argument with a fear that it could undermine concepts such as free will and personal responsibility. Brain imaging, Morse (2012, 355) concludes, should not be used to make definitive claims about criminal responsibility without considering the broader psychological and social factors at play. Forensic psychiatrists and other legal professionals must critically evaluate neuroimaging evidence and ensure that it is used appropriately in the courtroom, recognising its limitations and avoiding the temptation to overstate its relevance. The use of brain imaging in forensic psychiatry does not seem to point to a revolution in the criminal justice system; as Greene and Cohen (2006) have suggested, it seems rather to be heading in the same direction as non-forensic psychiatry. Like in psychiatry, as discussed above, brain imaging shows a potential to aid and perfect diagnosis, in the courtroom it might 'help rationalize the law further' (Morse 2012, 356).

Conclusions

Within the broader cultural history of visualising mental disorders, brain imaging is not exempt from 'othering' the mentally ill. From the early days of phrenology, where the bumps on a skull were thought to reveal the hidden traits of the mind, to modern-day brain imaging, there is a persistent trend of using visual representations to label those with mental illness as different or abnormal. In this chapter I have shown how brain imaging, despite its advanced technology and scientific underpinnings, continues this legacy by offering a seemingly objective method of making the invisible visible; mental disorders are projected onto the brain's surface as something that can be measured, observed and ultimately judged. The scientific and medical benefits of brain and neuroimaging, as well as its utility in diagnosing and treating mental disorders, are undeniable. The ability to visualise brain activity has provided crucial insights into the workings of the brain and has opened up new avenues for understanding and treating a number of conditions, including, albeit to a lesser extent, psychiatric ones. Yet, these advancements come at a significant ethical and epistemological cost. The interpretation of brain imaging data is complex, and the reduction of the cause of mental disorders to simply brain abnormalities can obscure the broader psychosocial factors that contribute to mental health. The continuity between older practices, like phrenology, and contemporary neuroimaging has already been noted and is indeed striking. Both approaches rely on the assumption that mental states, personality traits and/or disorders can be localised and visualised within the brain. While phrenology has long been discredited, its influence lingers in the way brain imaging is used today, particularly in forensic contexts where it can be employed to argue for, or against, criminal responsibility, risking the simplifying of complex behaviours into brain scans that are presented as objective evidence. Interestingly, like phrenology, its use in courtrooms is amply discussed and depicted in the media, but in practice its use is quite limited.

Brain imaging shapes public perceptions and cultural narratives surrounding mental illness. The media's portrayal of such scans often carries an illusion of transparency and truth, suggesting that these images can definitively capture the essence of mental disorders. This has the potential to reinforce stereotypes and promote stigma, as seen in the way schizophrenia or depression might be depicted through stark, colour-coded images that suggest abnormality.

Ultimately, in this chapter I have argued that while brain imaging offers a powerful tool for medicine, when employed in psychiatry it perpetuates the historical tendency to 'other' those suffering from a mental disorder. The visual representation of the brain in neuroimaging is not a neutral or purely scientific act, it is deeply embedded in cultural, social and political contexts that influence how these images are perceived and used. The challenge in the future is to critically engage with these images, acknowledging both their potential and their limitations, and to aim for a more nuanced understanding of mental health that integrates biological, psychological and social perspectives.

PART FOUR

Madness Inside-Out

CHAPTER SEVEN

'Anti-Psychiatry' and the Inversion of Visual Tropes

Madness Inside-Out: The Permeability of the Cage

IN THIS CHAPTER, I analyse how the visual tropes studied thus far are purposefully inversed or appropriated in the movements collectively known as 'anti-psychiatry', which sought to challenge traditional psychiatric practices and the very foundations of institutionalised mental health care. While this movement found favour in numerous nations, including Britain and the United States, and often went hand in hand with politics of deinstitutionalisation, Italy provides an excellent example of an influential 'anti-psychiatric' movement, one that had a profound and long-lasting impact on policies, politics and society. In particular, it provides a prime example of how visual culture was put at the centre not only of communication strategies but also, and perhaps most importantly, at the centre of the very strategies of protest. At the same time, the outputs of these strategies in turn became very influential on visual culture and shaped the way we visualise and understand mental disorders.

This chapter builds upon our exploration of the permeability of the cage/asylum, the borders troubled by madness, which I discussed in chapter three. These boundaries, we found, are not impervious; they are porous, allowing for interactions, movements and the eventual spilling over of the institution's reality into public consciousness. The permeability of the asylum is not just a spatial or physical metaphor but also an ideological and representational one. It is through this permeability that the asylum, initially depicted as an orderly institution of cure and control, begins to reveal its contradictions and darker realities.

Building upon these insights, this chapter will look at how the notion of permeability becomes central to the visual strategies of communication employed by the anti-psychiatry movement in Italy. By appropriating and subverting established visual and performative tropes, anti-psychiatry advocates sought to 'unmask' the purportedly therapeutic façade of asylums, revealing underlying systems of oppression and control. Through a critical analysis of various mediums—including poignant photobooks but also dynamic performative acts, such as the emblematic journey of Marco Cavallo in 1973—I will uncover how these approaches not only critiqued existing structures but also conceived alternative paradigms for understanding and addressing mental distress.

Central to this discussion is the contrast between depictions of the asylum as an orderly, curative space, on the one hand, and representations that highlight disorder, diversity and communal engagement on the other. In chapter three, we saw how dance and convulsive movements emerged as a powerful polysemic visualisation which can serve as a representation of mental disorder and its cure, as a symbol of that which needs to be suppressed and as a liberation from constraints. Similarly, anti-psychiatry's visual and performative communications harnessed this symbolism of movement and collective action to challenge such entrenched narratives. The 'insane', the inpatients of the asylum, overflow the walls, pour into the cities, invade the streets, but at the same time the walls are abated, the population of the 'sane' can roam freely into the space of the asylum, which, as part of the reform, starts to offer concerts and even a bar. Marco Cavallo—the large blue papier-mâché horse that became a symbol of freedom and hope for patients in the psychiatric hospital in Trieste—exemplifies how performative acts can transcend physical barriers and provoke societal reflection. This act of bringing art and performance into and out of the asylum's confines makes clear the transformative potential of permeability: turning spaces of confinement into arenas for dialogue and change.

The use of photography also played a critical role in anti-psychiatry's 'unmasking' strategy. Photobooks published candid images that created visual narratives from within asylums to confront the public with the shocking realities of institutional life, debunking sanitised or idealised perceptions. These visual narratives, much like performances, operated on the principle of revealing hidden truths and mobilising action.

From the Unmasking of Psychiatry to the Destruction of the Asylum

The Italian reform of psychiatric health care marked a revolutionary shift in the treatment of mental disorders. Until the 1950s, Italy lagged significantly behind countries such as Britain and France in psychiatric care; severe mental disorders were predominantly managed through institutionalisation, and involuntary commitment to asylums often became a lifelong sentence. This practice was governed by an 1894 law on 'mental alienation', which was modified only during the Fascist era, when it was decided that involuntary psychiatric hospitalisation would result in a permanent note on one's criminal record. 'Milder' mental disorders—effectively those affecting individuals who could afford better care—were treated in university and private clinics, and there was no nationwide social or community-based approach. Psychotherapeutic methods were also virtually absent, with a prevailing pessimistic and rigid 'organicism' dominating the field. From the mid-1950s onward, several psychiatrists, most notably Franco Basaglia, who worked as director of the asylums in Gorizia (1961–69), Colorno (1969–71) and Trieste (1971–78), began challenging this status quo through various initiatives. These included: abolishing white coats and 'shock therapies', such as ECT; partially opening closed wards; organising controlled outings for inpatients; and using documentary photography and cinema to raise awareness. These efforts gradually gained traction among the general public and within the political sphere, culminating in the passing of Law 180 in 1978. This law quickly placed Italy at the forefront of psychiatric health care by banning all public residential facilities for involuntary treatment: not only asylums but also psychiatric wards in general hospitals. Involuntary treatment was subjected to strict regulation. Italy now implements the shortest period for such treatment globally: this can now last only a maximum of seven days before requiring renewal through the same procedure as the initial commitment. This law effectively brought psychiatric treatment out into the community, transforming the approach to mental health care in Italy (Donnelly 2003; Crossley 2006).

The work that led to such a groundbreaking reform was accompanied by a strategy of communication/propaganda which was eminently visual. Even more importantly, such a strategy was guided and informed by a notion that was equally visual: that of 'unmasking' (*smascheramento* in Italian). As the foremost of the militant psychiatrists, Franco Basaglia, put it, 'every action of renewal [...] initially has this meaning: to unmask the violence of the psychiatric institution'

(Basaglia 2023b, 568). This is because, he said, the psychiatric institution actively conceals 'issues that have nothing to do with illness or science' (Basaglia 2023d, 515). According to Basaglia, these issues are ultimately embodied in the psychiatric hospital as a convenient place to 'dump' socio-economic deviants and remove them from 'civil' society rather than it functioning as a medical practice—in other words, it hides them from sight. Unmasking—making truth visible—is therefore the first line of action needed to dismantle the institution of psychiatry and promote a new, holistic view of mental disorders based on a bio-socio-psychological approach. Reform can only begin by revealing that the psychiatric hospital is an instrument of social control, aimed at containing and marginalising the deviant behaviour of the subaltern social classes, masking this marginalisation as a medical intervention. 'Unmasking' is therefore an integral part of the political strategy to be adopted in 'destroying the asylum', which Basaglia (2023d) regarded as the only possible aim in a reform of psychiatry. The term itself, 'unmasking', evokes a field of vision and reveals the centrality of both 'seeing' and 'making visible' in the strategy of reform of institutional psychiatry. Unmasking, however, is not a grand revelation that happens all at once. This is because 'the danger of hiding the new contradictions of reality under a new ideology that explains or covers them is present in any action of renewal' (Basaglia 2023b, 569). Unmasking is thus best understood as an attitude rather than an action that can be completed all at once; it is an ethics of the gaze, a way of looking, seeing and showing; a way of not only making visible, but of maintaining visibility. Without this continuous unmasking, 'which has an essentially political meaning, any technical solution is reduced to a cover-up of problems that have nothing to do with illness and with science' (Basaglia 2023c, 516). It is in light of such a notion of unmasking that we should study, as I will do in the following section, the two photobooks used as part of the reforms: *Morire di classe* and *Gli esclusi*.

Basaglia (2023d, 263) famously concluded that 'the destruction of the asylum is urgently necessary if not simply obvious fact', because it was behind its very wall that institutional psychiatry could hide its mandate of social control and regulation. The destruction of the asylum—tearing down the walls that separate it from 'sane' society—meant to return what was once concealed within to the place in which, according to reformist psychiatrists, it belongs—that is to say, the community. It was an action that was political and social as much as it was visual, and governed by the principle of the unmasking. The gates of the asylums were progressively opened to the general public, fostering a merger between two spaces, the city and the asylum, that had been separated for decades. A crucial part of the initiatives that accompanied this was to make the general public aware of what was happening behind the locked doors of asylums; partly tearing down the walls, partly unmasking, these were large-scale initiatives such as marches and demonstrations. The most famous is certainly the march of Marco Cavallo in Trieste in 1973, from which originated the symbol of open-door social psychiatry: the sculpture of a blue horse. Marco Cavallo was a blue papier-mâché horse built within the asylum of Trieste during Basaglia's tenure as director. It was designed to be brought out of the asylum, symbolically carrying in its belly—like an inverted Trojan horse—the desires and needs of the patients. Photos of the Marco Cavallo march display very well the inversion of visual tropes of the representation of mental disorders: psychiatrists, nurses and patients were not wearing uniforms and cannot be distinguished from each other. The containment of the asylum overflows, it 'spreads' into the city, much like imagery of the feast of fools, and in contrast to the orderly images of psychiatric hospitals we have seen in chapter three.

Gli esclusi and *Morire di classe*

First, I will turn my attention to a comparison of the strategies of visual representation employed in the two photobooks of 1969: *Gli esclusi. Fotoreportage da un'istituzione totale* (D'Alessandro and Piro 1969) and *Morire di classe. La condizione manicomiale fotografata da Carla Cerati e Gianni Berengo Gardin* (Basaglia and Ongaro Basaglia 1969).[1] These photobooks were the visual protagonists in the reform of

1 Both *Gli esclusi* and *Morire di classe* are now highly valued collectible photobooks but are difficult to access. A scanned version of *Gli esclusi* can be accessed via Webarchive at https://web.archive.org/web/20090207170253/http:/www.lucianodalessandro.com/esclusi/prespiro.html [accessed 23 Aug. 2024]. *Morire di classe* can be retrieved in an anastatic reproduction edited by *Agenzia sociale Duemilauno* at https://www.2001agsoc.it/materiale/sconfinamenti/Sconfinamenti.N14.pdf [accessed 23 Aug. 2024]. It has been republished by *Il Saggiatore* very recently (Basaglia and Ongaro Basaglia 2024). Neither *Gli esclusi* nor *Morire di classe* have page numbers, so to facilitate referencing I have employed the following page-numbering system: in *Gli esclusi* the first page with a picture is page 1, then the numbering follows continuously; in *Morire di classe* the title page is number 1, the original introduction begins at page 2 and ends at page 5, and the numbering then follows continuously.

psychiatric health care that, fed by the upheavals of the late 1960s, brought about the closure of psychiatric asylums in 1978. Even though they employed radically different strategies of representation, these photobooks aimed at translating into visual terms the philosophical coordinates that guided the reforms of psychiatric health care. What is more, both photobooks engage with the traditional iconography of madness, either by exploiting it or subverting it, and are thus part of the history of the visualisation of mental disorders that I am here detailing.

Gli esclusi. Fotoreportage da un'istituzione totale (*The Excluded: Photoreportage from a Total Institution*) is a photobook featuring 98 images by Luciano D'Alessandro (1933–2016), a renowned Neapolitan photojournalist who contributed to prominent Italian and international publications such as *Corriere della Sera* and *Life*, to mention just two. The photographs in *Gli esclusi* were taken during a documentary project at the Materdomini psychiatric institution in Nocera Superiore from 1965 to 1967. This project was begun by Sergio Piro, a phenomenological and reformist psychiatrist, as part of his anti-institutional efforts, paralleling the work of Basaglia in Gorizia with Berengo Gardin and Cerati for the other book *Morire di classe*. *Gli esclusi* was published by Il Diaframma in 1969, just weeks after Piro was dismissed due to his reformist stance. *Morire di classe. La condizione manicomiale fotografata da Carla Cerati e Gianni Berengo Gardin* (*Death by Class: The Condition in the Asylum Photographed by Carla Cerati and Gianni Berengo Gardin*), published by Einaudi in 1969, is a collection of photographs taken by Carla Cerati (1926–2016) and Gianni Berengo Gardin (1930–2025) in the asylums of Gorizia, Colorno, Florence and Ferrara. These works of photoreportage were commissioned by Franco Basaglia and his wife, Franca Ongaro, with the explicit goal of producing an 'anti-institutional' photobook.

I refer the reader to two of my previous works (Sforza Tarabochia 2018, 2019) for a comprehensive contextualisation of *Gli esclusi* and *Morire di classe*, but it is fair to say that D'Alessandro's *Gli esclusi* has always been overshadowed by *Morire di classe* and the former has received limited scholarly attention. Even though it was well received by critics at the time (Stefanile 1969), *Gli esclusi* has always been mentioned only in passing by scholars, who count it together with *Morire di classe* as 'the other' photobook of the psychiatric reform movement. So, while *Gli esclusi* has been overlooked by scholars, many maintain that *Morire di classe* actively contributed to the reform of psychiatric health care of 1978, albeit to different extents and in different ways (see for instance: Berengo Gardin and Cerati 1998;

Pitrelli 2004; Manzoli 2004; Giannichedda 2005; Curti 2013). Foot recognises *Morire di classe* as the co-initiator with *Gli esclusi* of the wave of 'asylum photography' (Foot 2015b, 29–30), but also maintains that its influence cannot be measured. If anything, it may have been overstated, since the photobook only sold approximately 11,000 copies and went out of print in the early 1980s (Foot 2015b, 28). Forgacs (2014, 232) also doubts whether the photobooks had any impact on the reforms.

Gli esclusi

In 1967, a selection of 21 of D'Alessandro's photographs was featured in the 117th issue of *Popular Photography Italiana* under the title 'Il mondo degli esclusi' (D'Alessandro 1967). The collection was introduced by a brief presentation by D'Alessandro himself, alongside an article by Piro titled 'Fotografia e alienità' (Piro 1967). This initial selection delved into what D'Alessandro described as the 'solitude of the mentally ill in relation to the world they originate from, and in relation to others, a solitude arising from the illness itself' (D'Alessandro 1967, 54). This perspective aligns closely with Basaglia's early phenomeno-existentialist views, where he considered mental illness as a 'shrinking' of the subject's existential structure: 'Shrinking of the *Dasein* signifies a narrowing of existential possibilities towards a predetermined one' (Basaglia 2023a, 57). D'Alessandro's images indeed focus on these 'shrunk' subjects, who remain disconnected from each other. To this extent he focuses the attention of the camera to hands and silent gestures devoid of reciprocity. Piro, in his accompanying article, emphasises this aspect, noting that

> The hands [are] of great spiritual importance, as they enable the manipulation of the world [...] but the hands of those living in alienation are abandoned, inert, contorted, and violently hooked [...] they express, in their hidden way, the language of solitude, isolation, abandonment, the impotence to live [...] total surrender. (Piro 1967, 88)

D'Alessandro's initial collection of photographs avoids acknowledging the institutional environment, entirely omitting the spaces, instead focusing on the isolated, shrunken lives of the individuals portrayed.

Two years later, D'Alessandro publishes *Gli esclusi*, whose subtitle now explicitly references the work of sociologist Erving Goffman. *Gli esclusi* is a *Fotoreportage da un'istituzione totale*. The asylum is the 'total institution', an all-encompassing institution: 'a place of residence and work where a large number of similarly situated individuals, isolated from the broader society for a significant period, lead an enclosed, formally administered round of life together' (Goffman 1961, xiii). This book presents a broader selection of images—98 instead of 21—imbued with a clearer political significance, perhaps influenced by Sergio Piro's preface, which frames them differently compared to 'Il mondo degli esclusi'. Piro observes that 'the emptiness is fully captured in the images', yet clarifies, 'but this is not the emptiness of illness as an inescapable biological fate; it is the emptiness of the apathy, inertia, and abandonment inflicted upon those excluded from any movement or dynamic' (Piro 1969). This represents, he argues, institutional violence: 'if the human space was already restricted by their alienation, it is further constrained by the violence and abandonment' (Piro 1969). By 1969, the destructive impact of asylum internment on psychiatric patients had been recognised and given a name. Burton referred to it as 'institutional neurosis', while Basaglia termed it 'institutionalisation', defining it as a 'behaviour bound to the process of the "shrinking" of the ego that the mentally ill endure from the moment they enter the asylum' (Basaglia 2023d, 271). The 'shrinking' Basaglia initially attributed to mental illness is now understood as an outcome of the institution itself, which 'shrinks' the subject's existence.

These insights translate into D'Alessandro's photographic language in fascinating ways. In *Gli esclusi*, as in 'Il mondo degli esclusi', D'Alessandro largely excludes the spatial and institutional context. His approach remains intimate, drawing on artistic and portrait photography. Except for two 'establishing shots' of the male and female ward courtyards, the images are individual or small group portraits. The 27 non-portrait images focus on details of hands. Unlike *Morire di classe*, which I will address later, *Gli esclusi* lacks a textual component to caption the images, aside from Piro's preface. D'Alessandro conveys the 'existential shrinking' imposed by the institution not through a direct message or by establishing a connection between the body of the inmate and the space or physical constraints, but rather through an intimist style reminiscent of early photographic neorealism; he emphasises expressions, hand gestures and body postures. The gazes of the subjects vary: some look directly at the camera (e.g., pp. 4, 26, 27, 37), some tilt their heads (e.g., pp. 7, 23), while others appear distracted (e.g., pp. 36, 73) or gaze beyond the frame (e.g., pp. 73, 92). Postures are less diverse; when hands and gestures are not the focus, subjects are often depicted with crossed arms or hands hidden between their legs. They are seated, lying down or crouching (e.g.,

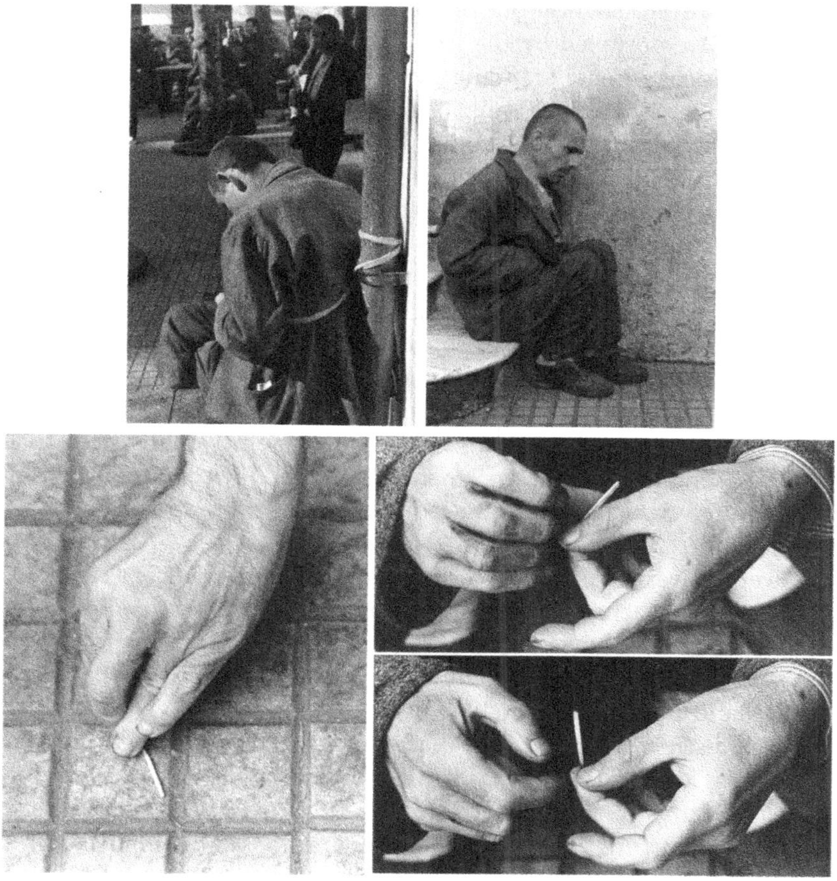

Figure 47: Luciano D'Alessandro. Selection of photos from Gli esclusi (1969). © Archivio Luciano D'Alessandro. Courtesy of Studio Bibliografico Marini.

pp. 64, 77, 86–87). Their gestures and postures echo the traditional iconography of melancholy, which I have discussed in chapter four: hands are hidden or in a pensive position, crouched or lying down, inactive (Fig. 47).

The dominant feeling that emerges from D'Alessandro's selection of photographs is one of idleness, which in *Gli esclusi* is portrayed as a consequence of institutionalisation rather than a symptom of mental illness. Hands and gestures are often used to convey this feeling. The very first image after Piro's introduction is a vertical shot of a courtyard wall. The whole left third of the image is occupied by an inmate standing, slightly out of focus. The remaining two-thirds of the frame are occupied by the wall. The top right quadrant features an out-of-focus inmate standing; the viewer's eyes are led to him by the vanishing point of the wall. The inmate in the foreground has his eyes closed, head tilted upwards, possibly basking in the sun. The arms meet each other at the hands; the left hand holds the back of the right hand. It is a peaceful posture, but also a very inert, passive one. The photo on page 5 features an inmate sitting on the floor of the courtyard, ankles locked, legs stretched, looking at his shoes. He keeps his hands between his thighs in a humble, self-restraining, posture. The image does not suggest serenity but inertia, idleness, boredom. In the background of the image, where the lead lines of the tiles direct the viewer's gaze, other inmates lie on the floor, idle. The traditional iconography of melancholy often overlaps with that of acedia or idleness: the melancholic person (in iconography most commonly a woman) is often acedious and idle, as we have seen in chapter four.

A very powerful sequence starts at page 17. The picture is a close-up, *plongeé*, of a crouched inmate in the courtyard. His left hand, slightly motion-blurred, reaches out for something on the floor. The following pages reveal that he was reaching for a used matchstick. The detail of his hand taking the match at page 18 is followed by two smaller pictures featuring the detail of both hands handling it; pages 20 and 21 feature a spread with the detail of both hands playing with the match, which is concealed by the fingers (Fig. 47). These images insist on a trivial gesture: by proposing a sequence of very similar pictures it seems to mimic a film reel, giving the viewer a sequential sense of movement. The movements, however, are minor: they describe an unimportant, unassuming and purposeless activity that suggests the boredom, idleness and ultimately the meaninglessness of time. The match also evokes the ubiquitous staff of madness, which I explored in the first chapter and which frequently appears in representations of melancholy as well. This can be seen, for example, in Lucas Cranach's 1532 painting *Melancholia*, where an angelic woman stares vacantly at playing putti while absently carving her thin stick.

In the following pages other details of hand gestures and inmates' postures give similar impressions. An inmate holds his hands in his trousers, in a very asexual posture, seemingly to warm them up (pp. 23 and 24–25); on page 28 an inmate looks at his hands; on the same page the picture is followed by two close-ups of hands rubbing. The spread on pages 30–31 details two wrinkled hands handling a crumpled piece of newspaper, establishing strong visual similes (wrinkled–crumpled; old–wasteful; abandoned–thrown), almost a visual iteration of the Heideggerian thrownness that characterises all human existences, but affects, redoubled, those abandoned in the asylum.

D'Alessandro conveys idleness not only through details of hands. Already the two establishing shots portray inmates either sitting or standing, but not engaged in any activity. Most other group or individual portraits feature idle subjects. The male establishing shot is followed by seven pages of idle subjects, interrupted by a possible conversation on page 11 and by the images of the patient writing on the wall, discussed later. The female establishing shot is followed by nine pages of idle subjects, interrupted at page 67 by the detail of a hand with a piece of bread.

D'Alessandro seems to use traditional iconographic themes of melancholy and idleness to depict the neglect experienced by those confined in asylums. 'Institutionalisation' becomes apparent through its impact on bodies, gestures and postures rather than through any relationship between spaces and bodies or the portrayal of the spaces' atrocities. The absence of a textual element draws viewers into an empathetic engagement, bringing them closer to the inmates and allowing them to intimately share their spaces. Through his photography, D'Alessandro performs a form of 'unmasking', revealing a process of discovery. This process is evident in the evolution of his photographic selection from 'Il mondo degli esclusi' to *Gli esclusi*. It is a journey through which the photographer uncovers the lives of the mentally ill and the realities of life within the asylum, and simultaneously exposes what truly happens to individuals, to us, when confined to the old asylum system.

Morire di classe

Morire di classe features a very different approach. Translated as *Death by Class*, *Morire di Classe* was edited by Franco Basaglia and his wife, Franca Ongaro, and published by Einaudi in 1969. It included photos taken in the preceding years by Carla Cerati—an already established portrait photographer—and the then-emerging Gianni Berengo Gardin in Italian asylums. Some of these hospitals were being reformed, such as Gorizia, some were still very traditionalist, such as Florence. As I have discussed elsewhere (Sforza Tarabochia 2018), Cerati and Berengo Gardin represent the asylum in a style that straddles the divide between photographic neorealism and Italian 'concerned photography'—which they co-initiated by signing its manifesto publication 'Fotografia di impegno civile' (Berengo Gardin et al. 1973, 18–19). In *Morire di classe* socio-political criticism is much more patent and the photographic assemblage displays a clear narrative intention. This is evidenced by Cerati and Berengo Gardin's preference for: small and large group portraits, rather than individual ones; the presence of pictures of structures and wide-angle shots that portray not only people but also the contextual space; and by the presence of photos that were not taken in the asylum (advertisements, images of protests, etc.). These contribute to the construction of a visual narrative and a sequential montage that we could define as protocinematographic. As opposed to *Gli esclusi, Morire di classe* features a complex textual apparatus that includes citations from psychiatry textbooks, texts that criticise psychiatry, poems, literature and theatre. Citations are formatted and laid out in a rather varied way and are always in some kind of relationship with the photos they caption. The association is not always immediately evident though, which seems to encourage readers to develop a critical awareness and their own interpretation.

Whereas *Gli esclusi* declaredly explores the neglect and the 'existential shrinking' of those interned in the asylum, and is thus an individual journey of existential unmasking, *Morire di classe,* in contrast, aims at 'unmasking institutional violence' as the first (or at least the most important) political step in a reform of psychiatry. As Basaglia and Ongaro write in their introduction to *Morire di classe,*

> Any action of renewal in a specific field has, initially, this meaning: to unmask the violence of the psychiatric institution [...]. This essentially pragmatic attitude, has enabled us to unveil the naked face of the mentally ill, beyond any label that science imposed on them and beyond any superstructure that the institution had provoked. (Basaglia 2023b, 568)

We also see this approach in Sontag's words, when she discusses the intrinsic relationship between photography and realism: 'all that photography's program of realism actually implies is the belief that reality is hidden. And, being hidden, is something to be unveiled. Whatever the camera records is a disclosure' (Sontag 2005, 94). The very subtitle of *Morire di classe, La condizione manicomiale fotografata,* 'the condition of the asylum photographed', hints precisely at this: Cerati and Berengo Gardin were to *reveal,* through photography, the reality that was structurally and ideologically hidden behind the walls of the old asylum.

In this way, *Morire di classe* can be regarded as part of Basaglia's political strategy and thought: the first attack against the institution in the form of a *smascheramento*. It is the unmasking of that paradoxical world which was becoming the *denied institution* (*istituzione negata*) (Basaglia 2023e), since they were reforming it from the inside, but that, in the context portrayed in *Morire di classe*, was still a concealed, *masked* institution.

Foot notices that *Morire di classe* is indeed a 'Basaglian book', in which 'various aspects of Basaglian philosophy ran', namely: an 'analysis of total institutions', an unravelling of the 'violent and long-term effects of [...] institutionalization' and an 'unambiguous social analysis of the asylum system' (Foot 2015b, 25–26). To these we should add the notion of *smascheramento* (unmasking), which binds together the first step of political activism in relation to institutional psychiatry, the ethics of the gaze and the practice of seeing deployed by the photographers and, last but not least, Basaglia's philosophy and reformist stance.

Morire di classe's contribution to the work of reform that 'radical psychiatry' and Basaglia especially were starting to implement between the 1960s and 1970s was thus the *unmasking* of the institution through photography. In an institution that conceals—willingly or not—the first revolutionary act is to reveal. This shift in perspective enables us to understand Cerati and Berengo Gardin's work in a different light. Far from being curious observers peering into a habitat, they aptly represent the gaze of the concerned photographer, committed to the unmasking of the inhuman conditions of life in the asylum.

As we have seen in chapters four and five, in reference to portraiture and visual signs, photography made madness visible to the gaze of the psychiatrists by capturing how mental disorder etched itself on the faces and bodies of the insane. *Morire di classe*, in contrast, inverts the relationship between the tools of visualisation and 'psychiatric power', as Foucault called it. Photography is no longer called upon to make mental illness visible to the gaze of the psychiatrist; rather, it is employed as a tool to unmask, to reveal what institutional psychiatry—practised behind the walls and gates of the asylum, far from public visibility—conceals.

In *Morire di classe*, there are of course several images of neglect and loneliness, individual or small group portraits, that do still recall traditional iconographic tropes much like *Gli esclusi* (see for instance pp. 10, 13, 15, 16, 18, 19). The photobooks are different though for two pivotal reasons that evidence, in the photographic language, the two different premises of *Gli esclusi* and *Morire di classe*. The first difference is that *Morire di classe*'s images are always shot with wide-angle lenses: 35mm or 28mm. Groups and individuals are always framed within the spatial context within which these images are captured. What emerges is no longer just the neglect, loneliness and desperation of the individual, but also the decrepit structures, the means of constraint, the insurmountable walls, the hospital-like aisles. Some of the pictures in *Morire di classe* are lifeless images: they depict the baths, the toilets, the empty courtyard (pp. 48, 49, 50, 52). The second difference is that all pictures but one in *Morire di classe* are taken at the level of the eyes of the subjects portrayed, whereas in *Gli esclusi* several images are high-angle, *plongée* shots. High-angle shots put the photographed subject in a subordinate position to the photographer, or, at least, they suggest a shrinking of the subject. Clearly, this is controlled intentionally by D'Alessandro, who wants to communicate in this way the 'existential shrinking' that is imposed on inmates. Cerati and Berengo Gardin do not, however, take the risk of using a visual code that, while effectively communicating the misery of the lives of those interned in the asylum, at the same time risks putting the photographer, and thus also the viewer, in a position of superiority towards the patients.

The only *plongée* shot in *Morire di classe*, taken by Cerati, is very important in the overall economy of the photobook (pp. 20–21). The image is paired with a citation from the *Manuale per gli infermieri di ospedale psichiatrico* by Umberto De Giacomo (1959) (Fig. 48). The citation describes what should be done in case of bites, either by insects, animals or inmates. The subject photographed is very attentive and present, thus the reader might be left puzzled by this association, if it is not interpreted in a contrastive manner: why would one assume that a person should bite? In an interview released to Francesca Orsi, Cerati herself revealed that the photographed subject actually did jump at her and bit her, right after she had taken the picture. Cerati comments: 'I thought he was right. How dare I photograph someone who did not agree to it?' (Cerati in Orsi 2025, 43). The photo alludes to this in the photographic grammar. The photographer, having used a wide-angle lens, must have got rather close, and she must have done it from above, to capture the only *plongée* shot that was selected to be included in *Morire di classe*: a photographic gesture that the photographer herself regards as aggressive.

Pages 26 and 27 are another peculiar combination that exemplifies both the narrative and the protocinematographic approaches (Fig. 49). The image on the left portrays a group of female inmates in an asylum courtyard; they lie on the floor, crouched, crossed arms, gazing to the floor, with a tattered look. One of them, crouched on the floor, is in a

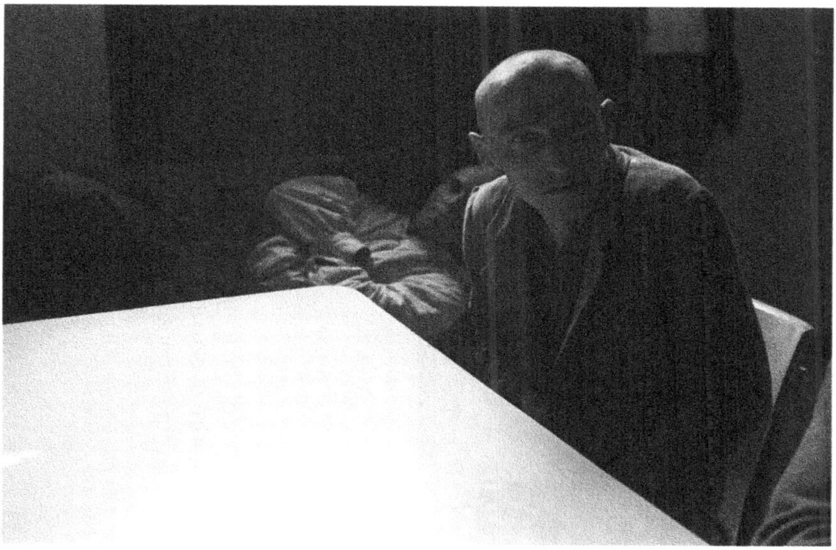

Figure 48: A photo by Carla Cerati from Morire di Classe. The photo is paired with a quote from a Textbook for psychiatric nurses detailing what to do in case of bites. From Morire di classe © il Saggiatore Srl, Milano 2024. Photo by Carla Cerati, © Carla Cerati / Archivio Elena Ceratti.

straitjacket. The image on the right portrays what is probably a bourgeois *soirée*. A group of elegantly dressed young people chats on a sofa in front of a marble coffee table; they smoke and drink wine from stem glasses and two paintings loom over them. This picture is captioned by a citation from the play *Marat/Sade: The Persecution and Assassination of Marat as Performed by the Inmates of the Asylum of Charenton under the Direction of the Marquis de Sade* by Peter Weiss (1964). This is a complex mis-en-abyme that references the Marquis de Sade, interned in the Charenton asylum, while he directs a play on Marat's assassination. The citation is an exclamation by Coulmier, the director of the Charenton asylum, who interrupts Sade's *Marat* rehearsals saying: 'I must protest / here we agreed to cut'. If we read this in protocinematographic terms this sentence binds together the two pictures. Foucault, one of the main points of reference to Basaglia and to critics of institutional psychiatry, had stated that internment in the asylum ultimately served the purpose of maintaining the bourgeois social order, through the removal from society of unproductive individuals. This seems to be the reason for Coulmier's protest in the context of *Morire di classe*: the photographers decide to 'cut' from the asylum courtyard to the

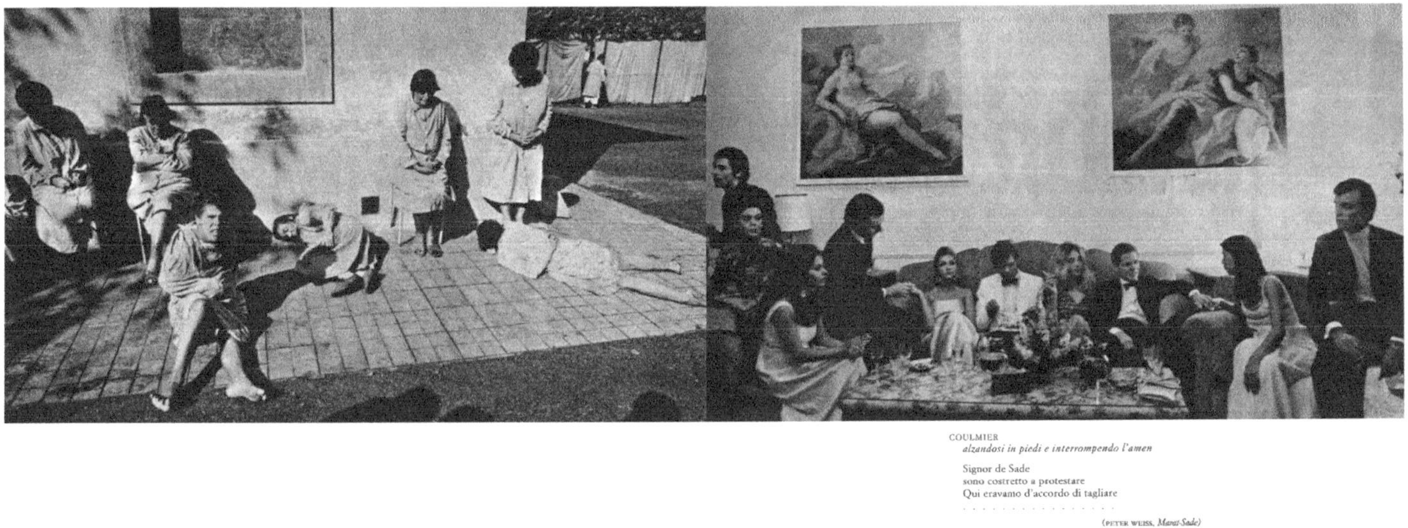
COULMIER
alzandosi in piedi e interrompendo l'amen
Signor de Sade
sono costretto a protestare
Qui eravamo d'accordo di tagliare
(PETER WEISS, *Marat-Sade*)

Figure 49: A two-page spread from Morire di classe. The spread pairs a wide angle shot of the female ward courtyard of an asylum with a bourgeoise soiree. The quote is from Peter Weiss's Marat/Sade. From Morire di classe © il Saggiatore Srl, Milano 2024, photos by Gianni Berengo Gardin, © Gianni Berengo Gardin / Contrasto.

bourgeois *soiree*, revealing that these are two sides of the same coin. But this, says the fictional director of the Charenton asylum, should not have been revealed: the film should have been 'cut' before revealing that psychiatry serves the purpose of maintaining the bourgeois social order.

Gli esclusi focuses on the signs that madness and internment in the asylum leave on the bodies of inmates: their expressions, gestures, posture. In *Morire di classe* the signs of madness and segregation are external, to emphasise the marginalisation of inmates and their social condition as being rejects of society: 'wrecks, husks of humans' says Rilke in his *Quaderni*, as quoted in *Morire di classe*. Numerous photographs are taken from behind a fence (e.g., p. 16), a gate (e.g., p. 59) or bars (e.g., p. 61). Images often reveal tall (and decrepit) walls behind the inmates (e.g., p. 15). The condition of madness is that of being caged or imprisoned, segregated, marginalised. We have seen earlier how, in his paintings, Goya had already used a similar strategy of visual composition to convey a comparable meaning, such as in *Casa de locos* where we can see that the whole upper half of the painting is a wall, with a window with bars; or in the *Corral de locos* where the central portion is entirely occupied by a featureless wall that separates the lunatics (bottom third) from the light (upper third).

Gli esclusi and *Morire di classe* visually contribute to the cultural climate that surrounds the Italian psychiatric reforms between the 1960s and 1970s, and they do so in different ways. In *Gli esclusi*, D'Alessandro deploys a neorealist and intimistic approach to convey the phenomeno-existentialist considerations of Sergio Piro, who employed him to document life in the asylum. *Gli esclusi* thus portrays the loneliness and the individual neglect that inmates live because of the psychiatric institution, and this adds to the suffering created by the mental disorder. *Morire di classe*, on the contrary, perhaps because it was commissioned by the very militant Franco Basaglia and Franca Ongaro, takes a much clearer political direction. The complex narrative and communicative strategies adopted, along with the protocinematographic editing, create a multifaceted narrative that aims at revealing the hidden realities of institutional psychiatry. Both *Gli esclusi* and *Morire di classe* deploy a form of unmasking: the former makes visible the individual suffering and the effect on the individual of institutionalisation, while the latter unmasks the hidden institutional violence.

Marco Cavallo and the Visual Destruction of the Asylum

Photography was not the only medium that was called upon for the task of unmasking the institution. The communication strategy of the reform movement and the strategy itself employed other visual means in order to invert and dismantle the traditional boundaries between the inside and the outside of the closed asylum. Many were practical and performative rather than representational. Basaglia's approach sought to bring society face-to-face with the issues it had long tried to hide away behind asylum walls. As Mollica (1985, 31) aptly noted, 'society had to be brought into collision with the problems it had tried to lock away in the asylum'. Basaglia (2023e, 458) himself articulated this shift when he stated that 'the protest against the institutional system transcends the psychiatric sphere and transfers to the social structures that sustain it', meaning that institutional psychiatry cannot be reformed from within, revolution needs to deal with the very society that has produced and sustains institutional psychiatry. To reform psychiatry is to reform society; issues once thought to be relevant only to the enclosed space of the asylum are now *made visible,* and should be recognised as a societal issue.

This inversion of the asylum's closed-off nature involved a series of initiatives aimed at breaking down the barriers between the psychiatric institution and the broader community. One of the most symbolic of these actions was the creation and march of Marco Cavallo, a giant blue papier-mâché horse. The story of Marco Cavallo is a pivotal moment in Basaglia's campaign, to the point that it became the very symbol of deinstitutionalisation, and the horse is still used as a travelling prop for deinstitutionalising practices all over the world. The project began when Basaglia, the newly appointed director of the Trieste asylum in 1972, invited a group of artists, including his cousin Vittorio Basaglia and the poet and playwright Giuliano Scabia, to work within the asylum. Scabia was known in particular for his 'teatro a partecipazione', a form of theatre that performed away from conventional spaces, blending social drama, performance and political activism. This innovative approach aligned with Basaglia's vision of transforming the oppressive environment of the asylum into a space where patients could express themselves freely and reconnect with the outside world.

This group of artists, unlike previous initiatives such as the 'Collettivo Arcobaleno', was not there to provide therapeutic support in a traditional sense. Instead, their goal was to create a form of communication that was unstructured and would evolve organically over time. As Scabia (1976, ix) himself put it, 'we wanted to operate a form of communication that was neither codified nor codifiable and that would structure itself over time'. They entered the asylum in January 1973 with complete freedom to explore and express their creativity. Their project was structured around the collective creation of large objects and puppets, alongside a permanent information service that kept all the asylum's wards informed about the progress of their work. This effort to link the partially open wards of the asylum symbolised the gradual dismantling of the barriers that had long separated the institution from the outside world. The artists established their base in 'Laboratorio P', formerly the P ward of the asylum, which housed non-violent male patients. This area was significant because it was one of the first wards to be opened as part of Basaglia's policy of gradually dismantling the asylum's closed structure. The choice of this location for the project also reflected the broader goal of integrating the institution with the outside world, both physically and symbolically.

In the context of this programme, the decision was taken to build a giant horse. This idea emerged during one of the regular meetings held at 5 p.m. each day, where artists, doctors, nurses and patients would gather to discuss their progress. The inspiration for the horse came from a drawing by Angelina Vitez, a former patient, who depicted a large horse carrying various objects in its belly. This led the group to conceive of the horse as a symbolic Trojan horse that could carry the desires and needs of the patients and staff out of the asylum and into the wider community. The horse was named Marco Cavallo after the real horse that had once hauled the laundry cart through the asylum's wards. The horse called Marco had been saved from slaughter by a petition from the patients and staff, and he had been sold to a farm in Udine where he could live out the rest of his days peacefully. The new Marco Cavallo, built from papier-mâché, became a symbol of the first collaborative effort of the patients toward their freedom and a connection with the outside world (Fig. 50).

After two months of group effort, the giant blue horse was ready to leave the confines of the asylum. This moment was the culmination of a broader strategy by Basaglia and his team to engage the public in the process of reforming psychiatric care. On the day of Marco Cavallo's intended departure from the asylum, a group of staff members blocked its passage. Their concern was that the horse's grand exit might be seen as the culmination of Basaglia's efforts, rather than the beginning of a long and difficult journey toward meaningful reform. They

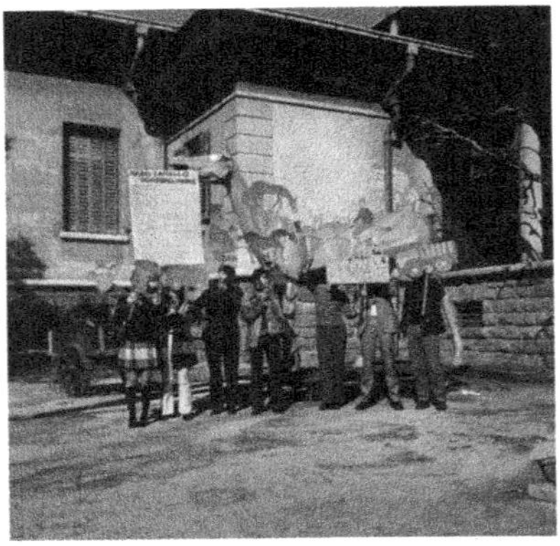

Figure 50: Marco Cavallo in front of the Laboratorio P. Photo by Mark Edward Smith. Courtesy of Dipartimento di Salute Mentale, Trieste.

feared that the march, rather than highlighting the ongoing struggles within the asylum, would be misinterpreted as a triumphal display, masking the continued violence, oppression and inadequacies of the psychiatric system. As Dell'Acqua (2007, 154) put it, 'the worry was that the festive outing, the symbol, could conceal to everyone's eyes the difficulties, the deficiencies, the miseries, the violence, the oppression that were still present in the asylum'. Despite these concerns, the decision was made to proceed with the march, but with a clear message to the public. A leaflet distributed during the event talked about the need for radical social transformation and highlighted the poor working conditions within the asylum, as well as the lack of prospects for former patients. The march itself was almost finished before it began when it became apparent that the asylum's gates were too low to allow Marco Cavallo to pass through. In a symbolic act of defiance, Basaglia and his team, including the above-cited Dell'Acqua, attempted to smash the top of the gate down with a bench. A photo by Neva Gasparo perfectly captures this defiant moment, which resonates almost as the visual founding myth of the destruction of the asylum, even though the top of the gate did not give in and Marco Cavallo had to be moved out sideways. Leaflets distributed ahead and during the march were visually very telling: they showed a procession of people lead by Marco Cavallo breaching the walls of the asylum with hands holding each other, creating a bridge over the brick wall to let Marco Cavallo out. The images on the leaflets resemble the depictions of the feast of fools, with the fools invading the cities of the 'sane' (Fig. 51).

This march was more than just a public spectacle; it was the inaugural act of the final phase of Basaglia's strategy. He had come to realise that reforming the asylum from within was insufficient; the institution needed to be rendered obsolete by shifting psychiatric

I DEGENTI E IL PERSONALE DELL'OSPEDALE PSICHIATRICO DI S.GIOVANNI,IL COMITATO DI QUARTIERE CON L'ADESIONE DELLA CONSULTA RIONALE DI S.VITO-CITTA'VECCHIA E GLI ARTISTI DEL LABORATORIO "P" ANNUNCIANO CHE DOMENICA 25 DALLE ORE 15 ALLE 21 AL RICREATORIO COMUNALE - (VIA COLAUTTI N. 5) AVRA' LUOGO

LA FESTA DI MARCO CAVALLO

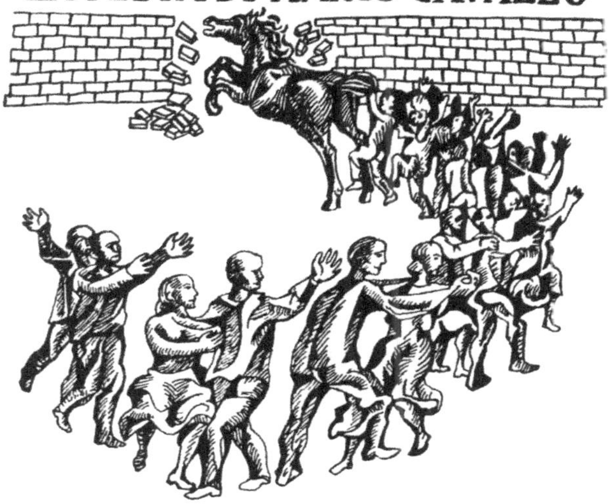

LA"FESTA" VOLUTA DAL COMITATO DI RIONE DI S.VITO - CITTA'VECCHIA RIENTRA NEL QUADRO DELLE MANIFESTAZIONI (LA PRIMA DELLE QUALI SI E'SVOLTA,CON LA PARTECIPAZIONE DEL DOTT.D.CASAGRANDE,AL CINEMA ALCIONE LO SCORSO MESE) ATTE AD APRIRE NEL QUARTIERE UN DISCORSO SUL "QUARTO MONDO",QUELLODEGLI ESCLUSI,CON LO SCOPO DI RENDERE COSCIENTE IL CITTADINO CHE L'ISTITUZIONE MANICOMIALE INTERESSA E COINVOLGE NOI TUTTI ED IN PARTICOLARE MODO LE CLASSI MENO ABBIENTI.

L'ESPERIENZA GORIZIANA HA RESO EVIDENTE CHE L'AMMALATO MENTALE E'UN UOMO CHE SI DEVE RECUPERARE ALLA SOCIETA' PERCHE' E'RECUPERABILE; CHE DEVE ESSERE RESPONSABILIZZATO E RESO PARTECIPE DELLA PROPRIA CURA COINVOLGENDO A TAL FINE I MEDICI,INFERMIERI E CITTADINI.

LA FESTA DI MARCO CAVALLO E'UN INCONTRO FRA DUE REALTA'DIVERSE:FRA CITTADINI E DEGENTI DELL'OSPEDALE PSICHIATRICO. LA PRESENZA DI MARCO CAVALLO VUOL ESSERE ANCHE UNA PRIMA PRESENTAZIONE NEL"MONDO FUORI" DEL LAVORO SVOLTO DAI DEGENTI INSIEME AL GRUPPO DI ARTISTI DEL LABORATORIO "P",APERTO DA UN MESE E MEZZO PRESSO L'OSPEDALE PSICHIATRICO DI S;GIOVANNI.

DURANTE LA FESTA AVRA'LUOGO UNA CONFERENZA STAMPA TENUTA DAL GRUPPO ARTISTI DEL LABORATORIO "P".

Figure 51: Flyer distributed on the occasion of the Marco Cavallo march, explaining the grounds of the initiative (1973). Photographic reproduction by Massimo Silvano. Courtesy of Dipartimento di Salute Mentale, Trieste.

care out into the community. This marked a departure from earlier efforts in the first asylum he directed, Gorizia, from where he had commissioned *Morire di classe*. There, Basaglia had implemented principles based on the 'therapeutic community', but had ultimately found that even well-intentioned reforms could not escape the institution's inherent power dynamics. The goal in Trieste was not just to humanise the asylum but to eliminate the need for such institutions altogether, to destroy the asylum itself, something Basaglia had only theorised while in Gorizia. Marco Cavallo's journey through the city symbolised a breaking down of barriers between the asylum and society, initiating a series of actions aimed at reintegrating former patients into the community. This process of deinstitutionalisation included the establishment of workers' cooperatives to empower former patients economically, as well as a search for city apartments to house those leaving the asylum (Foot 2015a). These efforts were not just about providing better care but about giving back responsibility and agency to the patients, ensuring that they could participate in social and civic life. Other symbolic initiatives included a flight organised by Alitalia on 16 September 1975, which took patients on a journey beyond the confines of the institution, and the renting of Villa Fulcis in Belluno later that year, where patients were able to experience life outside the hospital environment in a holiday setting. The purpose behind these activities was not only to raise public awareness but also to challenge and change societal perceptions of mental illness.

The deinstitutionalisation process was bidirectional: as the asylum opened up to the city, the city itself began to flow into the asylum. This was done through a series of public concerts and theatrical performances held within the asylum grounds, featuring famous figures such as Dario Fo and Gino Paoli. The former inpatients of the asylum also created a bar, *Il posto delle fragole*, which still operates at the time of writing (2025). For the first time, a space in an asylum was reclaimed as a place for community interaction, breaking down the walls that had long separated the 'sane' from the 'insane' and challenging society to reconsider its treatment of the mentally ill. The aim was to make, as Scabia (1976, 8) put it, 'the "inside" (the insane and the world of the asylum) reappropriate the "outside", the external world from which it is separated'. Pitrelli, later, better captured the bidirectionality of the process. In his words these initiatives were, collectively, 'a reciprocal restitution of spaces and people between the city and the psychiatric hospital' (Pitrelli 2004, 94).

Through these actions, Basaglia sought to dismantle the rigid boundaries that had kept patients confined and out of sight, promoting instead a vision of psychiatric care that was integrated with and visible to the broader community. Several argued that the outcome of Basaglia's strategy, the passing of Law 180, only embedded the dismantling of the boundaries without providing for the construction of a vision of community care. This consideration is worth mentioning, but, of course, goes beyond the purpose of the present study, and is very similar to criticisms given to all processes of deinstitutionalisation across the globe.

Conclusions

In a cultural history of the visualisation of mental disorders, the communication strategies of the movements we could collectively label 'anti-psychiatry' (albeit not entirely appropriately) display clearly how the existing visual tropes that 'other' the mentally ill can be subverted and appropriated. Certainly, the means are sometimes very different and the subversion is quite radical. The visual is employed in a symbolic way: it becomes a strategy of making visible, of unmasking. Visual artefacts are sometimes the byproduct of performances that stage this unmasking, as was the case with Marco Cavallo. There is a concretely visual component too: that of photobooks and photoreportage that engage with the traditional iconography of the othering of the insane, and subvert or appropriate it. The anti-psychiatric movement, particularly in Italy, turned these visual strategies of othering on their head, using them not to reinforce separation but to challenge and dismantle it. By examining the visual and performative strategies of the Italian radical psychiatry movement—such as the symbolic march of Marco Cavallo and the contrasting photobooks *Gli esclusi* and *Morire di classe*—this chapter shows how these acts not only critiqued existing psychiatric institutions, but also reimagined the relationship between society and those labelled as mad. The movement took the very tools that had been used to 'other' the insane—images of confinement, isolation and despair—and reappropriated them to reveal the oppressive nature of psychiatric institutions, and to advocate for a more humane, community-based approach to mental health care. This chapter also illustrates how the permeability of the walls of asylum—visually, physically and ideologically—enables a shifting of the othering narrative. By breaking down the barriers between the inside and outside of these institutions, the movement not only exposed the harsh realities of life within asylums, but also invited society to engage with these issues directly, thus fostering a dialogue that was essential for the subsequent reforms. This was visual as much as it was social and political: the strategy of 'unmasking' as the first step of the reform was a way of making madness visible, but not with the aim of pointing at the mad and making them recognisable. It was not meant to tell the sane from the insane. Unmasking meant to make madness visible to society as a whole, to show that mental disorder is part of society, it is everyone's problem—and perhaps it should not always be regarded as a problem. It was meant to make madness visible in terms of showing what institutional psychiatry did with madness, to make visible the practices of marginalisation and othering. Making madness visible becomes a powerful means of social and political change: madness troubles borders, even the ones created by the high walls of asylums.

In the next chapter, I will discuss another form of visual subversion of the othering of madness, that is to say the emergence of psychotic art, *art brut* and outsider art.

CHAPTER EIGHT

Psychotic Art, *Art Brut*, Outsider Art

SO FAR, we have explored how society and its dominant cultural forces have crafted various visual representations of those considered insane. In all these representations I have highlighted how visual strategies have been deployed to other the insane, to make them look different, to be able to tell the sane from the insane. In chapter seven I started to shift the focus, showing, through the Italian example, how these strategies can and have been subverted. What I have shown, however, was still a visual discourse *on* the insane, rather than a visual discourse *by* the insane. To this extent this chapter marks a further shift in focus: from the representations of the insane to how the insane begin to represent themselves, through forms of visual representation that would slowly be recognised as outsider art. A word of warning is needed from the outset though. The leading argument of this monograph is the visualisation of mental disorders as the othering of the insane. While with the recognition of outsider art we are undeniably witnessing the emergence of the self-representation of those suffering from a mental disorder, I will be foregrounding how this possibility of self-representation emerged within a discourse of othering. This chapter is not therefore on the art of the insane, but on its initial recognition, on that liminal space and time where and when, within a visual discourse of othering, the production of the insane found a way, albeit slowly, to make madness visible in the first person.

Even though it is also known as *art brut*, I will use primarily the term 'outsider art'. 'Outsider art' was a term coined by Roger Cardinal, in 1972, to translate Dubuffet's notion of *art brut* (Cardinal 1972). Like *art brut*, outsider art encompassed works from individuals who existed outside the social, cultural and psychological norms of the art world, particularly the mentally ill. These artists were often seen as isolated from society, operating within their own personal, internal worlds. While this isolation was romanticised as a source of artistic purity, it also perpetuated the idea that the mentally ill were separate from the rest of humanity, reinforcing their status as 'outsiders' (Maclagan 2010, 7). I will use 'psychotic art' or 'the art of the insane', instead, to refer to the earliest recognised works of outsider art, that, invariably, were acknowledged in psychiatric hospitals. I am well aware that in calling it 'psychotic' or 'of the insane' we are subscribing to an implicit politics of labelling. This is intentional, as it refers to the very first artefacts produced by asylum inpatients and recognised as potential works of art. The recognition of outsider art as a legitimate form of artistic expression, rooted in the Romantic conception of madness and genius, marks a crucial moment in the history of both art and psychiatry. This chapter will trace how the creative works of the insane, initially seen as mere curiosities or clinical evidence (i.e., visual evidence of madness), gradually gained acceptance as contributions to the world of art. The focus will not be, however, outsider art itself, although I will indeed refer to some notable examples. These works are already singled out for having been produced by artists alleged, according to dominant psychiatric paradigms, to be suffering from mental disorders. My perspective centres not only on what is being represented but on the conditions, practices and cultural frameworks that make those representations possible. Within this framework, reading into *outsider art*—that is, interpreting the content or aesthetics of such art in isolation—might divert attention from the broader cultural, historical and institutional factors that are essential in understanding how a self-representation of the insane managed to emerge between the cracks of a discourse of othering. I also want to avoid retrospective diagnosis, that is to say projecting current assumptions about creativity, mental disorders and authenticity onto past works. For the purpose of this study, it is thus more central to focus on the *definition* of outsider art. In its history and developments we will see how a space opened up in which the conditions for the recognition of the self-expression of the insane emerged. While indeed this emergence is a crucial milestone that legitimises the expression of those suffering from a mental disorder, at the same time, I will show, the very definition of the art of the insane *as* outsider participates in the visual othering I have been describing so far. Thus, rather than focusing on potential tropes, motifs and themes *of* outsider art, I will discuss the space of emergence of outsider art itself as a macro-trope, as it were, in the narrative of the othering of the insane and its potential subversion.

Madness and Genius: From the Romantics to the Modern Era

The nineteenth century was rife with 'mad' artists and representations of madness. Johann Heinrich Füssli (1741–1825), better known as Henry Fuseli, contributed a scene from the Santo Spirito hospital in Rome to the French translation of Lavater's treatise on physiognomy that we have encountered earlier (Fig. 52). The illustration depicted the raging mad, contorted in expressions of insanity and acts of violence (1781). William Blake (1757–1827), who 'provided an admirable Romantic figure around whom the legend of the insane genius might crystallize' (MacGregor 1989, 116), depicted in 1795 Nebuchadnezzar going mad and transforming into a beast. Blake was, however, 'far too sane' (MacGregor 1989, 116) to be relevant here. We have already discussed Goya's representations of the mad in the *Corral* and the *Casa de locos*. Towards the end of the century, we find Vincent Van Gogh (1853–90), a prolific artist and one of the pillars of modern art. Van Gogh struggled with mental health, famously cut one of his earlobes, was committed to mental asylums on several occasions and eventually took his own life. Among his many subjects he also depicted extreme emotional states (e.g., *At Eternity's Gate,* 1890) and scenes from the asylum (e.g., *Men's Ward at Arles,* 1889). If Blake had been, despite his 'perfect' health, the predecessor of the Romantic artist, Van Gogh was its perfect embodiment: tormented, suffering from severe mental disorders, and capable of harnessing this madness and channelling it onto the canvas. I will not focus on them, the famous, creative 'mad'. The overlap between Romanticism and the birth of 'modern' psychiatry produced a unique cultural climate during which madness took the centre stage and garnered much attention: certainly thanks as well to the artists I have just mentioned. Arguably, of course, anyone suffering from a mental disorder or deviating from behaviour defined as standard within the hegemonic culture could have created *something* at any point in history: doodles, graffiti on walls, nursery rhymes or poems, sculptures with available materials, etc. Such creations were, however, to the best of our knowledge, never the object of anyone else's attention and have not survived. It is during the time discussed here, though, that such creations, even when produced by people without formal training in the arts and not recognised as artists before being diagnosed with a mental disorder, start to pique the interest of the representatives of the hegemonic culture, i.e., psychiatrists. Also, such creations start to be preserved, collected, sometimes even reproduced and published. People—psychiatrists but also the general public—start

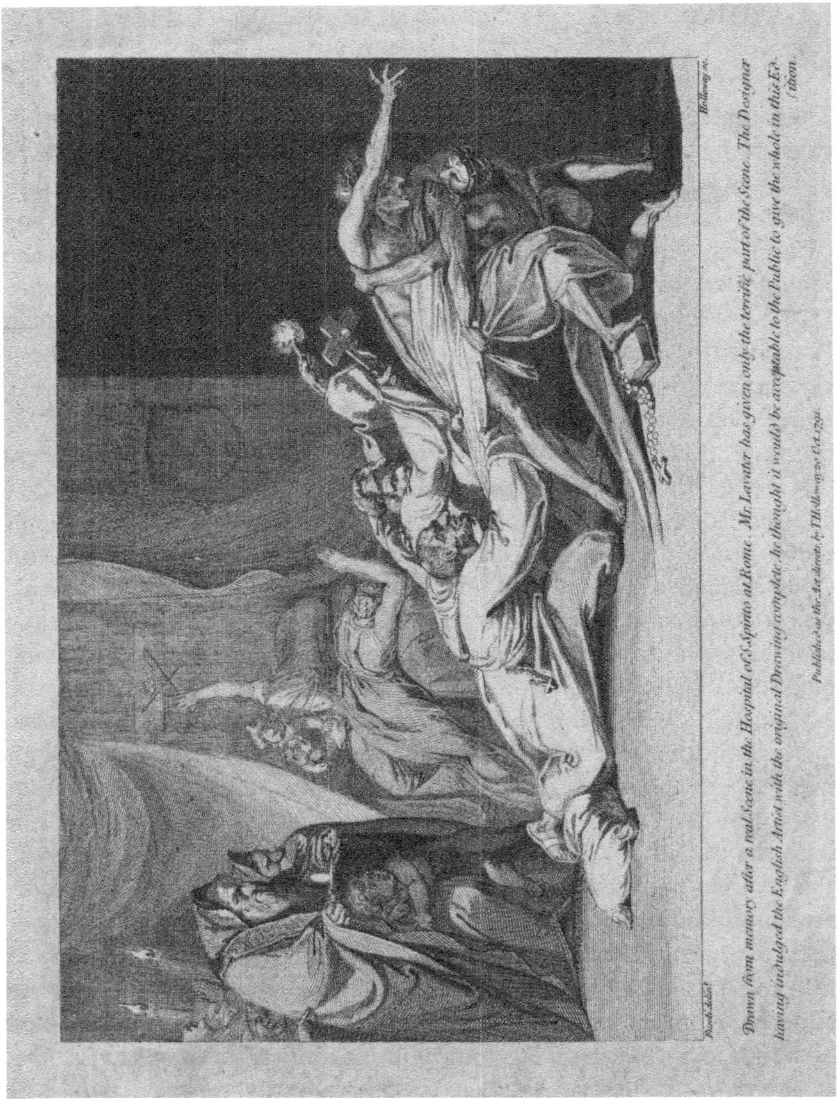
Drawn from memory after a real Scene in the Hospital of S. Spirito at Rome. Mr. Lavater has given only the terrific part of the Scene. The Designer
having indulged the English Artist with the original Drawing complete he thought it would be acceptable to the Public to give the whole in this
Published as the Act directs, by T. Holloway 20 Oct. 1791.

Figure 52: Henry Füssli. The Escapee: A Real Scene in the Hospital of San Spirito at Rome, December 1791 (Drawn from memory). Etching with engraving, from J.C. Lavater, *Essays on Physiognomy*, London 1789–98, vol. II, p. 288. Medical Historical Library, Harvey Cushing/John Hay Whitney Medical Library, Yale University.

talking about the creations of the insane. This creates the conditions for the recognition of what will be called, in the twentieth century, outsider art. Visual artefacts (and out of these mostly drawings and paintings) are the central item of outsider art, even though of course spontaneous artistic productions from inpatients might have included poems or oral or musical outputs. A large majority of inpatients, however, would have been illiterate and would not have been able to write—with a few notable exceptions which I will indeed discuss—so it is visual artefacts that started to be preserved, and laid the ground for the recognition of outsider art.

The very notion of *outsider* art brings us back to the leitmotif of this monograph. The history of the visualisation of mental disorders we have seen so far is a history of the visual *othering* of madness. This comes with several overlaps between the insane and the outsider, showing how madness troubles borders and makes barriers permeable. While it is undeniable that a counterhegemonic component is present in the very 'discovery' or 'definition' of outsider art, the opposite might also be true. As Maclagan (2010, 58) remarks, 'while bizarre and unclassifiable work will continue to be discovered, we have to ask ourselves what purposes are actually served by calling it "Outsider"'. Maclagan makes this statement one of the central tenets of his study of outsider art, and it is crucial to bear it in mind in this chapter as well. At the same time, we should be aware that outsider art is made by artists, and only labelled as art and as 'outsider' by an external eye. As Maclagan (2010, 64) continues, 'there is a double-sided creativity at work: on the one hand, the work of isolated and eccentric creators, and on the other the "eye" with which their art is recognized and rescued from obscurity by collectors'. This chapter will therefore deal with this 'eye' that defined and essentially generated outsider art. The very notion of outsider art blurs boundaries and complicates them, because it always presupposes an inside; even though the art of the insane is recognised as art, it is recognised as *outsider* art, art that is other to canonical art, art that is produced by outsiders, art that is outside of the gallery. Madness troubles boundaries even when it comes to representation and self-representation. This ambivalence is key to understanding if and how defining the art of the insane as 'outsider' art can be regarded as yet another form of visual *othering* of madness.

Romanticism, the European philosophical, literary and artistic movement that peaked in the early nineteenth century, could be said to centre on the proximity between madness and genius (Becker 1978, 13) as the only, or at least best, source of artistic creativity. The association between madness and genius is of course not new; it is one of the oldest and most persistent (and controversial) cultural notions (Jamison 1996, 50). A key figure in this discourse was Denis Diderot (1713–84), who argued that only strong passions could elevate the soul to greatness, with no room for rationality in achieving the sublime (Diderot 1916, 27). Diderot's conception of the mad genius, as explored in his *Encyclopaedia*, suggests that melancholic temperaments were prone to divine insights that bordered on madness: 'Oh, how close genius and madness are to each other!' (Diderot 1751, 260).

Romantic authors built on Diderot's ideas, often neglecting the distinction between pathological and creative forms of madness. They accepted all forms of insanity with enthusiasm, cultivating the concept of the creative personality as disturbed or eccentric. This Romantic view of madness was less about real experience and more about fantasy: madness as a treasure trove of imagination, free from reason (MacGregor 1989, 74 and 76). Byron famously epitomised this Romantic ideal. He claimed that all poets and writers were 'crazy', himself more than the rest (Lovell 1969, 115). Others, such as Coleridge, criticised Dryden's famous line 'Great wit to madness sure is near allied' and argued that genius involves a balance between profound sensibility and sharpness of thought (Coleridge 2014, 31).

The connection between madness and artistic genius was also a staple of Romantic philosophy. Arthur Schopenhauer (1788–1860), in *The World as Will and Representation*, argued that artistic creation transcends will and cognition. According to him, geniuses exhibit weaknesses verging on madness, as they abandon the cognition of relationships to grasp the essence of ideas. This proximity to madness is central to the creative process, allowing geniuses to transcend reality, providing them with the ability to impart the genuine essence of ideas (Schopenhauer 2010, 217). Friedrich Nietzsche (1844–1900) famously argued that madness is the only source of creativity and genius. In *The Birth of Tragedy*, he contrasted the Apollonian spirit of reason and form with the Dionysian spirit of irrationality and ecstasy, which he believed was crucial for artistic creation. Nietzsche questioned whether madness was really a symptom of degeneration at all, but was instead a force that brought great gifts to cultures (Nietzsche 1910, 7–8). Schelling (1775–1854) had already suggested that madness was the highest state of clairvoyance and the profound essence of the human spirit (Schelling 1994, 238), an idea that was echoed in the works of Johann Wolfgang von Goethe (1749–1832), who associated the unconscious (*unbewusst*) with unknown sources of artistic creativity and inspiration (Nicholls 2010, 107). It is thus not incidental that the Romantic fascination with the 'inaccessible area of the human mind, subtracted to the control of rational will' (Aloisi and Camilletti 2021, 2) paved the way for the discovery of the unconscious by Sigmund Freud at the turn of the century.

At the same time, physicians, alienists and directors of lunatic asylums, such as Philippe Pinel, played a crucial role in this discovery of outsider art. Pinel, whom we have encountered earlier, recognised the importance of engaging patients in creative activities, primarily as a therapeutic tool rather than as an acknowledgement of their artistic talent. He observed that 'the taste of the individual for his former pursuit of science, literature or other subjects unfolds itself' during convalescence, and fostering these returning talents could accelerate the development of mental faculties (Pinel 1806, 195–96).

Although Pinel's recognition of the creativity of the insane was limited to pre-existing artistic tendencies, it was among the first medical mentions of the potential artistic creativity in psychiatric patients. The first reproduction of a work of art by an inpatient came from John Haslam, the apothecary of Bethlem Hospital in London. Haslam published *Illustrations of Madness* in 1810, which detailed the paranoid delusions of James Tilly Matthews, admitted to Bethlem in 1797. Haslam included in it an illustration by Matthews known as the 'air-loom' (Fig. 54). This was to counter the family's claim that Matthews was not insane and should be released, so was not intended to celebrate Matthews's artistic potential but rather to reinforce the diagnosis of madness. Benjamin Rush, one of the founders of the United States, also believed that artistic talent could emerge after the onset of mental illness. He noted that 'talents for eloquence, poetry, music and painting, and uncommon ingenuity in several of the mechanical arts, are often evolved in this state of madness' (Rush 1979, 153–54).

Cesare Lombroso is recognised as the father of criminology despite his infamous theory of the 'born criminal': some criminals and madmen were just born that way, an idea rooted in Benedict-Augustin Morel's even more infamous and controversial theory of degeneration. Lombroso was, however, also central in recognising the artistic potential of the insane. His collection and analysis of art created by asylum inmates laid the groundwork for the later recognition of outsider art. Lombroso observed that many patients displayed remarkable creativity, producing works that were original and unrestrained by conventional artistic norms. He also theorised profound affinities between madness and artistic creation. In *The Man of Genius* (*Genio e Follia*), Lombroso claimed that 'the resemblance between insanity and genius [...] proves at all events that one does not exclude the other in the same subject'. He listed several geniuses who manifested signs of insanity, including

Vico, Poe and Schopenhauer, and analysed the causes of both genius and insanity, such as climate, race, heredity and disease (Lombroso 1891, 66). In his expanded work, Lombroso included a section on the art of the insane, describing it as a pronounced characteristic in some varieties of insanity. He noted that 'their imagination, freed from all restraint, allows creations from which a more calculating mind would shrink for fear of absurdity' (Lombroso 1891, 184). Lombroso's analysis covered several recurring characteristics in the art of the insane, such as geographical distribution, originality, eccentricity, symbolism, minuteness of detail, atavism, and a tendency towards arabesques and ornaments. He recognised that these works conveyed meaning, often through personal symbolism, though he also described them as eccentric or even atavistic, comparing them to the art of children or of 'primitive' populations (Lombroso 1891, 179). Despite his controversial conclusions, Lombroso's work remains the earliest surviving collection of outsider art and is displayed in the Museum of Criminal Anthropology in Turin. According to Lombroso, certain pathological elements, such as an exaggerated predilection for symbols, were present in both insane and canonical art. He thus theorised that the art of the insane could influence mainstream art too (Lombroso 1891, 208). Luigi Frigerio, an Italian alienist and a student of Lombroso, founded a drawing school for inpatients at the Pesaro asylum and published several observations on their art. Frigerio believed that these artistic products could help in diagnosis and prognosis, adding another layer of understanding to the relationship between art and mental illness (Vecchiarelli 2017, 1.07).

Lombroso and the Italians were not the only ones to study the artistic production of the insane, of course. Ambroise-August Tardieu, a forensic physician, briefly examined the drawings of two of his patients in his 1872 book *Étude médico-légale sur la folie*, but his interest was limited to their use as courtroom evidence. Tardieu exaggerated the bizarre nature of these images, suggesting that they resembled nightmares, and his contribution to recognising the artistic significance of such works was minimal (Tardieu 1872, 94). Paul-Max Simon, also a French alienist, was probably the first person to establish a connection between the ideas and delusions of the patient and their graphic productions. In his work, Simon recognised that these drawings were meaningful, either as symbols or because they revealed the patient's mental state. Despite his belief that there was no genius in these productions, Simon acknowledged their diagnostic value in that 'the incoherent compositions reveal [...] a double series of ideas: mystical ideas and scientific ideas' (Simon 1876, 367).

In the United States, William Noyes collected the works of a patient known only as 'G' and published detailed studies of these visual artefacts. Noyes recognised that G's work, which included paintings, drawings and sculptures, was not meaningless but a complex representation of a coherent system of delusional thoughts (Noyes 1888). The nineteenth century closed with Aleš Hrdlička's article 'Art and Literature in the Mentally Abnormal' in 1899. While Hrdlička distanced himself from the notion of the insane genius, he continued to emphasise the symbolic and often crude nature of the art of the insane. Hrdlička's personal collection of these works, though not extensively analysed, marked a continuing interest in the visual production of psychiatric patients (Hrdlička 1899, 385).

The Art of the Insane at the Turn of the Century

The art created by asylum inmates was initially viewed through a clinical lens. It did make madness visible, but it could not escape the mechanics of othering that we have described so far. Those who collected and studied it did so seeing it as a sign and a symptom of the disorder, not a form of expression or self-representation. It was meaningful, but its meaning was only the mental disorder itself, of which it was considered a symptom. It is, however, thanks to these early acknowledgements that it gradually gained recognition for its artistic merit.

Outsider art, therefore, represents not just a form of self-expression of the insane but also a challenge to the conventional boundaries of the art world. By embracing these works, the art world began to acknowledge that creativity and artistic talent could emerge from the most unlikely of sources, and that these pieces of art were valuable in their own right, irrespective of the artist's mental state or social standing. Had it not been for these pioneers, early examples of outsider art would not have survived. Limited as these considerations sound to our contemporary ears—sometimes sexist, racist and almost entirely devoted to exploiting the art of the insane to pin individuals to their diagnosis—they were still the first recognition that mental asylum patients could produce something meaningful and, as such, planting in the soil the seed of outsider art.

The first depictions of asylum patients producing 'art' have already been mentioned. The first one is the engraving in the 1710 illustrated edition of Jonathan Swift's *A Tale of a Tub* representing the interior male ward in Bedlam (Fig. 25). Of the six patients represented, one is

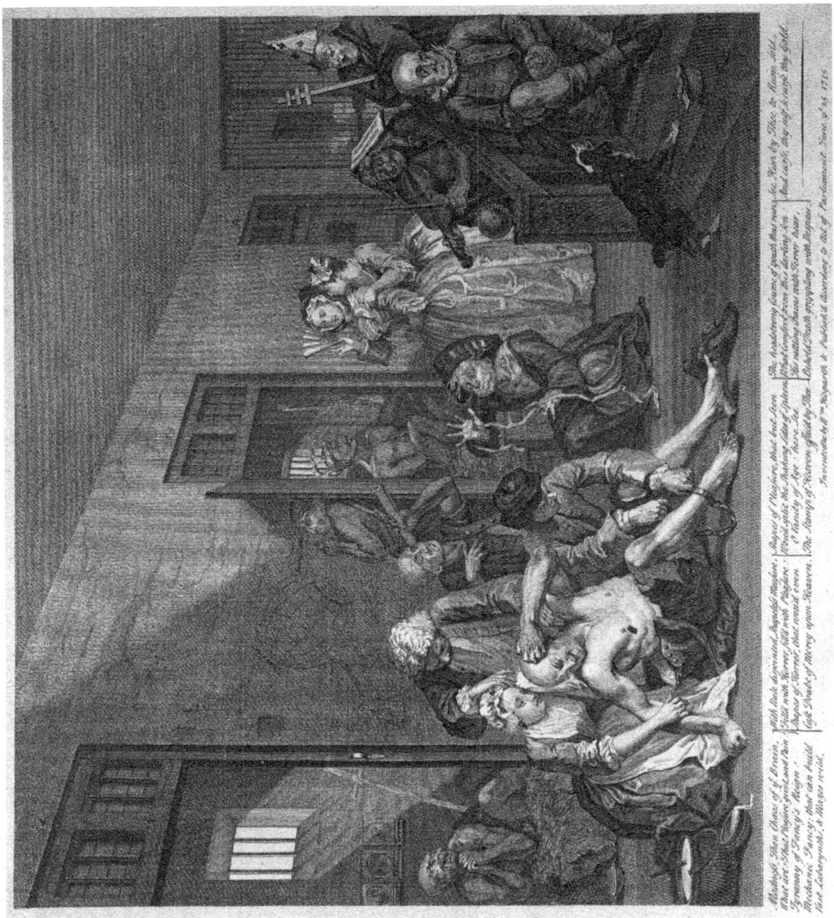

Figure 53: Hogarth's "The Rake's Progress"; plate VIII. M0008974. Source: Wellcome Collection.

looking at images painted on the wall; he is not drawing but it seems unlikely that the images on the wall could have been produced by anyone other than one of the inmates. Swift does not refer to madmen either drawing or staring at drawings on a wall, therefore this was a personal addition by the anonymous illustrator. In contrast, the final plate of William Hogarth's *A Rake's Progress* (1734) explicitly shows an inpatient drawing on a wall (Fig. 53).

This individual, half concealed behind a cell door, is drawing what looks like Whiston's 'crazy' plan of measuring the circumference of the earth using cannons and rockets. It is not just for the contents of the depictions themselves that these images are important (which have been discussed at length in relation to the representation of madness and *art brut,* for instance, by Gilman (2014) and MacGregor (1989)); these are of interest because they frame the production of outsider art within a clear spatial context: that of the asylum. Recognition of the existence of such a thing as outsider art within the psychiatric context depends, as I have shown in the previous section, on the social, cultural, medical and philosophical environment, but also on the concrete practices and limitations of its space of production.

This is another paradoxical expression of the permeability of the wall of the asylum (a concept I introduced in chapter three): for some it became a canvas and for others their works were able to escape the confinement that their creators themselves could not. The asylum as the context of this artistic production also dictates the materials employed in these artworks. Some of the artists that I will mention had access to paper and drawing and painting materials, making their works easier to preserve. Some of these works were engraved and reproduced in psychiatric publications, while other patients only had access to the walls, and their works will have been plastered over and forgotten. Others had access only to available materials, such as mops, rags, or food leftovers; some such artefacts have been preserved in Lombroso's museum, but the majority have been lost. Psychiatric institutions thus played a paradoxical role in the development of outsider art. On the one hand, they confined those (allegedly) suffering from a mental disorder, often restricting their creative expression. On the other, they provided the space and, occasionally, the materials necessary for artistic production. This dual role of the asylum, as both a space of oppression and a crucible for creativity, is evident in the works of many outsider artists, and continues to characterise and haunt outsider art to the present.

As we have seen above, Pinel was the first to mention the artistic potential of psychiatric patients. To our knowledge, however, there is only one set of surviving drawings by a patient of his, Alexis-Vincent-Charles Berbiguier de Terre Neuve du Thym. This was very likely a pseudonym, under which the patient published in 1821 an illustrated autobiography entitled *Les Farfadets or Not All Devils Come from the Other World*. Alexis saw Pinel only for one consultation and Pinel never commented on the drawings, even though he is portrayed in *Les Farfadets*, as a demon.

The first published work of outsider art is the plate that accompanies Haslam's work on Matthews's paranoid delusions. This is a reproduction of Matthews's own drawing of the terrifying 'air loom' (Fig. 54). The 'air loom' was, according to Matthews, the source of his problems as it was a machine that, by weaving air and gases into a 'wrap of magnetic fluid', allowed for the mesmeric control of the victim's mind. Matthews claimed that a gang of villains—illustrated in detail in his drawing—was controlling his mind through such a machine. This was only the tip of the iceberg of his paranoid schizophrenia, since, through a multitude of air looms scattered around London, villains were controlling the very politics of the nation, extending their magnetism all the way to the prime minister (Jay 2014).

One of Rush's patients—who signed himself 'Richard Nisbett, Mariner'—is possibly the first outsider artist whose work is preserved, along with Rush's own work, in Philadelphia (Gilman 1984). Nisbett (1753–1823) was a merchant and published writer before being committed for life to the Pennsylvania Hospital in Philadelphia. Some of the poems he wrote in the asylum were published while he was alive, although we have no record of his consent or awareness of this (Cavitch 2013, 367). Just before being admitted to the asylum, he wrote a farewell poem to his wife in a polished neoclassical style, which his close friends considered proof he was not mad and that confinement in the asylum was cruel (Coates n.d., 75–76). Perhaps because he was already a published writer, he was granted access to writing and painting materials and produced watercolours and maps to illustrate his poems. In his 1816 watercolour *An Antarctic Scenery*, Nisbett depicts a mythical nautical event during which waves shaped like angels decoy a fleet of pirates. His now famous *Mappa Mundi* (*c.*1819) features a very personal and chaotic landscape, with parts of the world crammed into the bottom two-thirds and the heavens populated by ancient Greek mythological characters, such as Pluto and Hecate (Fig. 55).

Jonathan Martin (1782–1838) was a long-term inmate of the Bedlam criminal lunatic ward (Haslam 1823, 18). We know Martin well, through his autobiographical writings, trial transcripts and

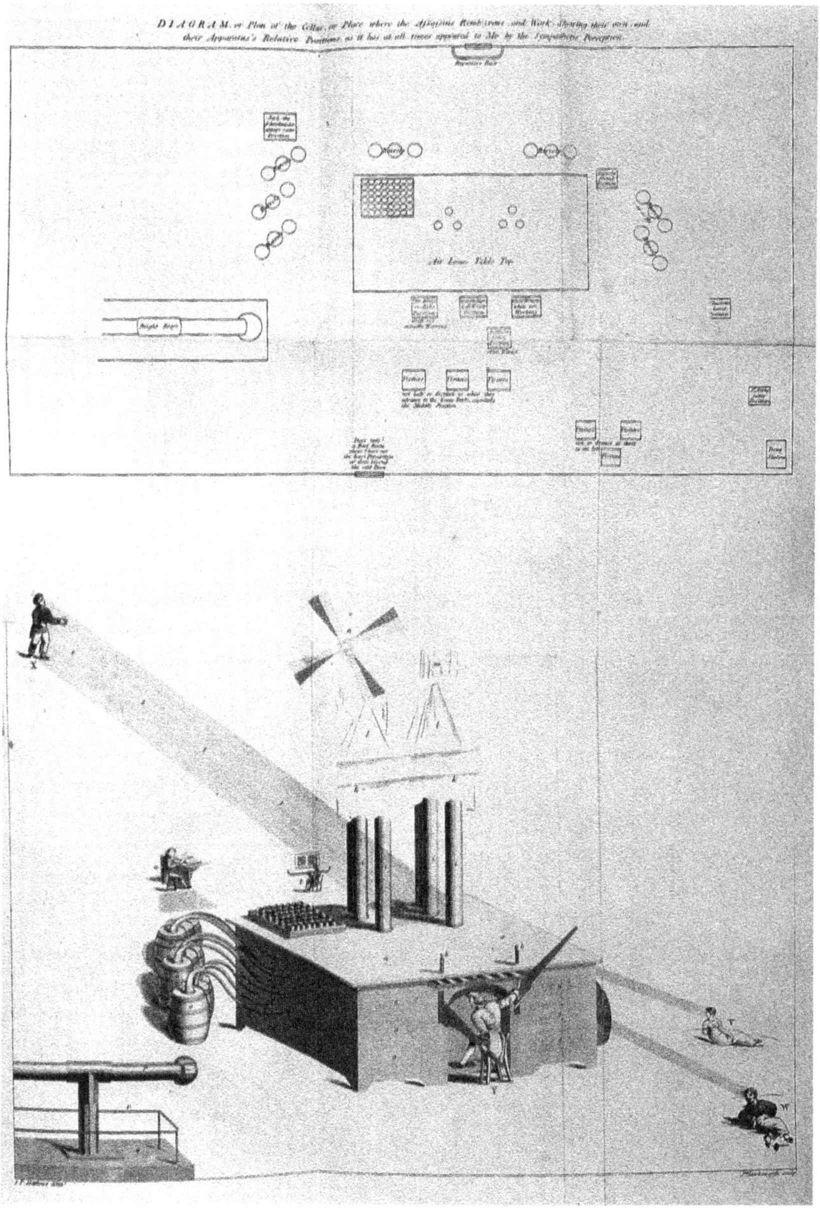

Figure 54: Illustrations of madness: exhibiting a singular case of insanity and a no less remarkable difference in medical opinion ... with a description of the tortures experienced [by the patient, James Tilly Matthews, in hallucinations] / By John Haslam. Source: Wellcome Collection.

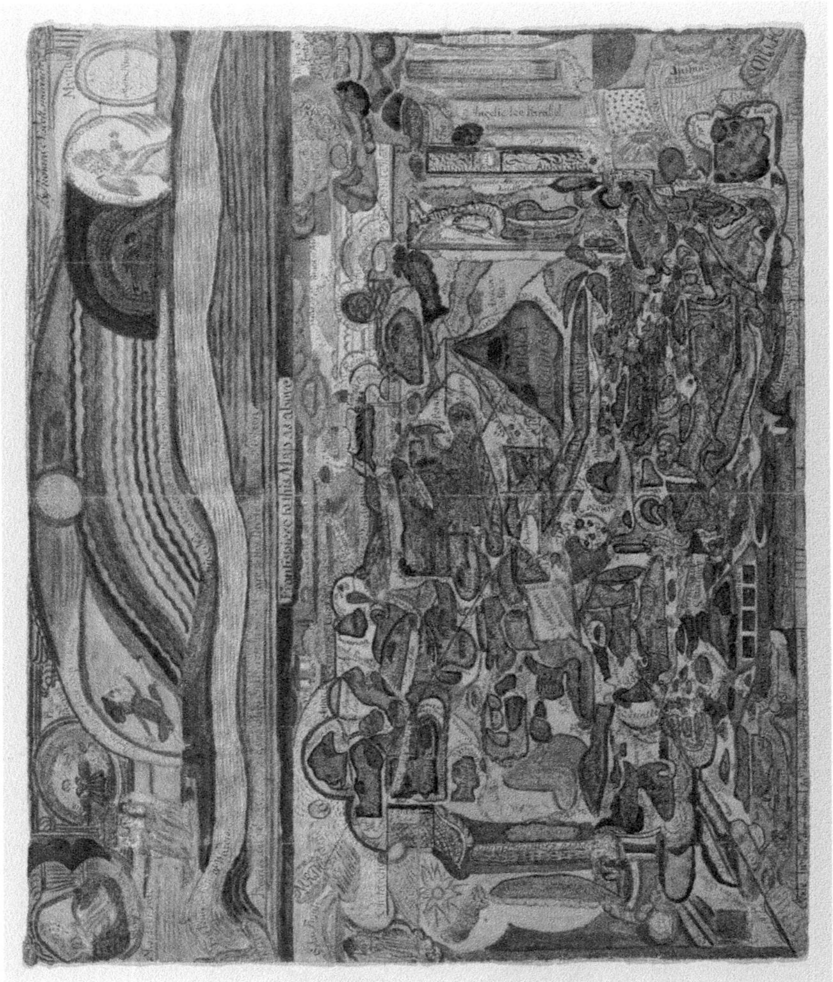

Figure 55: *Map of the World* by Richard Nisbett, ca. 1819, watercolor. Call number Of 010* 1819n. DAMS #15383, Historical Society of Pennsylvania.

accounts in the press. He had four brothers, two of whom were relatively famous: John Martin, a celebrated history painter; and William Martin, inventor and pamphleteer. Jonathan Martin spent some time in the navy, then worked as a tanner. He often disrupted church services and was committed to the private asylum of West Auckland first and then Gateshead, but then escaped and continued in his anticlerical mission. In 1825 he became an itinerant preacher, selling his autobiographical pamphlet *Life of Jonathan Martin*. When he arrived in York he started sending threatening letters to the clergy and finally set fire to York Minster, burning down its choir. Martin himself realised that this action made him famous: 'I have made as much noise as Buonaparte [*sic*] ever did' he commented in the *Yorkshire Gazette* on 28 March 1829. He was found insane at the trial for arson and committed to the criminal lunatic ward in Bedlam. Martin was not trained in the arts but always enjoyed drawing, to the point that, during his time in the navy, he escaped to source a 'box of colours for painting', a 'temptation' he 'could not resist' (Martin 1825, 12).

When he was imprisoned, after setting fire to York Minster but before being committed to Bedlam, his drawings were discussed in the press. The *York Herald* (11 April 1829, p. 2, col. 5) for instance mentioned him 'peacefully amusing himself [...] drawing and painting figures which his own disordered imagination alone can portray', and the *Yorkshire Gazette* showed some concerns about people seeking his autograph, his drawings being very popular at the time (18 April 1829, p. 2, col. 6). During his years in Bedlam, Martin drew only for the first two of his time there, but all of his works show incoherent compositions and odd shapes. Since Martin had already escaped from other asylums, he was kept in chains and could only draw in uncomfortable positions and only on one part of the large sheet of paper he had available. He was later prohibited from continuing to draw, however, since, according to Bedlam staff, this threw him into a state of 'very considerable excitement' (*The Times*, 7 June 1838, p. 6, col. 3).

Martin depicted battles between Good and Evil, and scenes such as the combat of Samson and the Lion and the son of Napoleon 'Buoneparte' (as Martin spelled Bonaparte's name) conquering England. In some of his drawings, Jonathan Martin interpreted and adapted the work of his famous brother John Martin, imbuing them with his own inner conflicts and sentiments. In *London's Overthrow* (Fig. 56), for instance, Jonathan Martin reproduces the composition of John Martin's *The Fall of Nineveh*. In Jonathan's drawing, Nineveh has become London, recognisable by Saint Paul's Cathedral and Westminster Abbey along the riverbanks of the Thames rather than the Tigris. Two inverted Union Jacks hang on Wren's monument to the Great Fire of London. The enemy army at whose hands Nineveh/ London falls is Bonaparte's French army. Rising as a new sun from the fires of the battle that is raging in the city is a lion, as Jonathan, portraying himself triumphant.

The influential and famous Romantic French writer Gérard Labrunie (1808–55; best known by his pen name, Gérard de Nerval), whom the surrealists recognised as their predecessor, was well known for suffering from an extreme form of bipolar disorder, at the time called manic-depressive psychosis. Gérard de Nerval was often hospitalised and eventually took his own life. While he is best remembered for his novels and poems, during his hospitalisations he started to paint and draw, especially on the walls with 'pieces of charcoal and brick' (De Nerval 2015, pt. 1, ch. VII, para. 5). The only testimonies that survive of these works are in the writing in de Nerval's own autobiography. The dominant figure in his wall art was Aurélia: the ideal woman, loosely based on his real-life obsession for Jenny Colon, narrator and protagonist of his autobiographical novel of the same name (published after his suicide in 1855). In de Nerval's own words, she is 'painted with the features of a goddess such as she had appeared to me in a dream' (De Nerval 2015, pt. 2, ch. XXX, para. 5). His wall paintings traced the hallucinations he saw on the walls themselves for he 'wanted to have a concrete sign of the apparition that came to console [him]' (De Nerval 2015, pt. 1, ch. VII, para. 3). Some of Gérard de Nerval's drawings on paper were collected by the French writer Maxime du Camp (1822–94), in whose *Souvenirs littéraires*, published in two volumes in 1882 and 1883, we find much information on de Nerval, as well as information on many other contemporary writers of the time. These surviving drawings are difficult to date though, and are difficult to attribute to him with any certainty. Little in them, however, gives away his condition: these are rather simple and well-organised drawings.

While de Nerval had no art training and is remembered almost exclusively for his written work, his contemporary Charles Meryon (1821–68) was considered 'the greatest French etcher of any time' (Burke 1974, 1) before being committed to the asylum of Charenton after a psychiatric crisis. The governor of Charenton allowed him to continue his etching activity within the hospital. Of the works he produced then, however, only one etching can be dated with certainty: *Ruines du Chateau de Pierrefonds*. This shows no signs of departure from Meryon's style before his hospitalisation, but when he left the asylum his style changed dramatically. He reworked several of his

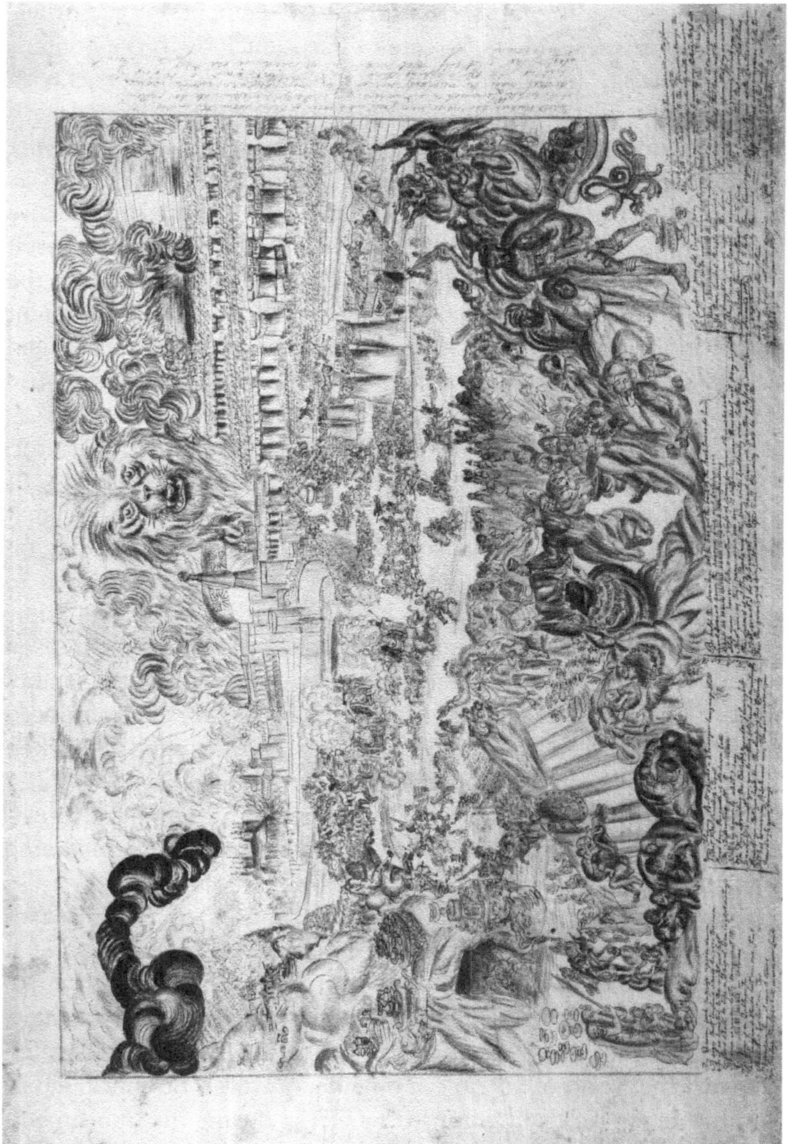

Figure 56: *London's Overthrow* by Jonathan Martin Pen and ink and wash on paper ca 1830. LDBTH703r. Courtesy of Bethlem Museum of the Mind.

previous etchings adding fantastic and bizarre elements to the otherwise realistic portrayals of the streets of Paris, such as in the 1866 *Le ministère de la marine,* in which the sky is filled with flying horses with riders, flying fish and what appear to be 'assault canoes' loaded with soldiers. Meryon's sudden departure from his previous style was met with very different reactions: his previous 'fans' and friends such as Burty seemed to disapprove of it, while the poet Charles Baudelaire was, unsurprisingly, fascinated by it (Aspenwall 1911). Meryon himself preferred these works to remain unknown: 'I have already had the occasion to express several times, an opinion that is carefully thought out, that it is fitting neither to show these pieces, nor to discuss them except extremely discreetly and prudently, because they can cause great disorders, even great evils' (Yarnall 1979, 291–92).

Richard Dadd (1817–86) was a Kentish painter and illustrator, known for works such as the frontispiece of *The Kentish Coronal* (1840) and the illustrations of *The Book of British Ballads* (1842). In August 1843, after being deemed of unsound mind, he killed his father on account of being convinced he was the Devil. Dadd then escaped to France, but while travelling to Paris he attempted to kill some fellow passengers and was apprehended by the police. He was hospitalised in Bedlam for about 20 years then was moved to Broadmoor Hospital, where he died a few years later. At the time, the work he produced before his hospitalisation captured the interest of the public only when (and because) he was apprehended for murder. The *Kentish Independent* for instance described Dadd as 'the murderer, an artist of acknowledging genius' (2 September 1843, p. 4). He started to be celebrated retrospectively as a genius who had gone mad because of an excess of imagination, which 'no doubt [...] predisposes to the diseases which has triumphed over him' (*Pictorial Times,* 9 September 1843, pp. 45–46). Evidence of his incipient insanity was sought in his works, although it was never convincingly found, perhaps unsurprisingly. During his roughly 20 years in lunatic asylums, Dadd had limited contact with the world of art on the outside; however, he continued to be a prolific artist, producing numerous works during his internment. His crimes and insanity elicited an extraordinary curiosity and, after internment, he became known as the mad painter of Bedlam. While initially his work was not reproduced, and so very few would have seen it, with time some paintings found their way out of the walls of the asylum, though we have no testimony as to how that happened. His painting *Caravanserai at Mylasa* (painted in 1845 in Bedlam) was the only painting from his asylum years to be shown at an exhibition: the Fine Art and Industrial Exhibition at Huddersfield in 1883. In the

Art Union his work was described as 'in parts eminently beautiful, but in other parts, in madness, without method'. Most importantly, the article foresaw 'how singular these outpourings of disease and mind will be to future collectors' (*Art Union*, February 1848, p. 66). In fact, in his 1902 *Reminiscences*, the painter Frederick Goodall (1902, 230) mentioned a Chalcographic Societies meeting that took place some years after 1843 during which he saw a 'remarkable collection of drawings' by Dadd, implying his work was indeed being collected and preserved. On 26 December 1877, the *World* even published a long interview with Dadd, in which the anonymous interviewer emphasised Dadd's active artistic production:

> He is surrounded by specimens of his own handiwork [...] Every detail is given with a marvellous minuteness and finish which could have been attained only by the use of the magnifying glass. [...] Art is thus his mistress still—it is to his beloved brush that he clings and wields continuously, with that enthusiasm and unwearying ardour the true painter can alone know. Many works will live after him, the product of these thirty odd years of absolute seclusion—melancholy monuments of a genius so early ship-wrecked, but which never went actually to ruin. (*World*, 26 December 1877, p. 13)

Dadd's masterpiece is *The Fairy Feller's Master-stroke* (Fig. 57), painted in Bedlam between 1855 and 1864. The painting was executed over the course of nine years, and features a stroke that MacGregor called 'microscopic' (MacGregor 1989, 127). The painting was commissioned by George Henry Haydon, head steward of Bedlam from 1852 to 1889. When Dadd was transferred to Broadmoor in 1864 he left the painting unfinished and wrote an explanatory poem, 'Elimination of a picture and its subject—called the Feller's Master Stroke', in which he describes in detail all the characters in the painting and their purpose. Apart from Shakespeare's Oberon and Titania in the top part of the painting, all the other figures are invented by Dadd. The largest one is obviously the Fairy Feller, priming a stroke to cut the chestnut from which Queen Mab's coach (from *Romeo and Juliet*) will be built. The figures at the top are the 'soldier, sailor, tinker, tailor, ploughboy, apothecary, thief' of the nursery rhyme; the apothecary additionally represents Dadd's father.

Along with fairy paintings, we have several portraits of physicians painted by Dadd, such as the portraits of Alexander Morison and of Charles Neville in Bedlam, and of William Orange in Broadmoor. These portraits testify to Dadd's ability to maintain a perfectly

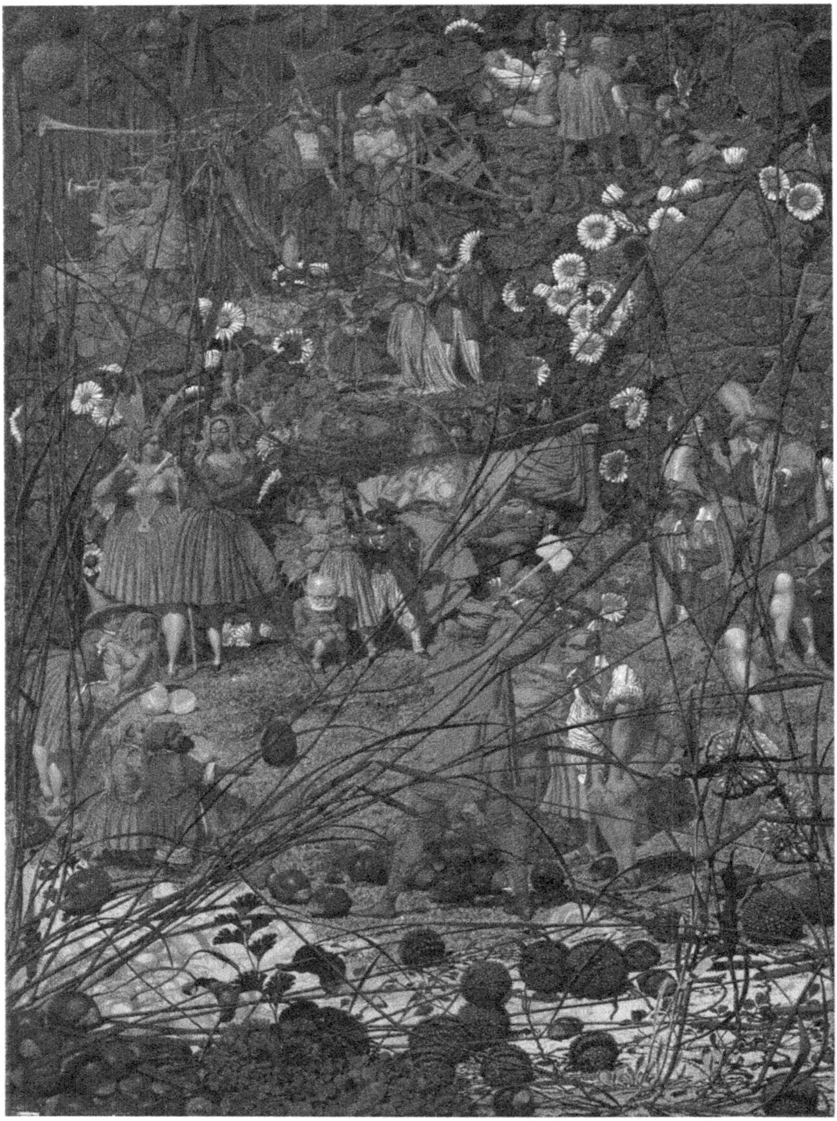

Figure 57: Fairy Fellers' Master-Stroke. Oil on Canvas 1855–1864 by Richard Dadd. Photo: Tate.

conventional style in parallel to his more original productions, such as the famous 1853 *Portrait of a Young Man* that depicts an unknown sitter in a rigid, almost photographic, pose, surrounded by disproportionate, tormented details: a large lawn roller, the contorted branches under the bench, and the mysterious combination of a fez, roses and towel on the right. Dadd was also commissioned works by the staff of the asylum; for example, he painted a now-destroyed gigantic version of *The Good Samaritan* in 1859, which hung in Bedlam's hallway, and also decorated Broadmoor theatre.

In Italy, in the meantime, Cesare Lombroso had been collecting various sorts of forensic finds since the beginning of his career in the mid-1850s (Montaldo 2015, 10). Among the skulls, death masks and photographs, he also brought together a collection of artefacts created by both criminals and the insane. It is on these that he based his initial observations in the abovementioned article 'The Art of the Insane', published in the inaugural volume of his journal *Archivio di psichiatria, scienze penali ed antropologia criminale* (1880). Some of these materials were also displayed at the 'Phreniatric Exhibition' in the same year in Reggio Emilia. In addition to numerous drawings and paintings, one find is of particular originality: the furniture etched by Eugenio Lenzi during his stay in the Royal Asylum of Lucca (*c.*1890), gifted to Lombroso by his friend and director of the Lucca asylum Andrea Cristiani. We do not know very much about Eugenio Lenzi, apart from the fact that he was a furniture carver before being admitted to Lucca based on a diagnosis of persecutory monomania (Lombroso 1906, 306). His secrétaire/table is a fine example of a melange of Baroque and Late Gothic carving with painted figures of exotic inspiration (Fig. 58). Lenzi's dressing table displays a similar mix of styles, and its 'mirror' is in fact a painting on wood. Also preserved in Lombroso's museum is a gigantic pipe, mounted on a tripod/table, decorated with naked riding figures possibly inspired by native American illustrations. All of Lenzi's works are of course only produced with the materials available to him, a variety of leftover and discarded timber, which creates a very effective rainbow of wooden colours.

Outsider art often reflects the cognitive and emotional experiences of mental illness, using visual strategies that differ significantly from mainstream art. Common themes, as already noted by Lombroso, include very personal symbolisms and mythologies, an obsession with detail, and an almost ritualistic repetition to the point where the whole canvas is filled without leaving any empty spaces, which Maclagan refers to as *horror vacui*. We can interpret these visual strategies as a way to understand the artists' mental states, offering us insights into

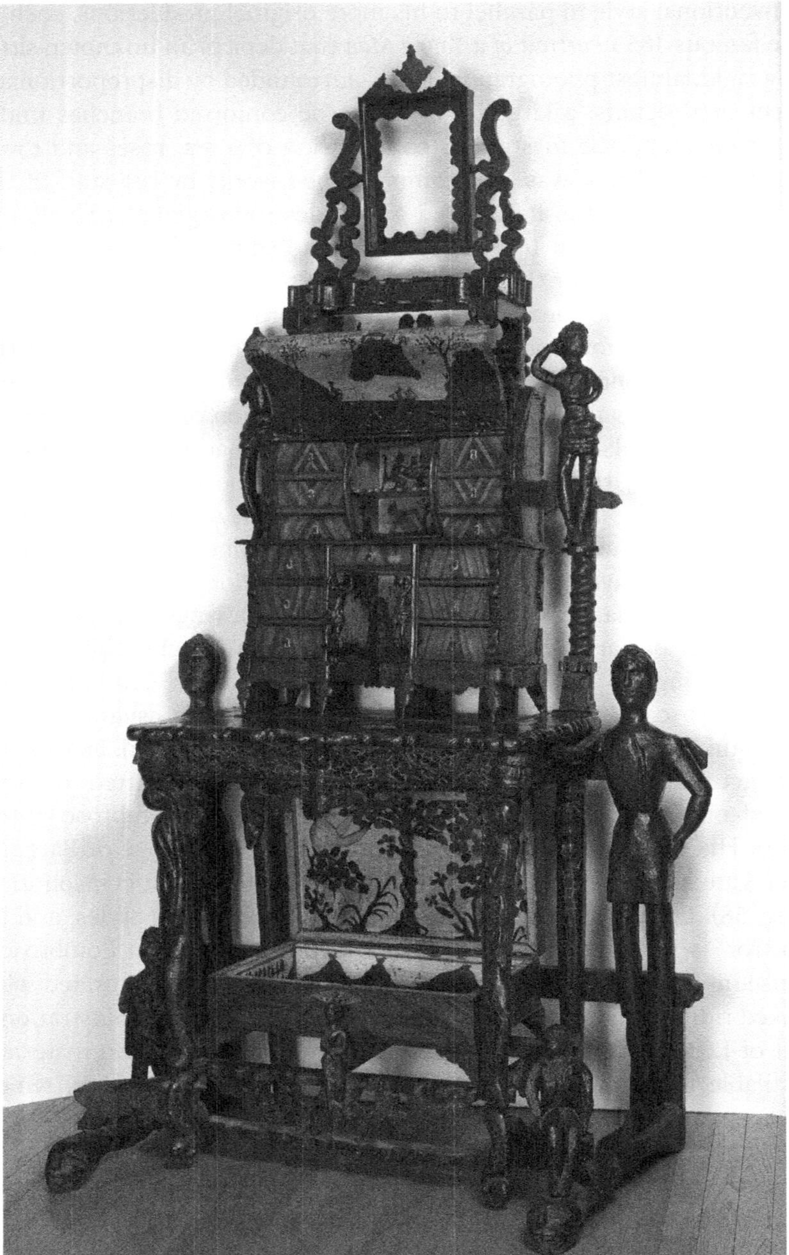

Figure 58: Eugenio Lenzi, Secretaire. Timber and paint on wood 1892. Courtesy of Museo di antropologia criminale "Cesare Lombroso", Università di Torino (Photo R. Goffi).

the experience of madness that are often inaccessible through other means, but this would replicate the mistake of early psychiatrists, who used 'outsider art' as a way to diagnose and treat mental disorders. However, we must bear in mind that it is only thanks to this mistaken strategy that the recognition of the art of the insane as an artistic form of expression was made possible in the early twentieth century.

Indeed, at this time, significant exhibitions of psychotic art were being held, beginning with ones at the Bethlem Hospital in London in 1900 and 1913, followed by exhibitions in Berlin (1913) and Moscow (1914). Auguste Marie also opened the first public 'mad museum' at the Villejuif Hospital in France in 1905, which further showcased the artistic works of mental patients. A first and rather radical step change towards recognising the aesthetic rather than the clinical value of such works came in 1907 when Paul Meunier, writing under the pseudonym Marcel Réja, published *L'Art chez les fous* (*Art by the Mad*). Réja argued that the works of the insane, though simple in form due to their lack of technical training, were driven by emotional necessity and an intellect shaped by their pathological state. He suggested that these creations shed light on the nature of artistic activity and provided a unique lens on the genesis of artistic expression (Réja 2014, 18).

Artists like Paul Klee and Wieland Herzfelde actively engaged with such psychotic art. Klee, in 1912, celebrated the art of the insane for its raw creativity. Two years later, Herzfelde, in the expressionist journal *Die Aktion*, argued that the mentally ill possessed a genuine artistic sensibility, even though it appeared strange and sometimes grotesque to others due to their different mental states. For expressionists, insanity became a symbol of artistic rebellion, an emblem of their vision for a new age (Röske 2003). They believed that the madness in their work would one day be recognised as a new form of truth, upending traditional notions of beauty and artistic norms (Rhodes 2023, 71–72).

Psychotic Art, Surrealism and Degenerate Art

André Breton and the surrealists played a key role in the recognition of outsider art. It is well known that surrealism sought to liberate the imagination from the constraints of rationality, and emphasised ways to liberate the expression of the unconscious, such as automatic writing and free association. In his first *Manifesto of Surrealism* (1924), Breton (1969, 5) emphasised the powerful imagination of the insane, describing them as 'victims of their imagination'. He argued that it was this unbridled imagination, rather than any inherent mental deficiency, that led to their institutionalisation. For Breton, the imagination of the insane was not a sign of a pathology but was rather a testament to a creative potential that society failed to understand and appreciate. This perspective laid the groundwork for surrealism's approach to creativity, where the boundaries between madness and artistic genius were deliberately blurred. For Breton, surrealism sought to 're-create a state akin to madness' (Breton 1969, 175) to foster creativity. Similar to, but more emphatically than, the Romantics, for the surrealists art originates from madness. Breton's critique was not theoretical, it had tangible impact on how the art of the insane was perceived and valued. Surrealism's embrace of the unconscious, the irrational and the spontaneous were very much in tune with psychotic art. By validating these forms of expression, the surrealists not only challenged the boundaries of what was considered legitimate art, but also questioned the societal norms that deemed such expressions as pathological. In parallel with surrealism, numerous exhibitions of art of the insane in mainstream art galleries were organised, such as the 1927–28 *Les imageries des fous* at the Vavin Gallery in France.

The surrealists' interest in the art of the insane was part of a broader movement within twentieth-century art to break away from the constraints of rationalism and bourgeois conventions. They sought to uncover deeper truths about the human psyche, which they believed were obscured by the demands of modern society. Psychotic art was considered as a raw, unfiltered depiction of the unconscious, which thus offered a powerful counterpoint to the polished, deliberate creations of academic art. For the surrealists, these works were profound expressions of the human condition, worthy of serious artistic consideration. Two works in particular play a key role in defining outsider art in the 1920s: one by Walter Morgenthaler (1921) and the other by Hans Prinzhorn (1922).

In 1921, Walter Morgenthaler published *Madness & Art: The Life and the Works of Adolf Wölfli*, the study that made Wölfli's work a central example of outsider art (Morgenthaler 1992). Morgenthaler's book was one of the first to focus on a psychiatric patient not only as a subject of medical interest but as a true artist in his own right. Wölfli, who spent over 30 years at the Waldau Hospital, produced thousands of intricate drawings and musical compositions, many of which were part of a vast autobiographical project. His work, including the visionary *From the Cradle to the Grave* (1908–12), explored his imaginary adventures before the death of his mother (Fig. 59). Morgenthaler noted the distinctive iconography in Wölfli's art, characterised by an obsessive *horror vacui*,

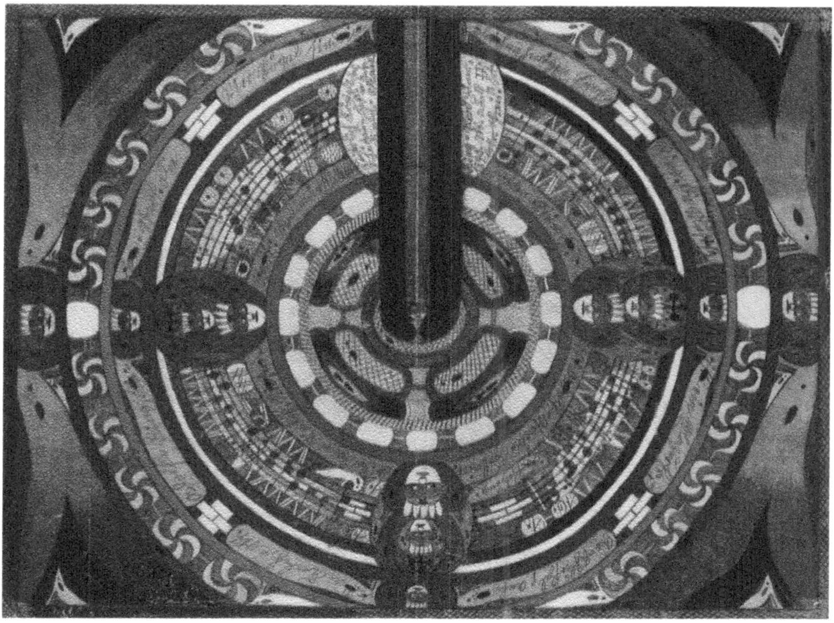

Figure 59: Adolf Wölfli, Keiserlich Königliches Schützen=Fest in Ada Kalch,=Skt. Adolf=Ring=Nord, 1919. Courtesy of Kunstmuseum, Basel, Sammlung Online, https://sammlungonline.kunstmuseumbasel.ch/eMP/eMuseumPlus?service=ExternalInterface&module=collection&objectId=10700&viewType=detailView.

where every space on the page is filled with imagery, musical notation or text. His drawings often featured symbolic 'little birds' as well, which Morgenthaler suggested were linked to Wölfli's sexual preoccupations, adding layers of meaning that shifted depending on context. Wölfli's art gained broader recognition when Swiss curator Harald Szeemann included his work in the *Documenta 5* exhibition in Kassel, Germany, in 1972, marking a key moment in outsider art's acceptance within the mainstream. Many of Wölfli's works are now held in the Adolf Wölfli Foundation at the Museum of Fine Arts in Bern, his so-called 'bread pictures'—created to sell in exchange for drawing materials—remain well represented in collections like Dubuffet's *Collection de l'Art Brut*.

In *Artistry of the Mentally Ill* (1922), Prinzhorn was cautious about categorising the creative output of mentally ill patients as 'art'. Instead, he suggested these works should be 'viewed psychologically' or he referred to them as *Bildnerei*: a term more accurately translated as

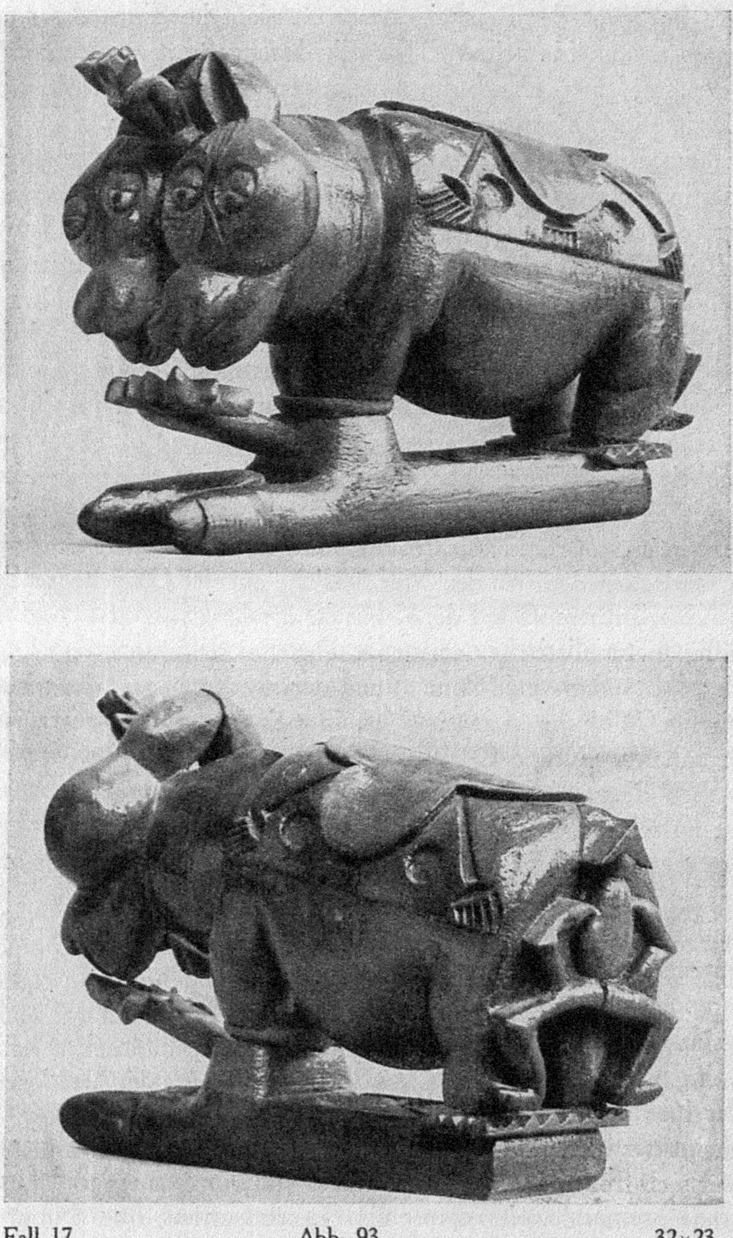

Fall 17. Abb. 93. 32×23.

„Nilpferd mit 2 Köpfen auf dem Stiefelknecht". Holz, bemalt.

Figure 60: Page from Prinzhorn's *Artistry of the Mentally ill*. Courtesy of Universitätsbibliothek, Heidelberg.

'image-making' rather than art in the conventional sense (Prinzhorn 1972, 1) (Fig. 60). Despite his reluctance to label these creations as art, Prinzhorn's work is a milestone in the recognition of outsider art. Just two years after the publication of his book, Prinzhorn co-curated an exhibition in Heidelberg showcasing the works of 'untrained mental patients' (Prinzhorn 1972, 3). Prinzhorn considered the art of the insane as spontaneous creations, arising from the patients' inner needs without external inspiration. He also noted, like Lombroso, a resemblance between these works and those produced by children or so-called primitive artists, and the importance of their supposed isolation and primitivity as the soil of their creativity (Prinzhorn 1972, 4). These ideas soon gained traction beyond Germany, and Prinzhorn's book amply circulated in French surrealist circles during the 1920s, largely thanks to Max Ernst. Although a French translation of the book would not be published until decades later, its images profoundly influenced surrealist thought. Prinzhorn's analysis of the art of the mentally ill was marked by a deep ambivalence. He referred to ten creators in particular (all male) as 'schizophrenic masters', recognising the powerful 'creative urge' behind their *Gestaltung*, a term Prinzhorn used to describe the unique configuration or organisation of their output (Prinzhorn 1972, xviii). According to Prinzhorn, psychotic art had to be 'direct, raw, and non-illusionistic' (Rhodes 2023, 74), and he saw in these works a testament to the patients' vitalist drive to create. However, he also viewed these creations through a normative lens, drawing a clear distinction between normal and pathological expressions. Prinzhorn drew on philosopher and psychologist Ludwig Klages, and argued that 'expression' is a fundamental human phenomenon, which allows internal psychological content to be conveyed. However, he observed that in the case of the mentally ill, this expression became 'self-sufficient', thus failing to serve as a means of communication with the external world. For Prinzhorn, this 'defect' in expression was a clear indication of the patient's abnormality (Prinzhorn 1972, 13). He recognised that a 'creative urge' resided in both 'normal' and 'abnormal' artists, yet he argued that only the creative drive of the 'normal' artist was linked to a willingness to engage with the shared world. In contrast, the schizophrenic artist, according to Prinzhorn, was detached from humanity, and unable and unwilling to reconnect. He stated that if a schizophrenic could re-establish this connection, they would be cured. He believed that the art of the mentally ill conveyed a sense of 'complete autistic isolation and gruesome solipsism', which further highlighted their detachment from the shared human experience (Prinzhorn 1972, 266).

This inherent distinction in Prinzhorn's work laid the groundwork for a very troubling legacy. His collection and theories became central to the infamous 1937 Nazi exhibition *Entartete Kunst* (Degenerate Art) in Munich, which used the concept of 'degeneration' to attack modernist artists. Although the Nazis extended Prinzhorn's ideas to also label mentally ill artists as 'degenerate', the seeds of this interpretation were already present in Prinzhorn's work. We do not know how much Prinzhorn would have subscribed to Nazi ideas because he died in 1933, but his ideas were further exploited by Carl Schneider, the psychiatrist and director of the Heidelberg Psychiatric Hospital, who delivered a lecture titled 'Degenerate Art and Mad Art'. In his 1939 article, Schneider utilised Prinzhorn's collection to argue that the art of the mentally ill was evidence of their abnormality and proposed a 'working therapy' to destroy these works and redirect patients toward 'normal tasks' (Schneider 1939, 160).

Outsider Art, *Art Brut*: Ambiguities and Issues

So far I have used the term 'outsider art' to define works that have been recognised as works of art but were produced outside of canonical art circles, and 'psychotic art' or the 'art of the insane' to distinguish outsider art specifically produced by those labelled as mentally ill. In the late 1940s, the first term to define outsider art was coined, namely *art brut*. It was the artist Jean Dubuffet who conceived the term to emphasise its disruptive potential; he was influenced by a trip to Swiss psychiatric hospitals with writer Paulhan and architect Le Corbusier to find masterpieces of such 'raw art'. In 1947, he established the *Foyer de l'art brut* at the René Drouin Gallery in Paris and, along with contemporaries like Breton, founded the *Compagnie de l'art brut* in 1948. Dubuffet defined *art brut* in 1948 as artistic works—be they paintings, drawings, sculptures or other objects—that were free from the influence of traditional art forms, whether it be from museums, salons or galleries. These works, according to Dubuffet, should emerge from the 'original human substance', and be driven solely by the creator's personal invention and emotional impulses. The key was that the works were produced without any concern for established conventions or external validation, even if they appeared rough or incomplete. Dubuffet maintained that the value of these creations lay in the pure, unfiltered manifestation of the individual's creative faculties, unmasked and unconstrained (Berne 1973, 205–6).

Dubuffet's *art brut* encompassed not only the creations of those labelled as 'mad' but also the works of children, 'primitives' and practitioners of folk art, because they had no formal connection to the art-historical canon and were untainted by the artistic traditions of the West. In Dubuffet's view, this made them more authentic, that is to say, less contaminated by cultural norms. *Art brut* contrasted with what he called the 'cultural arts', that is to say, works produced within traditional frameworks and thus diluted by societal expectations and norms (Dubuffet 1986, 32). Dubuffet sought to distance his notion of *art brut* from clinical or psychopathological interpretations. According to Maclagan (2010, 13), Dubuffet's collection

> superficially [...] resembled the heterogeneous collections that were assembled by turn-of-the-century psychiatrists such as Lombroso, Ladame and Morgenthaler; but one of the purposes of his collection was a quite contrary one: to free these works from any association with psychopathology and to recognize them instead as examples of uncompromisingly individual forms of creativity.

His goal was to liberate these works from the medical discourse that had previously defined them and to remove the pathological lens through which they were often viewed. Dubuffet's vision of *art brut* sought to celebrate unmediated personal expression and challenge traditional art frameworks. However, Dubuffet also aimed to position *art brut* as an alternative form of expression that disrupted conventional art institutions. It was certainly a step forward and it also gave *art brut* a potential for socio-political disruption, but he did not distance himself sufficiently from the essential premise—that is, to be disruptive it needs to be produced by individuals already labelled as different: *othered*. *Art brut* functions as the *other* of institutional art only because it is produced by those already *othered* by mainstream society. Crucial, in fact, to Dubuffet's definition of *art brut* were two premises: 'utter originality in form and content, and the social or psychological isolation of its creator' (Maclagan 2010, 14).

We have seen that from its origins, outsider art rests on an ambivalence around the relationship between madness and creativity. This ambivalence persists in *any* conception of outsider art. On the one hand, the mentally ill were celebrated for their spontaneous, uninhibited expression, but on the other, their work was viewed through a lens that was grounded on their initial exclusion from the mainstream. According to Maclagan (2010, 35), Dubuffet's approach to the art of psychiatric patients, while less overtly medicalised than those of earlier 'collectors' such as Lombroso or Prinzhorn, was still premised on the notion that the insane are other, and can thus tap into a more spontaneous creativity. Dubuffet's interpretation of works of *art brut* as valuable artistic expressions did not entirely escape Prinzhorn's framing, according to which outsider art was symptomatic of the patients' conditions. Instead, it reified the idea that creativity in the mentally ill was rooted in their detachment from societal norms (Maclagan 2010, 74).

As we have seen earlier, one of the defining moments of *art brut* was its collection: early collectors, such as Lombroso, brought together what they deemed worth preserving, but *mutatis mutandis* defined what outsider art was by deciding what to collect. Dubuffet's *Collection de l'Art Brut* was foundational in bringing attention to these works and shifting the conversation away from purely clinical interpretations. However, the act of collecting and curating this art—while ostensibly celebrating the marginalised—further positioned the mentally ill as 'other'. By institutionalising these works, curators and collectors reinforced the idea that the mentally ill existed in a world apart from mainstream society. While outsider art could be said to have been 'institutionalised' the moment it was defined as outsider art, similarly it entertains an ambiguous, almost paradoxical relationship with the institution of psychiatry itself, the asylum. This brings us back to the permeability of the walls of the psychiatric institutions: even in the context of outsider art, such places become the very condition of the creation of art. Asylums create the marginalised individuals who, cut off as they are from the world at large, and the world of art in particular, create art independently of its mainstream. They create the condition of isolation that Dubuffet claimed was central for the definition of *art brut*. At the same time, these asylums provided the materials (whether as part of art therapy or as salvaged materials) and the context to produce art. They were also where the eye of the collector (initially psychiatrists) could concentrate to find the art to collect. As Maclagan (2010, 106) has it, 'when the institutional context is taken into account, the balance shifts: in the end it still looks as if the definition of "psychotic art" is that of work created by people with designated psychological disorders, and this gives them a ready-made Outsider status'. The institutionalisation of outsider art is taken one step further in places like the House of Artists in Gugging (Austria) or the Living Museum in New York (USA). While these spaces provide opportunities for individuals with psychiatric conditions to create and exhibit their work, they also reinforce the notion that these individuals, and their art, belong in a separate category. The commercialisation of outsider art, where works are sold and collected in mainstream galleries, risks turning these creators into commodities, valued more for their difference than for their artistry (Maclagan 2010, 20).

It is impossible for anyone to be truly 'outside' the culture they inhabit. Even works that appear isolated or unmediated are still created within a broader social context that influences both the artist and the reception of their work. The very act of collecting and exhibiting outsider art in fact brings it into the institutional framework it was meant to resist. The distinction between inside and outside continues to be blurred, perhaps increasingly so. This blurring of boundaries is evident in the way outsider art has been integrated into the mainstream art market. Once collected and exhibited, these works are no longer entirely outside the cultural system at all, but instead occupy a liminal space. This creates a tension between a desire to celebrate outsider art for its originality, and the reality that its inclusion in galleries and museums inevitably subjects it to the same processes of commodification and institutionalisation that govern traditional art.

Conclusions

As the arts, including outsider art, became more commodified, the subversive potential of the art of the insane waned. The development of outsider art, while celebrating the creativity of those suffering from a mental disorder, has also contributed to the perpetuation of the othering of the insane. Dubuffet's insistence on the authenticity and originality of these works, while freeing them from clinical pathology, did not free their creators from the label of 'other'. While these works are celebrated for their raw, unfiltered creativity, they are also positioned as 'different', further placing madness in a world apart from the rest of society. The institutionalisation of outsider art, whether through collection or commercialisation, only deepens this divide, as outsider work risks being valued more for its difference than for its integration into the broader cultural landscape. Thus, the history of *art brut* and outsider art reflects the ongoing tension between celebration and exclusion in the visualisation of mental disorders.

However, the recognition of outsider art must not be downplayed. It is a milestone in the history of the representation of mental disorders, especially in terms of visualisation. The recognition of outsider art signifies the recognition that those who suffer from mental disorders can be creative, can be geniuses, or shows us simply that all human forms of expression and self-representation are valid and worthy of being valued and seen per se. Making the art of the insane visible means to make visible a once underrated and concealed aspect of mental disorders. Its recognition has had a subversive impact that has shaken the foundations of both psychiatric and artistic institutions, much akin to the 'unmasking' carried out by Italian radical psychiatry. To this extent, madness continues to trouble borders, especially those of institutions.

A Brief Concluding Note—Madness as Visual Otherness and Narratives of Madness Today

If sanity and insanity exist, how have we known them? Throughout these chapters I have shown that we have known them by visually othering the insane. Across the history of visualising mental disorders, I have observed persistent patterns of 'othering', tropes through which the visual representation of mental illness has served to delineate the boundaries between the 'sane' and the 'insane'. These boundaries are often blurred, and even when visualisation intervenes to define them, we encounter permeability and semantic exchanges. Mental disorders, however, have been rather invariably depicted as deviant, abnormal, different, as something to be contained and controlled, excluded and marginalised. This study has demonstrated how visual representations of mental disorders have not merely reflected prevailing medical and cultural understandings, but actively shaped them. Early anatomical drawings and institutional photography provided a pseudoscientific basis for psychiatric diagnoses, reinforcing pathologisation through visual evidence.

In the twentieth century, cinema and popular media further entrenched these stereotypes, often equating mental illness with violence, unpredictability or tragic vulnerability. In 1960, for the very first time in the history of cinema, spectators look through the eyes of a maniac murderer. Hitchcock's masterpiece *Psycho* (1961) features for the first time an inversion of the usual point of view: we are cast into the head of a mad serial killer. This is one of the mainstream tropes of the representation of madness in cinema: the psychopathic murderer, the serial killer. Most of us will have seen the masterful performances of actors such as Anthony Hopkins in *Silence of the Lambs* (1991) or Charlize Theron in *Monster* (2003). We do not need to look for extremes. According to Riles and colleagues (2021), up to 70 per cent of characters with mental disorders in cinema and television are associated with physical aggression, and there is often little differentiation between psychoses such as schizophrenia and psychopathy (i.e., lack of empathy and propensity for violence) (Goodwin 2014). Rare conditions such as dissociative identity disorder are not only over-represented but also represented in their most extreme manifestations, as in the trope of the split personality, for example, in *Fight Club* (1999), *Identity* (2003) and *Split* (2016). The (inevitable) descent into madness is also a prevalent trope in cinema. We see it at play in Hitchcock's *Vertigo* (1958), Scorsese's *Taxi Driver* (1976) and Hanneke's *Der siebente Kontinent* (1989), in which the daily life of an ordinary family starts to reveal its absurdity. The inversion of the perspective and madness is used as a means to show that it is the world that is mad (a trope with which we are certainly familiar by now—see chapter three). Madness in films often also engages with the trope of the bacchanal and collective insanity; such is the case for instance with Pasolini's *Salò* (1975). The descent into madness, however, is more commonly depicted on the silver screen as a consequence of isolation, for instance in Kubrick's *The Shining* (1980) or Eggers's *The Lighthouse* (2019). The entrance into the asylum is sometimes the consequence, sometimes the beginning and sometimes even the metaphor of the descent into madness. We see this in Fuller's *Shock Corridor* (1963), in Scorsese's *Shutter Island* (2010) and even in sci-fi films such as Gilliam's *12 Monkeys* (1995). Some of these tropes derive from the visual-cultural ones that I have explored in this book: the multitude of the insane, the entrance into the asylum and the permeability of its walls (madness as the world gone mad). Others, such as the over-representation of extreme disorders and the association with violence, seem to be the latest iteration of long-lasting tropes, such as the raging maniacs from the *Orlando Furioso* (1532) and Cibber's statues (1676) at the entrance of Bedlam. It has been reported numerous times that cinema and television tend to exacerbate stereotypes when it comes to depiction of mental disorders (e.g., Goodwin 2014; Riles 2020; O'Hara 2019; Nordahl-Hansen, Tøndevold and Fletcher-Watson 2018), showing how the tropes discussed in this monograph can have a very real effect on our understanding of madness.

The latest iteration of the visualisation of mental disorders and their othering is generative artificial intelligence (genAI). GenAI, despite perhaps common misconceptions, does not conjure images of mental disorders *ex nihilo*; it recombines and extrapolates them from vast datasets composed of millions of pre-existing images.

These datasets are often scraped indiscriminately and from 'less curated, lower-quality sections of the internet, expanding into more chaotic, unmoderated domains' (Flathers et al. 2024, 2). As such they are saturated with the visual conventions, cultural assumptions and historical tropes that have long shaped the depiction of 'madness', which we have explored in this monograph, making this historical analysis all the more relevant. AI-generated imagery is not a neutral or innovative way of seeing mental disorders, but rather a particularly efficient means of excavating—and perpetuating—the biases and stereotypes embedded in our collective visual culture (Papazova, Hasan and Khorikian-Ghazari 2025). Early research in this sense showed how prompting visual genAI with 'schizophrenia' returned images of horror-film-styled faces screaming (*à la* King's *It* or Wan's *Saw*) (King 2022). Flathers and colleagues (2024, 4) note how prompts for 'depression' return images of idle women in pensive position and dark colours, while prompts for 'schizophrenia' return raging and screaming males, akin to the iconography of melancholia and mania I discussed in chapter three.

As Flathers and colleagues (2024, 4) argue, genAI stands in continuity with earlier technologies: each leap forward in image production has initially been greeted as more objective and trustworthy than its predecessors, equipping those intent on classifying diagnoses by appearance with apparently more 'scientific' tools. Yet, as history has shown, such misplaced trust in the evidentiary power of the image reveals that the act of making madness visible is a socio-cultural act rather than a medical or scientific one. The danger today lies in the unprecedented reach and persuasive realism of genAI: the very mechanism that reveals entrenched stereotypes also amplifies and disseminates them globally, at the speed of the algorithm. In this way, genAI does not break with the historical logic of the visual 'othering' of the insane—it updates and scales it, making vigilance all the more urgent as we consider its implications for psychiatric concepts and public perceptions (Flathers et al. 2024, 4).

At the same time, new tropes emerge in visual culture, such as the ever-growing urbex (urban exploration) trend of photographing abandoned buildings, especially former mental hospitals: the decaying walls, the torn charts and signs on the dusty floors, the unavoidable wide-angle shot of a single chair or wheelchair in the foreground of a seemingly never-ending corridor, the gloomy photos of examination rooms and operating theatres (often, especially in the past decade, characterised by the enhanced sharpening and hyper-saturation afforded by HDR—high dynamic range—techniques). The list of potential photos, photographers and websites exemplifying this trend would be extremely long. I would encourage the reader to enter 'abandoned asylum photography', and variants thereof, into a search engine to discover an ever-growing number of such photographs and reportage. Such trends speak of morbid curiosity, certainly, but also of the desire to explore the historical roots of our current understanding of mental health, to ascertain that those places are indeed abandoned and decaying and do not still house our treatment of mental disorders. More complex works, rejecting the urbex trend, stand out. Such is the case with Giacomo Doni.[1] His work can be defined as one of conservation: conservation of memories, architectural spaces and their stories. Doni's photographic work focuses on preserving memory through the reconstruction of narratives: the spaces of former asylums are photographed and narrated directly in the first person, while patients emerge through testimonies, objects and even letters which inpatients addressed to the outside of the asylum but that were never posted, letters which he collects in his meticulous but also creative and humane archival work (Fig. 61).

Doni's work is one of the fissures in the historical patterns I have explored that are emerging in the contemporary landscape. Advocacy and recovery movements, patient-centred and intersectional approaches to mental health, 'mad studies' and evolving ethical standards in visual culture have indeed promoted more nuanced representations. Leveraging on the inversions operated by anti-psychiatry, and on the grounds of the recognition of outsider art, individuals with lived experience are reclaiming the narrative, using visual media not as a tool of othering but as a means of self-representation and empowerment. There are many such examples. Shawn Coss collected in the *It's All in Your Head* artbooks (2024) his 'Inktober Illness' and 'Feartober' illustrations, which feature DSM-5 diagnoses such as borderline personality disorder, in black and white with deep ink tones, reminiscent of horror comic books. Drawing on his experience as an ER nurse, Coss accompanies illustrations with a description of the disorder. 'It's hard to talk about mental illness, sometimes art speaks louder than words', he, quite rightly, claims in the promotional material to his second artbook.[2] Similarly, Toby Allen explores mental health through character design in his series 'Real Monsters' (2013–current).

1 Giacomo Doni's work can be found at https://www.giacomodoni.com/ [accessed 17 Mar. 2025].

2 See https://anymeansnecessary.com/collections/books/products/its-all-in-your-head-2nd-dose-edition [accessed 26 Aug. 2025].

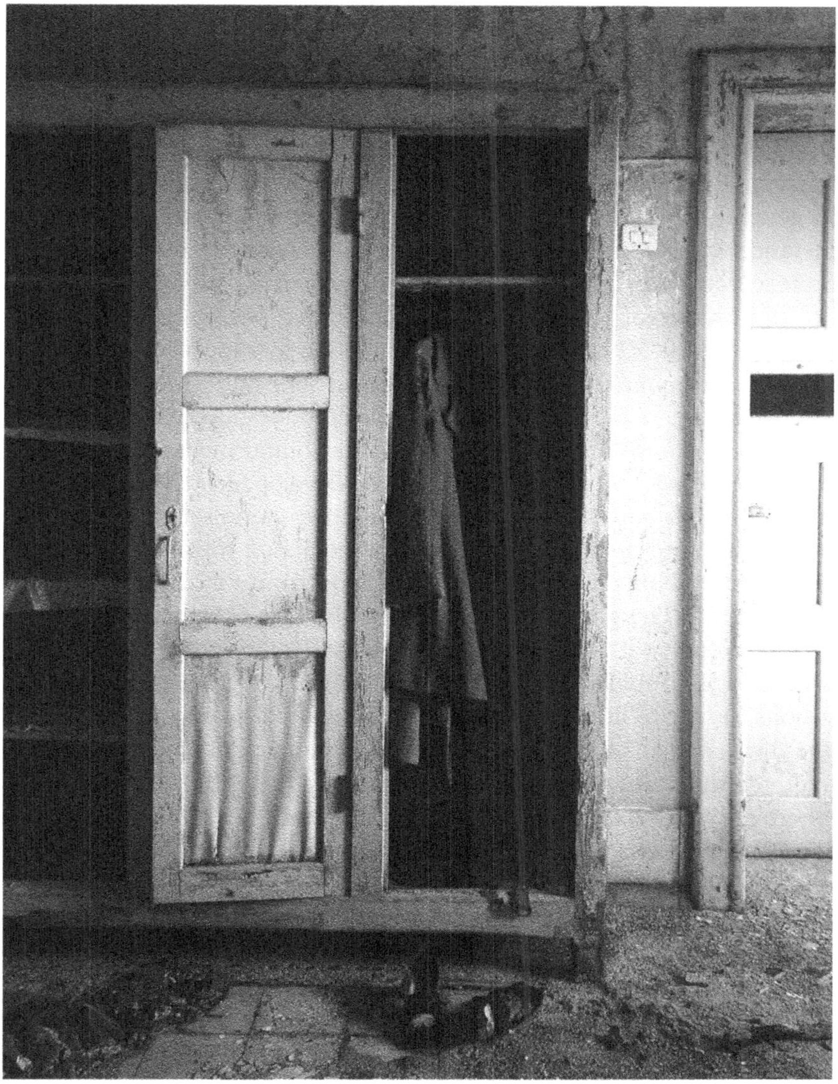

Figure 61: Giacomo Doni, *Identità*, ex manicomio di Cogoleto, 2007.
© Doni, www.giacomodoni.com.

He describes several DSM-5 diagnoses as if they were monsters in a role-playing game or Pokémon, and accompanies them with colourful illustrations, as if we were reading any of Dungeons & Dragons' many *Monster Manuals*.[3]

After Dubuffet's definition of *art brut*, numerous exhibitions and museums dedicated to outsider art, the art of the insane or insanity in general have been created all over the world. Such is the case for instance with the travelling *Museo della follia* that proposes a variety of representations of madness across the history of art, alongside outsider art and images of, and from, lunatic asylums.[4] Vision as a subject of mental distress is also thus acknowledged, further blurring the boundaries that iconography has tried to demarcate, but which have been just as troubled by such visualising attempts. Videogames explore, both visually and interactively, mental health and mental illness. The case of *Hellblade: Senua's Sacrifice* (2017), developed by Ninja Theory,[5] is emblematic: born as a puzzle action fantasy game set entirely in the mind of the protagonist, a Celtic girl called Senua who battles against the invading Norsemen, it became an opportunity to raise awareness of psychosis. The game was funded also by the Wellcome Trust, and was developed with the support of professors of psychology and advocacy groups to make Senua's experience of hearing voices and seeing visions as true to life as possible. The same year also saw the release of *The Town of Light*,[6] a first-person walking simulator in which the player explores the accurately mapped abandoned asylum of Volterra (Italy), where they find letters and notes by the former inpatients and visually reconstruct their story.

Championing an approach based on 'mad studies', Netchitailova (2019, 1514) suggests that 'unlike modern diagnoses, art gives us the possibility to explore, to venture into different views and interpretations'. A significant yet tangential strand to the central focus of this monograph is such use of visual arts in mental health care, for instance as promoted in the health humanities.[7] Here the visual is not employed to make madness visible in the historical sense I have explored here—to diagnose, categorise or 'other'—but to enable those living with mental disorders to narrate, process and sometimes

3 See https://www.zestydoesthings.com/realmonsters [accessed 20 Feb. 2025].
4 See https://museodellafollia.it/ [accessed 20 Feb. 2025].
5 See https://ninjatheory.com/ [accessed 20 Feb. 2025].
6 See http://www.thetownoflight.com/ [accessed 20 Feb. 2025].
7 See for instance http://www.healthhumanities.org/creative_practice_mutual_recovery/ [accessed 15 Aug. 2025].

reconfigure their own experiences. Such practices, which range from art therapy to community arts projects, can be seen as a continuity and culmination of the inversion traced in chapters seven and eight, respectively on anti-psychiatry and outsider art: the gaze is turned inward and reclaimed by the subject, the image becomes a tool of recovery rather than of control. The resulting works challenge stigma, build new identities and transform clinical and cultural spaces (Crawford et al. 2015). All scientific evidence supports rather than discredits such approaches, in that it demonstrates that culture, the arts and everyday experience have an important determining factor on our biology, even on our genetic material, for a long time considered to be an immutable destiny written before birth (see, e.g., Leigh 2010). While thanks to the health humanities and other efforts such approaches are gaining traction, biomedical research in psychiatry continues to perpetuate many of the visual tropes historically used to 'make madness visible', reinforcing rather than dismantling the objectifying gaze.

Every month that goes by new forms of visual representation—medical, scientific, artistic, othering, inclusive or otherwise—of mental disorders emerge, making the scope of the present work a never-ending process. The history of the visual representation of mental disorders ultimately forms a cultural history of visual 'othering'. This othering is an attempt to make sense of an invisible, chameleon-like, variable and potentially devastating occurrence, such as a mental disorder, by means of bringing it into the field of vision as something 'other'. A process of visual othering can be seen at work in references to many categories of 'outcasts' and 'unwanted'. The most recent of these is certainly that of 'asylum seekers', 'migrants': the multitude of such individuals depicted as overflowing—often, for obvious reasons, overflowing a *ship*—adrift in the sea, vagrants outside of their home; and the inverse visual need for containment, incarnated in the image of the wall, made of barbed wire, as long as entire national borders, as tall as that of a prison in containment centres. While the vision of the 'unwanted' turns to different subjects, at whatever point in time we decide to stop and take stock of the visual cultural production to date, the visual history of mental disorders reveals the power of the vision in shaping societal attitudes and cultures.

We cannot discount the centrality of visualisation, visual representation and the visual arts in shaping our understanding of the world in general and of mental disorders in particular. It is, however, an understanding which is afforded only through the unavoidable ideological prescriptions that the very gesture of making something manifest visually entails. While the legacy of othering and marginalisation remains deeply entrenched, new media and emerging approaches suggest the potential for visual culture to move in different directions, at least for mental health, enabling a reappropriation of discriminatory tropes and the overcoming of stigma.

References

Aggarwal, Niel K. 2009. "Neuroimaging, Culture, and Forensic Psychiatry." *Journal of the American Academy of Psychiatry and the Law* 37 (2): 239–44.

Agrimi, Jole. 1997. "La ricezione della 'fisiognomica' pseudoaristotelica nella facoltà delle arti." *Archives d'histoire doctrinale et littéraire du Moyen Âge* 64: 127–88.

Aloisi, Alessandra, and Fabio Camilletti. 2021. "Introduction." In *Archaeology of the Unconscious: Italian Perspectives*, edited by Alessandra Aloisi and Fabio Camilletti, 1–12. London: Routledge.

al-Rāzī, Abū Bakr Muḥammad ibn Zakarīyā. 1490. *Liber nonus ad Almansorem. Cum expositione Sillani de Negris. Receptae Petri de Tussignano supra nonum ad Almansorem*. Venice: Bonetus Locatellus impensis Octaviani Scoti.

Amateis, Margherita. 2015. "Ai confini dell'umano: Selvaggi, Folli, Orsi. Tradizioni amerindiane ed europee medievali." In *Uomini e orsi*, edited by Enrico Comba and Daniele Ormezzano, 212–91. Accademia University Press.

Antoine-König, Élisabeth. 2024. "Une balade de fou et de dames: L'amour, la luxure et la mort." In *Figures du fou: Du Moyen Age aux romantiques*, edited by Élisabeth Antoine-König and Le Pogame Pierre-Yves, 72–103. Paris: Gallimard.

Aretaeus. 1923. *On the Cure of Chronic Diseases. Book I*. In *The Extant Works of Aretaeus, the Cappadocian*, edited by Francis Adams. London: Sydenham Society.

Arnott, Robert, Stanley Finger and Chris Smith, eds. 2003. *Trepanation: History, Discovery, Theory*. Psychology Press.

Artico, Marco, Marialuisa Spoletini, Lorenzo Fumagalli, Francesca Biagioni, Larisa Ryskalin, Francesco Fornai, Maurizio Salvati, Alessandro Frati, Francesco Saverio Pastore and Samantha Taurone. 2017. "Egas Moniz: 90 Years (1927–2017) from Cerebral Angiography." *Frontiers in Neuroanatomy* 11: 81.

Aspenwall, Bradley. 1911. "Meryon and Baudelaire." *Print Collector's Quarterly* 1 (December): 587–609.

Assirelli, Marco. 1988. "L'immagine dello 'stolto' nel salmo 52." In *Il codice miniato: rapporti tra codice, testo e figurazione. Atti del III congresso di storia della miniatura. Cortona 20–23 ottobre 1988*, edited by Melania Ceccanti and Maria Cristina Castelli, 19–34. Florence: Olschki.

Attwell, David, and Costantino Iadecola. 2002. "The Neural Basis of Functional Brain Imaging Signals." *Trends in Neurosciences* 25 (12): 621–25.

Augustine. 1991. *Sermon 70A—Again from the same chapter of the gospel on humility*. In *The Works of Saint Augustine. A Translation for the 21st Century. Sermons III (51–94) on the New Testament*, edited by E. Hill, 243–45. New York: New York City Press.

Babiloni, Fabio, Claudio Babiloni, Filippo Carducci, Febo Cincotti and Paolo Maria Rossini. 2003. "'The Stone of Madness' and the Search for the Cortical Sources of Brain Diseases with Non-Invasive EEG Techniques." *Clinical Neurophysiology: Official Journal of the International Federation of Clinical Neurophysiology* 114 (10): 1775–80.

Backman, E. Louis. 1952. *Religious Dances in the Christian Church and in Popular Medicine*. George Allen and Unwin.

Bartholomew, Robert E., and Erich Goode. 2001. *Little Green Men, Meowing Nuns and Head-hunting Panics: A Study of Mass Psychogenic Illnesses and Social Delusion*. Illustrated edition. Jefferson: McFarland & Co.

Basaglia, Franco. 2023a. "Il mondo dell'incomprensibile schizofrenico." In *Scritti 1953–1980*, 47–70. Milan: Il Saggiatore.

—. 2023b. "Introduzione a *Morire di classe*." In *Scritti 1953–1980*, 567–72. Milan: Il Saggiatore.

—. 2023c. "La 'comunità terapeutica' come base in un servizio psichiatrico: Realtà e prospettive." In *Scritti 1953–1980*, 271–90. Milan: Il Saggiatore.

—. 2023d. "La distruzione dell'ospedale psichiatrico come luogo di istituzionalizzazione." In *Scritti 1953–1980*, 261–70. Milan: Il Saggiatore.

—. 2023e. "Presentazione a 'L'istituzione negata'." In *Scritti 1953–1980*, 455–58. Milan: Il Saggiatore.

Basaglia, Franco, and Franca Ongaro Basaglia, eds. 1969. *Morire di classe. La condizione manicomiale fotografata da Carla Cerati e Gianni Berengo Gardin*. Turin: Einaudi.

—, eds. 2024. *Morire di classe. La condizione manicomiale fotografata da Carla Cerati e Gianni Berengo Gardin. Ediz. illustrata*. Milan: Il Saggiatore.

Basser, Peter Joel, Joseph Mattiello and Denis Le Bihan. 1994. "MR Diffusion Tensor Spectroscopy and Imaging." *Biophysical Journal* 66 (1): 259–67.

Battanoli, Dalmazio. 1881. *Relazione statistica del M.C.M.: Quadriennio 1877–1880*. Venice: Antonio Francesconi.

Baxandall, Michael. 1988. *Painting and Experience in Fifteenth Century Italy: A Primer in the Social History of Pictorial Style*. 2nd edition. Oxford: Oxford University Press.

Beaulieu, Anne. 2002a. "Images Are Not the (Only) Truth: Brain Mapping, Visual Knowledge, and Iconoclasm." *Science, Technology, & Human Values* 27 (1): 53–86.

Beaulieu, Christian. 2002b. "The Basis of Anisotropic Water Diffusion in the Nervous System – a Technical Review." *NMR in Biomedicine* 15 (7–8): 435–55.

Becker, George. 1978. *The Mad Genius Controversy: A Study in the Sociology of Deviance*. London: Sage.

Bell, Charles. 1847. *The Anatomy and Philosophy of Expression as Connected to the Fine Arts*. London: John Murray.

Bell, Matthew. 2014. *Melancholia: The Western Malady*. Cambridge: Cambridge University Press.

Bennett, Craig M., Michael B. Miller and George L. Wolford. 2009. "Neural Correlates of Interspecies Perspective Taking in the Post-Mortem Atlantic Salmon: An Argument for Multiple Comparisons Correction." *Neuroimage* 1: 39–41.

Berengo Gardin, Gianni, and Carla Cerati. 1998. *Per non dimenticare: 1968 la realtà manicomiale di Morire di classe*, edited by Franca Ongaro Basaglia. Torino: Edizioni Gruppo Abele.

Berengo Gardin, Gianni, et al. 1973. "The Concerned Photographer: gruppo italiano." *Il diaframma: fotografia italiana*. Maggio: n.p.

Berne, Jacques, ed. 1973. *Jean Dubuffet. Cahier de l'Herne*. Paris: Éditions de l'Herne Murard.

Berrios, German E. 1984. "Epilepsy and Insanity During the Early 19th Century. A Conceptual History." *Archives of Neurology* 41 (9): 978–81.

Bertillon, Alphonse. 1890. *La photographie judiciaire avec un appendice sur la classification et l'identification anthropométriques*. Paris: Gautier-Villars et fils.

Blom, Jan Dirk. 2010. *A Dictionary of Hallucinations*. Cham: Springer.

Bloomfield, Peter S., Sudhakar Selvaraj, Mattia Veronese, Gaia Rizzo, Alessandra Bertoldo, David R. Owen, Michael A.P. Bloomfield, Ilaria Bonoldi, Nicola Kalk, Federico Turkheimer, Philip McGuire, Vincenzo de Paola and Oliver D. Howes. 2016. "Microglial Activity in People at Ultra High Risk of Psychosis and in Schizophrenia: An [11C]PBR28 PET Brain Imaging Study." *American Journal of Psychiatry* 173 (1): 44–52.

Bolis, Tomaso Mario. 2009. "Le ragioni di una mostra." In *"Nonostante la vostra cortese ospitalità..." Fotografia e disagio mentale oggi*, edited by Tommaso Mario Bolis and Claudio Marra, 9–18. Bologna: Quinlan.

Bollati, Giulio. 1979. "Note su fotografia e storia." In *Storia d'Italia. Annali 2. L'immagine fotografica 1845–1945*, edited by Carlo Bertelli and Giulio Bollati, 5–58. Turin: Einaudi.

Bos, Elisabeth Henriette, Rogier Hoenders and Peter de Jonge. 2012. "Wind Direction and Mental Health: A Time-Series Analysis of Weather Influences in a Patient with Anxiety Disorder." *Case Reports* 2012: bcr2012006300.

Boshears, Rhonda, and Harry Whitaker. 2013. "Phrenology and Physiognomy in Victorian Literature." *Progress in Brain Research* 205: 87–112.

Bourguignon, Erika Eichhorn. 1968. "World Distribution and Patterns of Possession States." In *Trance and Possession States*, edited by Raymond Prince, 3–34. Montreal: R.M. Bucke Memorial Society.

Brant, Sebastian. 1962. *The Ship of Fools*. Dover Publications.

Breton, André. 1969. *Manifestoes of Surrealism*. Ann Arbor: University of Michigan Press.

Bright, Molly G., Joseph R. Whittaker, Ian D. Driver and Kevin Murphy. 2020. "Vascular Physiology Drives Functional Brain Networks." *Neuroimage* 217: 116907.

Broca, Paul. 1876. "Sur l'âge des sujets soumis à la trépanation chirurgicale néolithique." *Bulletins et Mémoires de la Société d'Anthropologie de Paris* 11 (1): 572–76.

Brushfield, Thomas Nadauld. 1857. "Application of Photography to Lunacy." *Journal of the Photographic Society* 3: 289.

Bulbena, Antonio, Guillem Pailhez, Rosa Aceña, Jordi Cunillera, Adria Rius, Carles Garcia-Ribera, José Gutiérrez and Carla Rojo. 2005. "Panic Anxiety, Under the Weather?" *International Journal of Biometeorology* 49 (4): 238–43.

Burke, James D. 1974. *Charles Meryon: Prints & Drawings*. New Haven: Yale University Art Gallery.

Burton, Robert. 2004. *The Anatomy of Melancholy*. 1621.

Cagnetta, Franco, ed. 1981. *Nascita della fotografia psichiatrica*. Venice: La Biennale di Venezia.

Campanella, Tommaso. 2011. *Selected Philosophical Poems of Tommaso Campanella*, edited by Sherry Roush. Chicago: University of Chicago Press.

Campbell, Kirsten. 1999. "The Slide in the Sign; Lacan's Glissement and the Registers of Meaning." *Angelaki* 4 (3): 135–43.

Cardano, Girolamo. 2003. *Metoposcopia. Manuale per la lettura della fronte*. 2° edizione. Milano: Mimesis.

Cardinal, Roger. 1972. *Outsider Art*. London: Studio Vista.

Cardinali, Daniel Pedro. 2016. *Ma Vie en Noir: Fifty Years with Melatonin and the Stone of Madness*. New York: Springer.

Carey, Benedict. 2006. "Searching for the Person in the Brain." *New York Times*.

Catullus. 1913. *Carmina*. In *Catullus. Tibullus. Pervigilium Veneris*, translated by F.W. Cornish, J. Postgate, J.W. Mackail and G. Goold, edited by Jeffrey Henderson. Cambridge: Harvard University Press.

Cavitch, Max. 2013. "Clericus and the Lunatick." *The Papers of the Bibliographical Society of America* 107 (3): 367–76.

Charcot, Jean-Martin. 1889. *Clinical Lectures on Diseases of the Nervous System Delivered at the Infirmary of la Salpêtrière*, translated by Thomas Savill. London: The New Sydenham Society.

Cheyne, George. 1733. *The English Malady: or, A Treatise of Nervous Diseases of all Kinds as Spleen, Vapours, Lowness of Spirits, Hypochondriacal, and Hysterical Distempers, etc.* London: Strahan.

Clarke, Basil. 1975. *Mental Disorder in Earlier Britain: Exploratory Studies*. Cardiff: University of Wales Press.

Coates, Samuel. N.d. *Cases of Several Lunatics in the Pennsylvania Hospital and the Causes Thereof in Many of the Cases', ca. 1785–1825*. Philadelphia: Pennsylvania Hospital Historic Collections.

Cocles, Bartolommeo della Rocca. 1536. *Physionomiae et Chiromantiae Compendium*. Strasbourg: Albertus, J.

Cohen, Jonathan, and Aaron Meskin. 2004. "On the Epistemic Value of Photographs." *Journal of Aesthetics and Art Criticism* 62 (2): 197–210.

Colaizzi, Janet. 2005. "Seclusion & Restraint: A Historical Perspective." *Journal of Psychosocial Nursing and Mental Health Services* 43 (2): 31–37.

Coleridge, Samuel Taylor. 2014. *Biographia Literaria*. Edinburgh: Edinburgh University Press.

Conolly, John. 1858. "The Physiognomy of Insanity." *Medical Times and Gazette* 16: 2–4.

Corcoran, Kevin. 1997. "Mental Illness Defined." *The Times (Hammond, Indiana)*, 14 Sept. 1997, 64.

Coughlin, Sean. 2018. "Athenaeus of Attalia on the Psychological Causes of Bodily Health." In *Mental Illness in Ancient Medicine: From Celsus to Paul of Aegina*, edited by Chiara Thumiger and Peter N. Singer, 107–42.

Courtine, Jean-Jacques, and Claudine Haroche. 2007. *Histoire du visage: exprimer et taire ses émotions (du XVIe au début du XIXe siècle)*. Paris: Payot & Rivages.

Crawford, Paul, Brian Brown, Charley Baker, Victoria Tischler and Brian Abrams. 2015. *Health Humanities*. London: Palgrave.

Cross, Simon. 2010. *Mediating Madness: Mental Distress and Cultural Representation*. Basingstoke: Palgrave Macmillan.

Crossley, Nick. 2006. *Contesting Psychiatry: Social Movements in Mental Health*. Psychology Press.

Cserey, Éva. 1974. "Adatok a besztercebányai (Banská Bystrica) kalyhacsempékhez." *Folia archaeologica* 25: 205–17.

Cubero, José. 1998. *Histoire du vagabondage – Du Moyen Âge à nos jours*. Paris: Editions Imago.

Curti, Denis. 2013. *Gianni Berengo Gardin: Stories of a Photographer*. Venice: Marsilio.

D'Alessandro, Luciano. 1967. "Il mondo degli esclusi." *Popular Photography Italiana* 117: 51–54.

D'Alessandro, Luciano, and Sergio Piro. 1969. *Gli esclusi. Fotoreportage da un'istituzione totale*. Milan: Il Diaframma.

D'Autilia, Gabriele. 2012. *Storia della fotografia in Italia: dal 1839 a oggi*. Turin: Einaudi.

Dalla Palma, Sisto. 1981. "Nel labirinto della follia." In *Nascita della fotografia psichiatrica*, edited by Franco Cagnetta, 9–10. Venice: Marsilio.

Dandy, Walter E. 1918. "Ventriculography Following the Injection of Air Into the Cerebral Ventricles." *Annals of Surgery* 68 (1): 5–11.

Dani, Alessandro. 2018. *Vagabondi, zingari e mendicanti: leggi toscane sulla marginalità sociale tra 16o e 18o secolo*. Luxemburg: Editpress.

De Nerval, Gerard. 2015. *Aurelia: The Dream and the Life*, translated by J. O'Keefe. No City: Kindle Edition.

De Saussure, Ferdinand. 2013. *Course in General Linguistics. Bloomsbury Revelations*. London: Bloomsbury.

Deane, Susannah. 2019. "rLung, Mind, and Mental Health: The Notion of 'Wind' in Tibetan Conceptions of Mind and Mental Illness." *Journal of Religion and Health* 58 (3): 708–24.

Dell'Acqua, Giuseppe. 2007. *Non ho l'arma che uccide il leone*. Viterbo: Stampa Alternativa.

Della Porta, Giovan Battista. 1586. *De humana physiognomonia*. 4 vols. Vico Equense: Cacchi, Giuseppe.

—. 1599. *De humana physiognomonia*. 6 vols. Naples: Tarquinio Longo.

—. 1610. *Della Fisonomia dell' huomo*. Naples: Giacomo Carlino e Costantino Vitale.

DePaulo, J. Raymond. 2006. "Bipolar Disorder Treatment: An Evidence-Based Reality Check." *American Journal of Psychiatry* 163 (2): 175–76.

Descartes, René. 1995. *A Discourse on Method*, translated by John Veitch. Urbana, IL: Project Gutenberg. 1637.

Devlin, Hannah. 2020. "Schizophrenia Study Finds Evidence of Reduced Links Between Brain Cells." *Guardian*.

Di Marco, Silvia. 2015. "Tra simbolo e indice. Considerazioni sulla fotografia psichiatrica di H.W. Diamond." *PsicoArt—Rivista di arte e psicologia* 5 (5): 1–28.

Diderot, Denis. 1751. "Les Theosophes." *Encyclopaedia* Vol XVI: 253–61.

—. 1916. *Diderot's Early Philosophical Works*, translated by Margaret Emily Jourdain. Chicago: The Open Court Publishing Company.

Didi-Huberman, Georges. 2004. *Invention of Hysteria: Charcot and the Photographic Iconography of the Salpêtrière*, translated by Alisa Hartz. Cambridge: MIT Press.

Dobbs, David. 2005. "Fact or Phrenology?" *Scientific American Mind*, 16(1).

Donnelly, Michael. 2003. *The Politics of Mental Health in Italy*. London: Routledge.

Drew, Patrick J. 2019. "Vascular and Neural Basis of the BOLD Signal." *Current Opinion in Neurobiology* 58: 61–69.

Dubuffet, Jean. 1986. *Asphyxiante Culture*. Paris: Les Éditions de Minuit.
Dumit, Joseph. 2004. *Picturing Personhood: Brain Scans and Biomedical Identity*. Princeton: Princeton University Press.
Eisenberger, Naomi I., Matthew D. Lieberman and Kipling D. Williams. 2003. "Does Rejection Hurt? An FMRI Study of Social Exclusion." *New York* 302 (5643): 290–92.
Engel, Johann Jacob. 1785. *Ideen zu einer Mimik*. Berlin: Mylius.
Enoch, David, Basant K. Puri and Hadrian Ball. 2020. *Uncommon Psychiatric Syndromes*. London: Routledge.
Erle, Sibylle. 2010. *Blake, Lavater, and Physiognomy*. London: Legenda.
Esquirol, Jean-Etienne-Dominique. 1838. *Des maladies mentales considérées sous les rapports médical, hygiénique et médico-légal*. Paris: J.-B. Baillière.
Falkai, Peter, Andrea Schmitt and Nancy Andreasen. 2018. "Forty Years of Structural Brain Imaging in Mental Disorders: Is it Clinically Useful or Not?" *Dialogues in Clinical Neuroscience* 20 (3): 179–86.
Faria, Miguel A. 2013. "Violence, Mental Illness, and the Brain—A Brief History of Psychosurgery: Part 1—From Trephination to Lobotomy." *Surgical Neurology International* 4: 49.
Finger, Stanley, and William Clower. 2003. "On the Birth of Trepanation: The Thoughts of Paul Broca and Victor Horsley." In *Trepanation: History, Discovery, Theory*, edited by Robert Arnott, Stanley Finger and Chris Smith. Psychology Press.
Finger, Stanley, and Paul Eling. 2019. *Franz Joseph Gall: Naturalist of the Mind, Visionary of the Brain*. Oxford: Oxford University Press.
First, Michael B., Wayne C. Drevets, Cameron Carter, Daniel P. Dickstein, Lauren Kasoff, Kerri L. Kim, Jonathan McConathy, Scott Rauch, Ziad S. Saad, Jonathan Savitz, Karen E. Seymour, Yvette I. Sheline and Jon-Kar Zubieta. 2018. "Clinical Applications of Neuroimaging in Psychiatric Disorders." *American Journal of Psychiatry* 175 (9): 915–16.
Flathers, Matthew, Griffin Smith, Ellen Wagner, Carl Erik Fisher and John Torous. 2024. "AI Depictions of Psychiatric Diagnoses: A Preliminary Study of Generative Image Outputs in Midjourney V.6 and DALL-E 3." *BMJ Mental Health* 27 (1): e301298.
Foot, John. 2015a. *The Man Who Closed the Asylums: Franco Basaglia and the Revolution in Mental Health Care*. London: Verso.
—. 2015b. "Photography and Radical Psychiatry in Italy in the 1960s. The Case of the Photobook *Morire di Classe* (1969)." *History of Psychiatry* 26 (1): 19–35.
Forgacs, David. 2014. *Italy's Margins: Social Exclusion and Nation Formation Since 1861*. Cambridge: Cambridge University Press.
Fornaciari, Verusca. 2005. "Fotografando il manicomio. L'archivio fotografico dell'istituto psichiatrico San Lazzaro di Reggio Emilia." In *Il volto della follia. Cent'anni di immagini del dolore*, edited by Sandro Parmiggiani, 107–11. Milan: Skira.
Foucault, Michel. 2002. *Archaeology of Knowledge*. London: Routledge.
—. 2009. *History of Madness*. London: Routledge.
Fraser, Kathrin. 1998. "The Photographic Insane." *Cinémas* 9 (1): 139–51.
Frugard, Roger. 2002. *The Chirurgia of Roger Frugard*, edited by Leonard D. Rosenman. Philadelphia, PA: Xlibris Corp.

Gall, Franz Joseph, and Johann Gaspar Spurzheim. 1810. *Anatomie et physiologie du système nerveux en général, et du cerveau en particulier, : Avec des observations sur la possibilité de reconnoître plusieurs dispositions intellectuelles et morales de l'homme et des animaux, par la configuration de leurs têtes*. Paris: F. Schoell.

Galzigna, Mario. 2007. "San Servolo: Dal convento al manicomio. Materiali per una storia." In *Museo del Manicomio di San Servolo. La follia reclusa*, 7–32. Venice: Arsenale.

Georget, Étienne-Jean. 1820. *De la folie, ou aliénation mentale*. Paris: Crevet.

—. 1823. *De la folie, ou aliénation mentale*. Paris: Rignoux.

Geremek, Bronisław. 1994. *Poverty: A History*, translated by Agnieszka Kołakowska. Oxford: Blackwell.

—. 2014. "L'emarginato." In *L'uomo medievale*, edited by Jacques Le Goff. Kindle. Bari: Laterza.

Giannichedda, Maria Grazia. 2005. "Introduzione." In *L'utopia della realtà*, edited by Franca Ongaro, vii–lii. Turin: Einaudi.

Gifford, Douglas Juan. 1974. "Iconographical Notes Towards a Definition of the Medieval Fool." *Journal of the Warburg and Courtauld Institutes* 37 (1): 336–42.

Gillihan, Seth J. 2016. "Using Brain Scans to Diagnose Mental Disorders." *Psychology Today*. Available at https://www.psychologytoday.com/gb/blog/think-act-be/201605/using-brain-scans-to-diagnose-mental-disorders

Gilman, Sander L. 1984. "Madness and Representation: Hans Prinzhorn's Study of Madness and Art in its Historical Context." In *The Prinzhorn Collection: Selected Work from the Prinzhorn Collection of the Art of the Mentally Ill: Krannert Art Museum, University of Illinois, Urbana/Champaign, Champaign, Illinois, November 10, 1984 to January 6, 1985 …* edited by Stephen Prokopff and Gisbert Freiherr zu Putlitz, 7–14. Urbana-Champaign, IL: Krannert Art Museum.

—. 1988. *Disease and Representation: Images of Illness from Madness to AIDS*. Ithaca: Cornell University Press.

—. 2014. *Seeing the Insane*. Brattleboro, VT: Echo Point Books & Media.

—. 2015. *The Face of Madness: Hugh W. Diamond and the Origin of Psychiatric Photography*. Brattleboro: Echo Point Books and Media. 1976.

Glasser, Otto. 1993. *Wilhelm Conrad Röntgen and the Early History of the Roentgen Rays*. San Francisco: Norman Publishing.

Godbey, Emily. 2000. "Picture Me Sane: Photography and the Magic Lantern in a Nineeenth-Century Asylum." *American Studies Journal* 41 (1): 31–69.

Goffman, Erving. 1961. *Asylums: Essays on the Social Situation of Mental Patients and Other Inmates*. 1st edition. New York: Anchor Books.

Goldstein, Jan E. 2001. *Console and Classify: The French Psychiatric Profession in the Nineteenth Century*. Chicago: University of Chicago Press.

Goodall, Frederick. 1902. *The Reminiscences of Frederick Goodall*. London: Walter Scott.

Goodwin, John. 2014. "The Horror of Stigma: Psychosis and Mental Health Care Environments in Twenty-First-Century Horror Film (part II)." *Perspectives in Psychiatric Care* 50 (4): 224–34.

Govi, Gilberto. 1851. "Académie des sciences." *La Lumière: Revue de la photographie* 12 (2): 5.

Greene, Joshua, and Jonathan Cohen. 2006. "For the Law, Neuroscience Changes Nothing and Everything." In *Law and the Brain*, edited by Semir Zeki and Oliver Goodenough, 207–26. Oxford: Oxford University Press.

Gross, Angelika. 1999. "Das Bild des Narren: Von Psalm 52 zu Sebastian Brant." In *Bild und Abbild vom Menschen im Mittelalter: Akten der Akademie Friesach "Stadt und Kultur im Mittelalter", Friesach (Kärnten), 9. – 13. September 1998*, edited by Elisabeth Vavra, 273–91. Klagenfurt: Wiser Verlag.

Gruia, Ana Maria. 2008. "Fools, Devils and Alchemy. Secular Image in the Monastery." *Studia Patzinaka* 2: 129–45.

Guazzo, Francesco Maria. 1988. *Compendium Maleficarum: The Montague Summers Edition*. Chelmsford: Courier Corporation.

Hamilton, Jon. 2022. Brain Scans May Reveal a Lot About Mental Illness, But Not Until Studies Get Bigger. *MPR News*. Available at https://www.npr.org/sections/health-shots/2022/04/26/1094319294/mri-brain-scan-mental-illness-brain-research [accessed 26 Apr. 2025].

Harpin, Anna, and Juliet Foster. 2014. "Introduction: Locating Madness and Performance." In *Performance, Madness and Psychiatry: Isolated Acts*, edited by Anna Harpin and Juliet Foster. London: Palgrave Macmillan.

Harrington, Anne. 2019. *Mind Fixers: Psychiatry's Troubled Search for the Biology of Mental Illness*. New York: W.W. Norton & Co.

Harris, Max. 2014. *Sacred Folly: A New History of the Feast of Fools*. Ithaca: Cornell University Press.

Hartman, John J., Sarah M. White, James G. Ravin and Gerald P. Hodge. 1976. "The Stones of Madness." *American Imago* 33 (3): 266–95.

Harvey, E. Ruth. 1975. *The Inward Wits: Psychological Theory in the Middle Ages and the Renaissance*. London: Warburg Institute, University of London.

Haseloff, Günther. 1938. "Die Psalterillustration im 13. Jahrhundert: Studien zur Geschichte der Buchmalerei in England, Frankreich und den Niederlanden." PhD, Göttingen.

Haslam, John. 1823. *Sketches in Bedlam: Or Characteristic Traits of Insanity as Displayed in the Cases of One Hundred and Forty Patients of Both Sexes, Now, or Recently, Confined in New Bethlem. By a Constant Observer*. London: Sherwood, Jones.

Hausken, Liv. 2015. "The Visual Culture of Brain Imaging." *Leonardo* 48 (1): 68–69.

Henderson, Theodore A., Muriel J. van Lierop, Mary McLean, John Michael Uszler, John F. Thornton, Yin-Hui Siow, Dan G. Pavel, Joe Cardaci and Phil Cohen. 2020. "Functional Neuroimaging in Psychiatry—Aiding in Diagnosis and Guiding Treatment. What the American Psychiatric Association Does Not Know." *Frontiers in Psychiatry* 11: 276.

Hetherington, Kevin, and Rolland Munro. 1997. *Ideas of Difference: Social Spaces and the Labour of Division. Sociological review monograph*. Oxford: Blackwell Publishers/The Sociological Review.

Hinrichs, TJ, and Linda L. Barnes, eds. 2013. *Chinese Medicine and Healing: An Illustrated History*. Cambridge: Harvard University Press.

Hippocrates. 1923. *Breaths*. In *Prognostic. Regimen in Acute Diseases. The Sacred Disease. The Art. Breaths. Law. Decorum. Physician (Ch. 1). Dentition (Loeb Classical Library 148)*, translated by W.H.S. Jones, edited by W.H.S. Jones, 219–54. Cambridge: Harvard University Press.

Hoccleve, Thomas. 1982. *Selected Poems*, edited by Bernard O'Donoghue. Manchester: Fyfield Books, Carcanet.

Holbein, Hans. 1869. *Holbein's Icones historiarum Veteris Testamenti*, edited by Henry Green and Alfred Woltmann. Manchester: Published for the Holbein Society by A. Brothers; Trübner & Co.

Horsley, Victor. 1888. "Trephining in the Neolithic Period." *Journal of the Anthropological Institute of Great Britain and Ireland* 17: 100–6.

Hounsfield, G.N. 1973. "Computerized Transverse Axial Scanning (Tomography). 1. Description of System." *British Journal of Radiology* 46 (552): 1016–22.

Hrdlička, Aleš. 1899. "Art and Literature in the Mentally Abnormal." *American Journal of Psychiatry* 55: 385–404.

Hundt, Magnus. 1501. *Antropologium de hominis dignitate, natura, et proprietatibus; de elementis, partibus et membris humani corporis.* Liptzick: Baccalarium Wolfgangum Monacensem.

Iadecola, Costantino. 2017. "The Neurovascular Unit Coming of Age: A Journey Through Neurovascular Coupling in Health and Disease." *Neuron* 96 (1): 17–42.

Insel, Thomas. 2013. "Transforming Diagnosis" Available at https://psychrights.org/2013/130429NIMHTransformingDiagnosis.htm [accessed 13 Feb. 2026].

—. 2022. *Healing: Our Path from Mental Illness to Mental Health.* London: Penguin.

Insel, Thomas, and Rémi Quirion. 2005. "Psychiatry as a Clinical Neuroscience Discipline." *JAMA* 294 (17): 2221–24.

Jamison, Kay R. 1996. *Touched with Fire: Manic-Depressive Illness and the Artistic Temperament.* New York: Free Press.

Jay, Mike. 2014. "Illustrations of Madness. James Tilly Matthews and the Air Loom." Available at https://publicdomainreview.org/essay/illustrations-of-madness-james-tilly-matthews-and-the-air-loom/ [accessed 13 Feb. 2026].

Jung, Carl Gustav. 2010. *Four Archetypes: Mother, Rebirth, Spirit, Trickster*, translated by R.F.C. Hull and Sonu Shamdasani, with a new foreword by Sonu Shamdasani. Princeton: Princeton Univeristy Press.

Kemp, Simon, and Kevin Williams. 1987. "Demonic Possession and Mental Disorder in Medieval and Early Modern Europe." *Psychological Medicine* 17 (1): 21–29.

Kevles, Bettyann H. 1997. *Naked to the Bone: Medical Imaging in the Twentieth Century.* New Brunswick: Rutgers University Press.

Kieser, Dietrich Georg. 1855. *Elemente der Psychiatrik.* Breslau and Bonn: Kaiserliche L.-C. Akademie.

King, Morgan. 2022. "Harmful Biases in Artificial Intelligence." *Lancet Psychiatry* 9 (11): e48.

Klibansky, Raymond, Erwin Panofsky and Fritz Saxl. 1964. *Saturn and Melancholy: Studies in the History of Natural Philosophy, Religion, and Art.* London: Nelson.

Kors, Alan Charles, and Edward Peters. 2001. *Witchcraft in Europe, 400–1700: A Documentary History.* Philadelphia: University of Pennsylvania Press.

Koutsouleris, Nikolaos, Stefan Borgwardt, Eva M. Meisenzahl, Ronald Bottlender, Hans-Jürgen Möller and Anita Riecher-Rössler. 2012. "Disease Prediction in the At-Risk Mental State for Psychosis Using Neuroanatomical Biomarkers: Results from the FePsy Study." *Schizophrenia Bullettin* 38 (6): 1234–46.

Koutsouleris, Nikolaos, Eva M. Meisenzahl, Stefan Borgwardt, Anita Riecher-Rössler, Thomas Frodl, Joseph Kambeitz, Yanis Köhler, Peter Falkai, Hans-Jürgen Möller, Maximilian Reiser and Christos Davatzikos. 2015. "Individualized Differential Diagnosis of Schizophrenia and Mood Disorders Using Neuroanatomical Biomarkers." *Brain* 138 (Pt. 7): 2059–73.

Krieger, Steffen Norbert, Markus Nikolar Streicher, Robert Trampel and Robert Turner. 2012. "Cerebral Blood Volume Changes During Brain Activation." *Journal of Cerebral Blood Flow & Metababolism* 32 (8): 1618–31.

Kromm, Jane. 2002. *The Art of Frenzy: Public Madness in the Visual Culture of Europe, 1500–1850*. London: Continuum.

—. 2010. "General introduction." In *A History of Visual Culture: Western Civilization from the 18th to the 21st Century*, edited by Jane Kromm and Susan Benforado Bakewell, 1–17. Oxford: Berg.

Kuhl, David E., and Roy Q. Edwards. 1963. "Image Separation Radioisotope Scanning." *Radiology* 80 (4): 653–62.

Lacan, Ernest. 1856. *Esquisses photographiques à propos de l'Exposition universelle et de la Guerre d'Orient*, edited by développements historique de la photographie, applications, biographies et portraits. Paris: Grassart.

Ladino, Lady Diana, Gary Hunter and José Francisco Téllez-Zenteno. 2013. "Art and Epilepsy Surgery." *Epilepsy & Behavior* 29 (1): 82–89.

Laharie, Muriel. 1991. *La folie au Moyen Âge: XIe-XIIIe siècles*. Paris: Léopard d'Or.

Lanska, Douglas. 2019. "The development and evolution of 'cerebral thermometry': The physiology underlying a nineteenth-century approach to cerebral localization and neurological diagnosis." *Journal of the History of the Neurosciences* 28: 1–31.

Lauterbur, Paul C. 1973. "Image Formation by Induced Local Interactions: Examples Employing Nuclear Magnetic Resonance." *Nature* 242 (5394): 190–91.

Lavater, Johann Caspar. 1775. *Physiognomische Fragmente, zur Beförderung der Menschenkenntniss und Menschenliebe*. Vol. 2. Leipzig und Winterthur: Bey Weidmanns Erben und Reich, und Heinrich Steiner und Compagnie.

—. 1794. *Essays on Physiognomy: For the Promotion of the Knowledge and the Love of Mankind*, translated by Thomas Holcroft. Boston: Printed for William Spotswood & David West.

Lavater, Johann Caspar, and Jacques-Louis Moreau de la Sarthe. 1809. *L'art de connaître les hommes par la physionomie*. Vol. 8. Paris: L. Prudhomme.

Leigh, Hoyle. 2010. *Genes, Memes, Culture, and Mental Illness: Toward an Integrative Model*. New York: Springer.

Levack, Brian P. 2013. *The Devil Within: Possession & Exorcism in the Christian West*. New Haven: Yale University Press.

Lieberman, Jeffrey A., T. Scott Stroup, Joseph P. McEvoy, Marvin S. Swartz, Robert A. Rosenheck, Diana O. Perkins, Richard S.E. Keefe, Sonia M. Davis, Clarence E. Davis, Barry D. Lebowitz, Joanne Severe and John K. Hsiao. 2005. "Effectiveness of Antipsychotic Drugs in Patients with Chronic Schizophrenia." *New England Journal of Medicine* 353 (12): 1209–23.

Lillie, Malcolm C. 1998. "Cranial Surgery Dates Back to Mesolithic." *Nature* 391 (6670): 854.

Lis, Catharina, James Coonan and Hugo Soly. 1979. *Poverty and Capitalism in Pre-Industrial Europe*. Hassocks: Harvester.

Logothetis, Nikos K. 2008. "What We Can Do and What We Cannot Do with fMRI." *Nature* 453 (7197): 869–78.

Lombroso, Cesare. 1890. *Pazzi e anomali*. Città di Castello: S. Lapi.

—. 1891. *The Man of Genius*. Translated by Walter Scott. London: Walter Scott.

—. 1906. "Il mio museo criminale." *L'illustrazione italiana* 33 (13): 306.

Lovell, Ernest J., ed. 1969. *Lady Blessington's Conversations of Lord Byron*. Princeton: Princeton University Press.

MacGregor, John M. 1989. *The Discovery of the Art of the Insane*. Princeton: Princeton University Press.

Maclagan, David. 2010. *Outsider Art: From the Margins to the Marketplace*. London: Reaktion Books.

Macmillan, Malcolm. 2001. "John Martyn Harlow: Obscure Country Physician?" *Journal of the History of the Neurosciences* 10 (2): 149–62.

—. 2004. "Inhibition and Phineas Gage: Repression and Sigmund Freud." *Neuropsychoanalysis* 6 (2): 181–92.

Macmillan, Malcolm, and Matthew L. Lena. 2010. "Rehabilitating Phineas Gage." *Neuropsychological Rehabilitation* 20 (5): 641–58.

Maher, Winifred B., and Brendan Maher. 1982. "The ship of fools: *Stultifera Navis* or *ignis fatuus*?" *American Psychologist* 37 (7): 756–61.

Mann, John. 2000. *Murder, Magic, and Medicine*. Oxford: Oxford University Press.

Manzoli, Federica. 2004. "La follia per immagini: Storia fotografica della fine dei manicomi." *Journal of Science Communication* 3 (2): 1–7.

Marien, Mary Warner. 2021. *Photography: A Cultural History*. London: Hachette UK.

Martin, Jonathan. 1825. *The Life of Jonathan Martin, Incendiary of York Minster: With Some Account of William and Richard Martin*. London: Jonathan Martin.

Martino, Paolo. 2008. "L'identità culturale europea negli studi linguistici e filologici." In *L'identità europea. Lingua e cultura. Atti dell'incontro europeo di docenti universitari in occasione del 50o anniversario dei trattati di Roma*, edited by Paolo Martino, 17–46. Rome: Edizioni Studium.

Mayberg, Helen S. 2014. "Neuroimaging and Psychiatry: The Long Road from Bench to Bedside." *Hastings Center Report* Spec No: S31-6.

Maynard, Patrick. 2018. *The Engine of Visualization: Thinking Through Photography*. 1st edition. Ithaca: Cornell University Press.

Mazzi, Maria Serena. 1991. "Gli inutili: miserabili e vagabondi." In *Vita materiale e ceti subalterni nel Medioevo*, edited by Maria Serena Mazzi, 159–80. Alessandria: Edizioni dell'Orso.

McAlister, Neil Harding. 1977. "The Dancing Pilgrims at Muelebeek." *Journal of the History of Medicine and Allied Sciences* XXXII (3): 315–19.

McCabe, David P., and Alan D. Castel. 2008. "Seeing is Believing: The Effect of Brain Images on Judgments of Scientific Reasoning." *Cognition* 107: 343–52.

McDonagh, Patrick. 2008. *Idiocy: A Cultural History*. Liverpool: Liverpool University Press.

Ménard, Philippe. 1977. "Les fous dans la société médiévale. Le témoignage de la littérature au XIIe et au XIIIe siècle." *Romania* 392 (4): 433–59.

Micale, Mark S. 1990. "Charcot and the Idea of Hysteria in the Male: Gender, Mental Science, and Medical Diagnosis in Late Nineteenth-Century France." *Medical History* 34 (4): 363–411.

Michael, Robert B., Eryn J. Newman, Matti Vuorre, Geoff Cumming and Maryanne Garry. 2013. "On the (Non)Persuasive Power of a Brain Image." *Psychonomic Bullettin & Review* 20 (4): 720–25.

Midelfort, H.C. Erik. 1999. *A History of Madness in Sixteenth-Century Germany*. Stanford: Stanford University Press.

Mirzoeff, Nicholas. 1999. *An Introduction to Visual Culture*. London: Routledge.

Missios, Symeon. 2007. "Hippocrates, Galen, and the Uses of Trepanation in the Ancient Classical World." *Neurosurgical Focus* 23 (1): E11.

Mitchell, William J.T. 1994. *Picture Theory: Essays on Verbal and Visual Representation*. Chicago: University of Chicago Press.

Mitelli, Giuseppe Maria. 1967. *Proverbj figurati di Giuseppe Maria Mitelli*, edited by Lorenzo Marinese and Alberto Manfredi. Lecco: Edizioni d'Arte Rotta.

Mizrahi, Vivian. 2021. "Seeing Through Photographs: Photography as a Transparent Visual Medium." *Journal of Aesthetics and Art Criticism* 79: 52–63.

Mollat, Michel. 1986. *The Poor in the Middle Ages: An Essay in Social History*. New Haven: Yale University Press.

Mollica, Richard F. 1985. "From Antonio Gramsci to Franco Basaglia: The Theory and Practice of the Italian Psychiatric Reform." *International Journal of Mental Health* 14 (1/2) (The Unfinished Revolution in Italian Psychiatry: An International Perspective): 22–41.

Monash University. 2023. "New Maps Reveal the Individual Brain Changes Linked to Different Mental Illness." *Science Daily* [accessed 4 Feb. 2025].

Monier-Williams, Monier. 1872. *A Sanskṛit-English Dictionary*. Oxford: Clarendon Press.

Montaldo, Silvano, ed. 2015. *Il Museo di antropologia criminale "Cesare Lombroso"*. Milan: Silvana Editoriale.

Morgenthaler, Walter. 1992. *Madness & Art: The Life and the Works of Adolf Wölfli*. Lincoln: University of Nebraska Press.

Mori, Susumu, and Jingyang Zhang. 2006. "Principles of Diffusion Tensor Imaging and Its Applications to Basic Neuroscience Research." *Neuron* 51 (5): 527–39.

Morison, Alexander. 1826. *Outlines of Lectures on Mental Diseases*. London: Longman, Rees, Orme, Brown & Green, and S. Highley.

—. 1840. *The Physiognomy of Mental Diseases*. London: Longman.

Morse, Stephen J. 2012. "Neuroimaging Evidence in Law: A Plea for Modesty and Relevance." In *Neuroimaging in Forensic Psychiatry: From the Clinic to the Courtroom*, edited by Joseph R. Simpson, 341–57. Oxford: Wiley-Blackwell.

Mosso, Angelo. 1880. "Sulla circolazione del sangue nel cervello dell'uomo." *Atti della Accademia Nazionale dei Lincei, Classe di Scienze Fisiche, Matematiche e Naturali* III: 237–358.

—. 1882. "Applicazione della bilancia allo studio della circolazione del sangue nell'uomo." *Atti della Reale Accademia delle Scienze di Torino* XVII: 534–35.

—. 1894. *La temperatura del cervello: studi termometrici*. Milan: Fratelli Treves.

Mostowlansky, Till, Andrea Rota, Joel Robbins, Rupert Stasch, Matei Candea, Andrew Sanchez, Sian Lazar, Hildegard Diemberger and Felix Stein. 2020. "Emic and Etic." *Cambridge Encyclopedia of Anthropology*. Available at https://doi.org/10.29164/20emicetic [accessed 13 Feb. 2026].

Muzzarelli, Federica. 2009. "Breve storia della fotografia manicomiale." In *"Nonostante la vostra cortese ospitalità..." Fotografia e disagio mentale oggi*, edited by Tomaso Mario Bolis and Claudio Marra, 19–49. Bologna: Quinlan.

Netchitailova, Ekaterina. 2019. "The Mystery of Madness through Art and Mad Studies." *Disability & Society* 34 (9–10): 1509–15.

Nicholls, Angus. 2010. "The Scientific Unconscious: Goethe's post-Kantian Epistemology." In *Thinking the Unconscious: Nineteenth-Century German Thought*, edited by Angus Nicholls and Martin Liebscher, 87–120. Cambridge: Cambridge University Press.

Nietzsche, Friedrich. 1910. *The Birth of Tragedy or Ellenism and Pessimism*. Edinburgh and London: T.N. Foulis.

Nordahl-Hansen, Anders, Magnus Tøndevold and Sue Fletcher-Watson. 2018. "Mental Health on Screen: A DSM-5 Dissection of Portrayals of Autism Spectrum Disorders in Film and TV." *Psychiatry Research* 262: 351–53.

Noyes, William. 1888. "Paranoia: A Study of the Evolution of Systematized Delusions of Grandeur." *American Journal of Psychology* 1 (3): 460–78.

Nutton, Vivian. 2004. *Ancient Medicine*. London: Taylor & Francis.

O'Hara, Mark. 2019. "Cinema of the Monstrous. Disability and the 'Eye-Feel'." *Journal of Curriculum Theorizing* 34 (5): 44–57.

Obrig, Hellmuth, and Arno Villringer. 2003. "Beyond the Visible: Imaging the Human Brain with Light." *Journal of Cerebral Blood Flow & Metababolism* 23 (1): 1–18.

Oesterreich, Traugott Konstantin. 1966. *Possession: Demoniacal and Other Among Primitive Races, in Antiquity, the Middle Ages, and Modern Times*. International Library of Psychology. London: Kegan Paul and Trench Trubner & Co.

Ogawa, Seiji, Teresa M. Lee, Alan R. Kay and David W. Tank. 1990. "Brain Magnetic Resonance Imaging with Contrast Dependent on Blood Oxygenation." *Proceedings of the National Academy of Sciences of the United States of America* 87 (24): 9868–72.

Onians, Richard Broxton. 2011. *The Origins of European Thought: About the Body, the Mind, the Soul, the World, Time, and Fate*. Cambridge: Cambridge University Press.

Onwordi, Ellis Chika, Els F. Halff, Thomas Whitehurst, Ayla Mansur, Marie-Caroline Cotel, Lisa Wells, Hannah Creeney, David Bonsall, Maria Rogdaki, Ekaterina Shatalina, Tiago Reis Marques, Eugenii A. Rabiner, Roger N. Gunn, Sridhar Natesan, Anthony C. Vernon and Oliver D. Howes. 2020. "Synaptic Density Marker SV2A Is Reduced in Schizophrenia Patients and Unaffected by Antipsychotics in Rats." *Nature Communications* 11 (1): 155.

Orsi, Francesca. 2025. *La nuova alleanza tra fotografia e psichiatria. Da Basaglia a oggi*. Milan: Mimesis.

Ortner, Donald J. 2003. *Identification of Pathological Conditions in Human Skeletal Remains*. Cambridge: Academic Press.

Padel, Ruth. 1992. *In and Out of the Mind: Greek Images of the Tragic Self*. Princeton: Princeton University Press.

Panofsky, Erwin. 1955. *Meaning in the Visual Arts: Papers in and on Art History*. New York: Doubleday.

Papazova, Irina, Alkomiet Hasan and Naiiri Khorikian-Ghazari. 2025. "Biased AI Generated Images of Mental Illness: Does AI Adopt Our Stigma?" *European Archives of Psychiatry and Clinical Neuroscience*.

Paracelsus. 1979. "The Diseases that Deprive Man of His Reason, Such as St Vitus' Dance, Falling Sickness, Melancholy, and Insanity, and Their Correct Treatment." In *Four Treatises of Theophrastus Von Hohenheim: Called Paracelsus*, 127–212. Baltimore: Johns Hopkins Press.

Pearl, Sharrona. 2009. "Through a Mediated Mirror: The Photographic Physiognomy of Dr Hugh Welch Diamond." *History of Photography* 33 (3): 288–305.

Penfield, Wilder. 1958. *The Excitable Cortex in Conscious Man*. Liverpool: Liverpool University Press.

Penfield, Wilder, and Edwin Boldrey. 1937. "Somatic Motor and Sensory Representation in the Cerebral Cortex of Man as Studied by Electrical Stimulation." *Brain* 60 (4): 389–443.

Pepper, Stephen C. 1942. *World Hypotheses: A Study in Evidence*. Berkeley: University of California Press.

Phelps, Michael E., Ellen J. Hoffman, Nizar A. Mullani and Michel M. Ter-Pogossian. 1975. "Application of Annihilation Coincidence Detection to Transaxial Reconstruction Tomography." *Journal of Nuclear Medicine* 16 (3): 210–24.

Pianigiani, Ottorino. 1907. *Vocabolario etimologico della lingua italiana*. Roma: Società editrice Dante Alighieri di Albrighi, Segati.

Pietrini, Sandra. 2002. "Medieval Fools in Biblical Iconography." *Medieval English Theatre* 24: 79–103.

Pinel, Philippe. 1806. *A Treatise on Insanity*. Sheffield: W. Todd.

Pinson, Yona. 2003. "Folly and Childishness Go Hand in Hand: Hans Holbein's 'Dixit Insipiens'." *Notes in the History of Art* 22 (3): 1–2.

Piro, Sergio. 1967. "Fotografia e alienità." *Popular Photography Italiana* 117: 55 and 88.

—. 1969. "Prefazione." In *Gli esclusi. Fotoreportage da un'istituzione totale*, n.p. Milan: Il diaframma.

Pitrelli, Nico. 2004. *L'uomo che restituí la parola ai matti: Franco Basaglia, la comunicazione e la fine dei manicomi*, edited by Peppe Dell'Acqua. *Saggi. Società*. Roma: Editori Riuniti.

Plato. 1914. *Phaedrus*. In *Euthyphro; Apology; Crito; Phaedo; Phaedrus*, translated by Harold North Fowler and W.R.M. Lamb, edited by Harold North Fowler, xx, 583. London and New York: W. Heinemann; Macmillan.

—. 1969. *Republic*. In *Plato in Twelve Volumes, Vols. 5 & 6*, edited by Paul Shorey. Cambridge: Harvard University Press.

Pócs, Éva, and András Zempléni, eds. 2022. *Spirit Possession: Multidisciplinary Approaches to a Worldwide Phenomenon*. Budapest: Central European University Press.

Podwalski, Piotr, Krzysztof Szczygieł, Ernest Tyburski, Leszek Sagan, Błażej Misiak and Jerzy Samochowiec. 2021. "Magnetic Resonance Diffusion Tensor Imaging in Psychiatry: A Narrative Review of Its Potential Role in Diagnosis." *Pharmacological Reports* 73 (1): 43–56.

Pormann, Peter E. 2013. "Medical Epistemology and Melancholy: Rufus of Ephesus and Miskawayh." In *Mental Disorders in the Classical World*, edited by William V. Harris, 223–43. Boston: Brill.

Porter, Roy. 2002. *Madness: A Brief History*. Oxford: Oxford University Press.

Prinzhorn, Hans. 1972. *Artistry of the Mentally Ill*. New York: Springer.

Pullan, Brian. 1978. "Poveri, mendicanti e vagabondi (secoli XIV–XVII)." In *Storia d'Italia: Dal feudalesimo al capitalismo*, edited by Ruggiero Romano and Corrado Vivanti, 811–1047. Turin: Einaudi.

Rabelais, François. 1653. *Five Books of the Lives, Heroic Deeds and Sayings of Gargantua and His Son Pantagruel*, translated by T. Urquhart and P. Motteux. No City: Kindle.

Racine, Eric, Ofek Bar-Ilan and Judy Illes. 2005. "fMRI in the Public Eye." *Nature Reviews Neuroscience* 6 (2): 159–64.

Raichle, Marcus E. 1998. "Behind the Scenes of Functional Brain Imaging: A Historical and Physiological Perspective." *Proceedings of the National Academy of Sciences of the United States of America* 95 (3): 765–72.

Réja, Marcel. 2014. *L'Art chez les fous (1907)*. Whitefish: Literary Licensing, LLC.

Renzi, Salvatore. 1853. *Collectio salernitana / vol. II*. Naples: Tipografia del Filiatre-Sebezio.

Rhodes, Colin. 2023. *Outsider Art: Art Brut and its Affinities*. London: Thames & Hudson.

Richterová, Julie. 1982. *Středověké kachle*. Prague: Muzea hlavního města.

Riis, Thomas. 1981. *Aspects of Poverty in Early Modern Europe*. Alphen aan den Rijn: Sijthoff.

Riles, Julius Matthew. 2020. "The Social Effect of Exposure to Mental Illness Media Portrayals: Influencing Interpersonal Interaction Intentions." *Psychology of Popular Media* 9 (2): 145–54.

Riles, Julius Matthew, Brandon Miller, Michelle Funk and Ethan Morrow. 2021. "The Modern Character of Mental Health Stigma: A 30-Year Examination of Popular Film." *Communication Studies* 72 (4): 668–83.

Ripa, Cesare. 1593. *Iconologia overo descrittione dell'imagini vniversali cavate dall'antichita et da altri lvoghi*. Rome: Heredi Gio Gigliotti.

Riverius, Lazarus. 1655. *The Practice of Physick, in seventeen books*, edited by Abdiah Cole, Nicholas Culpeper and William Rowland. London: Peter Cole.

Rivers, Christopher. 1994. *Face Value: Physiognomical Thought and the Legible Body in Marivaux, Lavater, Balzac, Gautier, and Zola*. Madison: University of Wisconsin Press.

Rocca, Julius. 2003. "Galen and the Uses of Trepanation." In *Trepanation: History, Discovery, Theory*, edited by Robert Arnott, Stanley Finger and Chris Smith, 253–71. Hove: Psychology Press.

Roepstorff, Andreas. 2004. "Mapping Brain Mappers: An Ethnographic Coda Human Brain Function." edited by Richard S.J. Frackowiak, Karl J. Friston, Christopher D. Frith, Raymond J. Dolan, Cathy J. Price, Semir Zeki, John T. Ashburner and William D. Penny, 1105–17. Burlington: Academic Press.

—. 2007. "Navigating the Brainscape: When Knowing becomes Seeing Skilled Visions. Between Apprenticeship and Standards." edited by Cristina Grasseni, 191–206. Oxford: Berghahn Books.

Rose, Gillian. 2016. *Visual Methodologies: An Introduction to Researching with Visual Materials*. London: Sage.

Rose, Nikolas. 2016. "Reading the Human Brain: How the Mind Became Legible." *Body & Society* 22 (2): 140–77.

—. 2018. *Our Psychiatric Future*. Cambridge: Polity.

Rose, Nikolas and Joelle M. Abi-Rached. 2013. *Neuro: The New Brain Sciences and the Management of the Mind*. Princeton: Princeton University Press.

Rosenhan, David L. 1973. "On Being Sane in Insane Places." *Science* 179 (4070): 250–58.

Röske, Thomas. 2003. "Expressionism and Insanity." *Raw Vision* 45: 32–39.

Roskies, Adina L. 2007. "Are Neuroimages Like Photographs of the Brain?" *Philosophy of Science* 74: 860–72.

Rush, A. John, Madhukar H. Trivedi, Stephen R. Wisniewski, Andrew A. Nierenberg, Johnathan W. Stewart, Diane Warden, George Niederehe, Michael E. Thase, Philip W. Lavori, Barry D. Lebowitz, Patrick J. McGrath, Jerrold F. Rosenbaum, Harold A. Sackeim, David J. Kupfer, James Luther and Maurizio Fava. 2006. "Acute and Longer-Term Outcomes in Depressed Outpatients Requiring One or Several Treatment Steps: A STAR*D Report." *American Journal of Psychiatry* 163 (11): 1905–17.

Rush, Benjamin. 1979. *Medical Inquiries and Observations on the Diseases of the Mind*. Special edition. Birmingham: Classics of Medicine Library. 1812.

Saade, Charbel, Elie Najem, Karl Asmar, Rida Salman, Bassam El Achkar and Lena Naffaa. 2019. "Intracranial Calcifications on CT: An Updated Review." *Journal of Radiology Case Reports* 13 (8): 1–18.

Saffioti, Tito. 2013. *Gli occhi della follia: giullari e buffoni di corte nella storia e nell'arte*. Milan: Book Time.

Sagarwala, Raza, and Henry A. Nasrallah. 2020. "White Matter Pathology Is Shared across Multiple Psychiatric Brain Disorders: Is Abnormal Diffusivity a Transdiagnostic Biomarker for Psychopathology?" *Biomarkers in Neuropsychiatry* 2: 100010.

Sandrone, Stefano, Marco Bacigaluppi, Marco R. Galloni and Gianvito Martino. 2012. "Angelo Mosso (1846–1910)." *J Neurol* 259 (11): 2513–14.

Sandrone, Stefano, Marco Bacigaluppi, Marco R. Galloni, Stefano F. Cappa, Andrea Moro, Marco Catani, Massimo Filippi, Martin M. Monti, Daniela Perani and Gianvito Martino. 2014. "Weighing Brain Activity with the Balance: Angelo Mosso's Original Manuscripts Come to Light." *Brain* 137 (Pt. 2): 621–33.

Sandrone, Stefano, and Lorenzo Lorusso. 2022. *The Birth of Modern Neuroscience in Turin*. Oxford: Oxford University Press.

Savalescu, Julian, L. Will Davies, Rebecca Roache, Will Davies and J. Pierre Loebel. 2020. *Psychiatry Reborn: Biopsychosocial Psychiatry in Modern Medicine*. Oxford: Oxford University Press.

Scabia, Giuliano. 1976. *Marco Cavallo. Una esperienza di animazione in un ospedale psichiatrico*. Turin: Einaudi.

Scharfe, Hartmut. 1999. "The Doctrine of the Three Humors in Traditional Indian Medicine and the Alleged Antiquity of Tamil Siddha Medicine." *Journal of the American Oriental Society* 119 (4): 609–29.

Schelling, Friedrich Wilhelm. 1994. "The Stuttgart Seminars." In *Idealism and the Endgame of Theory: Three Essays*. Albany: State University of New York Press.

Schenck, Johann Georg. 1608. *Lithogenesia sive de microcosmi membris petrefactis: et de calculis eidem microcosmo per varias matrices innatis: pathologia historica, per theorian & autopsian demonstrata. Accessit analogicum argumentum ex macrocosmo de calculis brutorum corporib. innatis*. Frankfurt: Matthias Becker für Theodor de Bry Erben.

Schinaia, Cosimo. 2004. "Fotografia e psichiatria." In *20: L'immagine fotografica, 1945–2000*, edited by Uliano Lucas, In Storia d'Italia. Annali, 459–76. Turin: Giulio Einaudi.

—. 2005. "Chiaroscuri. Sui rapporti tra fotografia e psichiatria." In *Il volto della follia. Cent'anni di immagini del dolore*, edited by Sandro Parmiggiani, 33–48. Milan: Skira.

Schneider, Carl. 1939. "Entartete Kunst und Irrenkunst." *Archiv für Psychiatrie und Nervenkrankheiten* 11o: 135–64.

Schomerus, Georg, Christian Schwahn, Astrid Holzinger, Patrick W. Corrigan, Hans J. Grabe, Mauro Giovanni Carta and Matthias C. Angermeyer. 2012. "Evolution of Public Attitudes about Mental Illness: A Systematic Review and Meta-Analysis." *Acta Psychiatrica Scandinavica* 125 (6): 440–52.

Schopenhauer, Arthur. 2010. *The World as Will and Representation*, translated by Judith Norman, Alistair Welchman and Christopher Janaway, edited by Judith Norman, Alistair Welchman and Christopher Janaway. Cambridge: Cambridge University Press.

—. 2015. "On Physiognomy." In *Schopenhauer: Parerga and Paralipomena: Short Philosophical Essays, The Cambridge Edition of the Works of Schopenhauer*, edited by Adrian Del Caro and Christopher Janaway, 568–74. Cambridge: Cambridge University Press.

Schumer, Maya C., Henry W. Chase, Renata Rozovsky, Simon B. Eickhoff and Mary L. Phillips. 2023. "Prefrontal, Parietal, and Limbic Condition-Dependent Differences in Bipolar Disorder: A Large-Scale Meta-Analysis of Functional Neuroimaging Studies." *Molecular Psychiatry* 28 (7): 2826–38.

Schupbach, William. 1978. "A New Look at *The Cure of Folly*." *Medical History* 22 (3): 267–81.

Scull, Andrew. 2007. *Madhouse: A Tragic Tale of Megalomania and Modern Medicine*. New Haven: Yale University Press.

—. 2011. *Hysteria: The Disturbing History*. Biographies of Disease. Oxford: Oxford University Press.

—. 2016. *Madness in Civilization: A Cultural History of Insanity from the Bible to Freud, from the Madhouse to Modern Medicine*. First paperback edition. London: Thames & Hudson.

Segal, Ashlea, Linden Parkes, Kevin Aquino, Seyed Mostafa Kia, Thomas Wolfers, Barbara Franke, Martine Hoogman, Christian F. Beckmann, Lars T. Westlye, Ole A. Andreassen, Andrew Zalesky, Ben J. Harrison, Christopher G. Davey, Carles Soriano-Mas, Narcís Cardoner, Jeggan Tiego, Murat Yücel, Leah Braganza, Chao Suo, Michael Berk, Sue Cotton, Mark A. Bellgrove, Andre F. Marquand and Alex Fornito. 2023. "Regional, circuit and network heterogeneity of brain abnormalities in psychiatric disorders." *Nature Neuroscience* 26 (9): 1613–29.

Sekula, Allan. 1986. "The Body and the Archive." *October* 39: 3–64.

Sforza Tarabochia, Alvise. 2018. "Photography, Psychiatry, and Impegno: *Morire di classe* (1969) Between Neorealism and Postmodernism." *Italianist* 38 (1): 48–69.

—. 2019. "Mental, Social and Visual Alienation in D'Alessandro's Photography." In *The Years of Alienation in Italy: Factory and Asylum Between the Economic Miracle and the Years of Lead*, edited by Alessandra Diazzi and Alvise Sforza Tarabochia, 211–28. London: Palgrave.

Shahade, Arati, and Orlando De Jesus. 2024. "Opisthotonus." StatPearls [Internet]. Available at https://www.statpearls.com/nursepractitioner/ce/activity/98673 [accessed 13 Sep. 2025].

Showalter, Elaine. 1980. "Victorian Women and Insanity." *Victorian Studies* 23 (2): 157–81.

Simon, Paul-Max. 1876. "L'imagination dans la folie: Etude sur les dessins, plans, descriptions, et costumes des aliénés." *Annales médico-psychologiques* 16: 358–90.

Simpson, Donald. 2005. "Phrenology and the Neurosciences: Contributions of F.J. Gall and J.G. Spurzheim." *ANZ Journal of Surgery* 75 (6): 475–82.

Simpson, Joseph R. 2012. *Neuroimaging in Forensic Psychiatry: From the Clinic to the Courtroom*, edited by Joseph R. Simpson. Oxford: Wiley-Blackwell.

SIUSA. 2014. Carte da legare. Available at https://siusa-archivi.cultura.gov.it/cgi-bin/siusa/pagina.pl?RicProgetto=carte [accessed 13 Sep. 2025].

Skeat, Walter W. 1888. *An Etymological Dictionary of the English Language*. 2nd edition, revised and corrected. Oxford: Clarendon Press.

Snell, Robert. 2018. *Portraits of the Insane: Theodore Gericault and the Subject of Psychotherapy*. London: Karnak.

Sontag, Susan. 2005. *On Photography*. New York: Rosetta Books.

Sprooten, Emma, Alexander Rasgon, Morgan Goodman, Ariella Carlin, Evan Leibu, Won Hee Lee and Sophia Frangou. 2017. "Addressing Reverse Inference in Psychiatric Neuroimaging: Meta-Analyses of Task-Related Brain Activation in Common Mental Disorders." *Human Brain Mapping* 38 (4): 1846–64.

Spurzheim, Johann Caspar. 1817. *Observations on the Deranged Manifestations of the Mind, or Insanity*. London: Baldwin, Cradock and Joy.

Stabile, Giorgio. 2008. "Sapor-sapientia: tatto e gusto tra cultura agraria, medicina e mistica." In *Natura, scienze e società medievali: Studi in onore di Agostino Paravicini Bagliani*, edited by Claudio Leonardi and Francesco Santi, 287–344. Florence: SISMEL Edizioni del Galluzzo.

Stefanile, Mario. 1969. "Un reportage fotografico di Luciano D'Alessandro." *Il Mattino*.

Stewart, Thomas Dale. 1958. "Stone Age Skull Surgery: A General Review, with Emphasis on the New World." In *Annual Report of the Smithsonian Institution 1957*, 469–91. Washington: US Government Printing Office.

Stone, Julie L., and Monica L. Miles. 1990. "Skull Trepanation Among the Early Indians of Canada and the United States." *Neurosurgery* 26 (6): 1015–19; discussion 1019–20.

Sturken, Marita, and Lisa Cartwright. 2017. *Practices of Looking: An Introduction to Visual Culture*. Oxford: Oxford University Press.

Tagg, John. 1988. *The Burden of Representation. Essays on Photographies and Histories*. London: Palgrave MacMillan.

Tagliabue, Luigi. 1993. "L'istituto S. Lazzaro: Lo psichiatra, il suo sguardo." In *Immagini dal manicomio. Le fotografie storiche del S. Lazzaro di Reggio Emilia 1892–1936*, edited by Paola Lalli, 20–33. Reggio Emilia: AGE Grafico-Editoriale.

Tamassia, Arrigo. 2011. "La fotografia del nostro manicomio." In *Parole e immagini dal manicomio. Studi e materiali dalle cartelle cliniche tra Otto e Novecento*, edited by Riccardo Panattoni, 11–15. Milan: Bruno Mondadori.

Tardieu, Ambroise. 1872. *Étude médico-légale sur la folie*. Paris: J.B. Baillière et fils.

Temkin, Owsei. 1971. *The Falling Sickness: A History of Epilepsy from the Greeks to the Beginnings of Modern Neurology*. Baltimore: Johns Hopkins University Press.

Tertullian. 1931. *Apologeticus*. In *Apology; De spectaculis*, translated by T.R. Glover, Gerald H. Rendall and Walter C.A. Ker, edited by T.R. Glover, Gerald H. Rendall and Walter C.A. Ker, 2–229. London: William Heinemann.

Terzian, Hrayr. 1981. "La fotografia psichiatrica." In *Nascita della fotografia psichiatrica*, edited by Franco Cagnetta, 21–24. Venice: Marsilio.

Thiher, Allen. 1999. *Revels in Madness: Insanity in Medicine and Literature*. Ann Arbor: University of Michigan Press.

Thivel, Anthoine. 2005. "Air, Pneuma and Breathing from Homer to Hippocrates." In *Hippocrates in Context: Papers Read at the XIth International Hippocrates Colloquium, University of Newcastle upon Tyne, 27–31 August 2002*, edited by Philip Van der Eijk, 239–50. Boston: Brill.

Trenery, Claire, and Peregrine Horden. 2017. "Madness in the Middle Ages." In *The Routledge History of Madness and Mental Health*, edited by Greg Eghigian, 62–80. London: Routledge.

Tytler, Graeme. 2014. *Physiognomy in the European Novel: Faces and Fortunes*. Princeton: Princeton University Press.

Valente, Luisa. 2018. "'Dixit insipiens in corde suo "non est deus"'. Mini-Archeologia del soggetto insipiente." In *Sujet libre: pour Alain de Libera*, edited by Jean-Baptiste Brenet and Laurent Cesalli, 327–34. Paris: Vrin.

van Loo, Hannah M., and Jan-Willem Romeijn. 2015. "Psychiatric Comorbidity: Fact or Artifact?" *Theoretical Medicine and Bioethics* 36 (1): 41–60.

Van Wyhe, John. 2004. *Phrenology and the Origins of Victorian Scientific Naturalism*. Aldershot: Ashgate.

Vecchiarelli, Roberto. 2017. *Cronache dal manicomio: Cesare Lombroso e il giornale dei pazzi del manicomio di Pesaro*. Sestri Levante: Oltre edizioni.

von Aue, Hartmann. 1979. *Iwein: The Knight with the Lion*, translated by Thomas J.W. Lincoln. University of Nebraska Press.

Vul, Edward, Christine Harris, Piotr Winkielman and Harold Pashler. 2009. "Puzzlingly High Correlations in fMRI Studies of Emotion, Personality, and Social Cognition." *Perspectives on Psychological Science* 4 (3): 274–90

Waller, John. 2008. *A Time to Dance, a Time to Die: The Extraordinary Story of the Dancing Plague of 1518*. London: Icon.

—. 2009. "A Forgotten Plague: Making Sense of Dancing Mania." *Lancet* 373 (9664): 624–25.

Wang, Xuan, Chao Yan, Peng-Yuan Yang, Zheng Xia, Xin-Lu Cai, Yi Wang, Sze Chai Kwok and Raymond C.K. Chan. 2024. "Unveiling the Potential of Machine Learning in Schizophrenia Diagnosis: A Meta-Analytic Study of Task-Based Neuroimaging Data." *Psychiatry and Clinical Neurosciences* 78 (3): 157–68.

Warden, Diane, A. John Rush, Madhukar H. Trivedi, Maurizio Fava and Stephen R. Wisniewski. 2007. "The STAR*D Project Results: A Comprehensive Review of Findings." *Current Psychiatry Reports* 9 (6): 449–59.

Wardlaw, Joanna M., Garret O'Connell, Kirsten Shuler, Janet DeWilde, Jane Haley, Oliver Escobar, Shaun Murray, Robert Rae, Donald Jarvie, Peter Sandercock and Burkhard Schafer. 2011. "'Can It Read My Mind?' – What Do the Public and Experts Think of the Current (Mis)uses of Neuroimaging?" *PLoS One* 6 (10): e25829.

Wauters, Wendy. 2018. "'Extracting the Stone of Madness' in Perspective." In *Jaarboek Koninklijk Museum voor Schone Kunsten Antwerpen 2015–2016*, 9–36. Antwerp: Garant.

Webb, Stephen G. 1988. "Two Possible Cases of Trephination from Australia." *American Journal of Physical Anthropology* 75: 541–48.

Weemans, Michel. 2024. "268 – L'extracteur de pierre de folie, ou La Sorcière de Malleghem." In *Figures du fou: Du Moyen Age aux romantiques*, edited by Elisabeth Antoine-König and Pierre-Yves Le Pogam, 413. Paris: Gallimard.

Wernick, Miles N., and John Aarsvold. 2004. *Emission Tomography: The Fundamentals of PET and SPECT*. Amsterdam: Elsevier.

Willeford, William. 1969. *The Fool and His Scepter: A Study in Clowns and Jesters and Their Audience*. Evanston: Northwestern University Press.

Willis, Thomas. 1683. *Two Discourses Concerning the Soul of Brutes Which Is that of the Vital and Sensitive of Man*. London: Thomas Ding.

Wright, Harold G. 1867. "Address on the Medical Uses of Photography." *Photographic Journal Being the Journal of the Photographic Society* 11 (178): 202–10.

Yarnall, James Leo. 1979. "Meryon's Mystical Transformations." *Art Bulletin* 61: 289–300.

Zago, Stefano, Roberta Ferrucci, Sara Marceglia and Alberto Priori. 2009. "The Mosso Method for Recording Brain Pulsation: The Forerunner of Functional Neuroimaging." *Neuroimage* 48 (4): 652–56.

Zempléni, András. 2022. "Introduction." In *Spirit Possession: Multidisciplinary Approaches to a Worldwide Phenomenon*, edited by Éva Pócs and András Zempléni. Budapest: Central European University Press.

Zink, Michel. 2024. "Fou d'amour et amour fou." In *Figures du fou: Du Moyen Age aux romantiques*, edited by Elisabeth Antoine-König and Pierre-Yves Le Pogam, 60–71. Paris: Gallimard.

Zugman, André, Laura Jett, Chase Antonacci, Anderson M. Winkler and Daniel S. Pine. 2023. "A Systematic Review and Meta-Analysis of Resting-State fMRI in Anxiety Disorders: Need for Data Sharing to Move the Field Forward." *Journal of Anxiety Disorders* 99: 102773.

Index

Printed and bound by CPI Group (UK) Ltd, Croydon, CR0 4YY

13/09/2026

14961098-0007